Praise for
Armin A. Brott

**"For fathers soon expecting the ultimate gift—a new member
of the family—*The Expectant Father* is his best friend."**
—CNN Interactive

The Expectant Father

"One would be hard put to find a question about having a baby that's not
dealt with here, all from the father's perspective."—*Library Journal*

"…a terrific gift, offering insight into pregnancy and the first few weeks of
parenthood."—BabyCenter.com

Also by Armin Brott in the New Father series

The New Father:
A Dad's Guide to the First Year

"This book would make a great gift for any new dad."
—Lawrence Kutner, Ph.D., columnist, *Parents* magazine

"Read a book? Who has time? But you'd be wise to find some so you can take
advantage of a fabulous resource…*The New Father*."
—*Sesame Street Parents*

Fathering Your Toddler:
A Dad's Guide to the Second and Third Years

"…Brott demystifies child development…and make[s] fathers…enjoy the
vital role they play in their kids' lives even more. A great addition to any
parenthood library." —*Child* magazine

Fathering Your School-Age Child,
A Dad's Guide to the Wonder Years: 3 to 9

"Brott…drolly delivers readable, practical guidance on fathering."
—*Library Journal*

The Military Father:
A Hands-on Guide for Deployed Dads

The Single Father:
A Dad's Guide to Parenting without a Partner

Father for Life:
A Journey of Joy, Challenge, and Change

THE
EXPECTANT
FATHER

THE ULTIMATE GUIDE FOR DADS-TO-BE

4th EDITION

ARMIN A. BROTT
AND JENNIFER ASH

Abbeville Press Publishers
New York · London

To Tirzah and Talya, who showed me how to do it the first and second times, and Zoë, who reminds me every day just how much fun being a dad can be.—A.A.B.

For Joe, Clarke, and Emmy, and my parents, Clarke and Agnes Ash, with love and affection.—J.A.

EDITOR: Jacqueline Decter
DESIGNER: Celia Fuller
PRODUCTION EDITOR: Nicole Lanctot
PRODUCTION MANAGER: Louise Kurtz

Fourth hardcover edition
10   9   8   7   6   5   4   3
ISBN 978-0-7892-1212-2
Fourth paperback edition
15   14   13   12   11   10   9   8
ISBN 978-0-7892-1213-9

Cover photograph by Geoff Spear. For cartoon credits, see page 334.

Library of Congress Cataloguing-in-Publication Data available upon request

For bulk and premium sales and for text adoption procedures, write to Customer Service Manager, Abbeville Press,116 West 23rd Street, New York, NY 10011, or call 1-800-ARTBOOK.

Visit Abbeville Press online at www.abbeville.com.

Contents

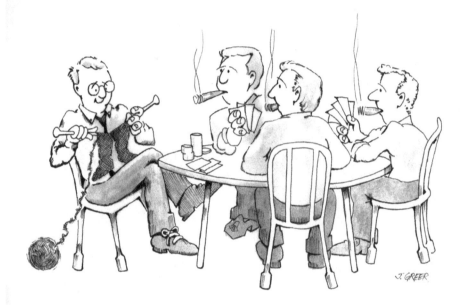

Introduction

When my wife got pregnant with our first child, I was the happiest I'd ever been. That pregnancy, labor, and the baby's birth was a time of incredible closeness, tenderness, and passion. Long before we'd married, my wife and I had made a commitment to participate equally in raising our children. And it seemed only natural that the process of shared parenting should begin during pregnancy.

Since neither of us had had children before, we were both rather ill prepared for pregnancy. Fortunately for my wife, there were literally hundreds of books and other resources designed to educate, encourage, support, and comfort women during their pregnancies. But when it finally hit me that I, too, was expecting (although in a very different kind of way), and that the pregnancy was bringing out feelings and emotions I didn't understand, there simply weren't any resources for me to turn to. I looked for answers in my wife's pregnancy books, but information about what expectant fathers go through (if it was discussed at all) was at best superficial, and consisted mostly of advice on how men could be supportive of their pregnant wives. To make things worse, my wife and I were the first couple in our circle of close friends to get pregnant, which meant that there was no one else I could talk to about what I was going through, no one who could reassure me that what I was feeling was normal and all right.

Until fairly recently, there has been precious little research on expectant fathers' emotional and psychological experiences during pregnancy. The very title of one of the first articles to appear on the subject should give you some idea of the medical and psychiatric communities' attitude toward the impact of pregnancy on men. Written by William H. Wainwright, M.D., and published in the July 1966 issue of the *American Journal of Psychiatry*, it was called "Fatherhood as a Precipitant of Mental Illness." (Another wonderful title that came out at about the same time was: "Psychoses in Males in Relation to Their Wives' Pregnancy and Childbirth.")

As you'll soon find out, though, an expectant father's experience during the transition to fatherhood is not confined simply to excitement—or mental illness; if it were, this book would never have been written. The reality is that men's emotional response to pregnancy is no less varied than women's; expectant fathers feel everything from relief to denial, fear to frustration, anger to joy. And for up to 80 percent of men, there are physical symptoms of pregnancy as well (more on this on pages 74–79).

So why haven't men's experiences been discussed more? In my opinion it's because we, as a society, value motherhood more than fatherhood, and we automatically assume that issues of pregnancy, childbirth, and child rearing are women's issues. But as you'll learn—both from reading this book and from your own experience—that's simply not the case.

WHO, EXACTLY, HAS WRITTEN THIS BOOK?

From the very beginning, my goal in writing *The Expectant Father* has been to help you—the father—understand and make sense of what you're going through during your pregnancy. The rationale was simple: the more you understand about what you're going through, the better prepared you'll be and the more likely you'll be to take an interest in—and stay involved throughout—the pregnancy. Research has shown that the earlier fathers get involved (and what could be earlier than pregnancy?), the more likely they are to be involved after their children are born. And that's good for your child, good for you, and good for your relationship with your child's mother.

All that's very nice, of course, but it's clearly dependent on your partner's *being* pregnant. So a good understanding of *her* perspective on the pregnancy—emotional as well as physical—is essential to understanding how *you* will react. It was precisely this perspective that Jennifer Ash, along with my wife and hundreds of other expectant and new mothers I've interviewed over the years, provided. Throughout the process of writing the book, all of these women contributed valuable information and comments, not only about what pregnant women are going through but also about the ways women most want men to be involved, and the impact that involvement has on the entire pregnancy experience.

A NOTE ON STRUCTURE

Throughout the book I try to present straightforward, practical information in an easy-to-absorb format. Each of the main chapters is divided into four sections, as follows:

What's Going On with Your Partner

Even though this is a book about what you as an expectant father are going through during pregnancy, and how you can best stay involved, it's critical that you understand what your partner is going through and when. For that reason, we felt that it was important to start each chapter with a summary of your partner's physical and emotional pregnancy experience.

What's Going On with the Baby

You can't very well have a pregnancy without a baby, right? This section lets you in on your future child's progress—from sperm and egg to living, breathing infant—and everything in between.

What's Going On with You

This section covers the wide range of feelings—good, bad, and indifferent—that you'll probably experience at some time during the pregnancy. It also describes such things as the physical changes you may go through, your dreams, your changing values, your relationships with other people, and the ways the pregnancy may affect your sex life.

Staying Involved

While the "What's Going On with You" section covers the emotional and physical side of pregnancy, this section gives you specific facts, tips, and advice on what you can *do* to make the pregnancy "yours" as well as your partner's. For instance, you'll find easy, nutritious recipes to prepare, information on how to start a college fund for the baby, valuable advice on getting the most out of your birth classes, great ways to start communicating with your baby before he or she is born, tips on finding work/family balance (hint: there's no such thing, but with planning, you may be able to get close). And sprinkled throughout, you'll find suggestions for how to be supportive of your partner and how to stay included at every stage of the pregnancy.

The Expectant Father covers more than the nine months of pregnancy. We've included a detailed chapter on labor and delivery and another on Cesarean section, both of which will prepare you for the big event and how best to help your partner through the birth itself. Perhaps even more important, these chapters prepare you for the often overwhelming emotions you may experience when your partner is in labor and your child is born.

We've also included a special chapter that addresses the major questions and concerns you may have about caring for and getting to know your child in the first few weeks after you bring him or her home. If someone hasn't bought them for you already, I'd recommend that you rush right out and get copies of *The New Father: A Dad's Guide to the First Year* and *Fathering Your Toddler: A Dad's Guide to the Second and Third Years*. These books pick up where this one leaves off and continue the process of giving you the skills, knowledge, confidence, and support you'll need to be the best possible dad. All of them are also available as e-books.

Toward the end of this book there is a chapter called "Fathering Today," in which you'll learn to recognize—and overcome—the many obstacles you may encounter along the road to becoming an actively involved dad.

As you go through *The Expectant Father*, remember that the process of becoming a dad is different for every man, and that none of us will react to the same situation in exactly the same way. You may find that some of what's described in the "What's Going On with You" section in the third-month chapter won't really ring true for you until the fifth month, or that you already experienced it in the first month. I've tried to tie the ideas and activities in the "Staying Involved" sections to specific stages of the pregnancy. But, hey, it's your baby, so if you want to do things in a different order, knock yourself out.

A NOTE ON TERMINOLOGY

Wife, Girlfriend, Lover, He, She . . .

In an attempt to avoid offending anyone (an approach I've discovered usually ends up offending everyone), we've decided to refer to the woman who's carrying the baby as "your partner." And because your partner is just as likely to be carrying a boy as a girl, we've alternated between "he" and "she" when referring to the baby (except where something applies specifically to boys or girls).

Hospitals, Doctors. . .

Not everyone who has a baby delivers in a hospital or is under the care of a medical doctor. Still, because that's the most frequent scenario, we've chosen to refer to the place where the baby will be born as "the hospital" and to the people attending the birth (besides you, of course) as "doctors," "nurses," "medical professionals," or "practitioners"—except, of course, in the sections that specifically deal with home birth and/or midwives.

As a rule, today's dads (and expectant dads) want to be much more involved with their children than their own fathers were able to be. It's my firm belief that the first step on the road toward full involvement is to take an active role in the pregnancy.

And it's our hope that when you're through reading *The Expectant Father*—which is the book Jennifer wishes she could have bought for her husband when she was pregnant and the one I wish I'd had when I was an expectant dad—you'll be much better prepared to participate in this important new phase of your life.

So why should you get involved now, before you actually become a dad? Simply put, because it's good for your child, your partner, and yourself. As mentioned above, involvement during pregnancy is a good predictor of involvement after the pregnancy. And children who grow up in homes where the dad is involved do better in math and science, are more sociable, are more tenacious when solving problems, and, thinking *waaaay* out into the future, are less likely to use drugs or alcohol or become teen parents.

When the dad-to-be is involved during the pregnancy, he and his partner are more likely to be together for their child's third birthday than partnerships in which dad isn't as involved. Pregnant women whose partners are involved prenatally are more likely to get prenatal care and, if they smoke, to quit. And according to researcher Jacinta Bronte-Tinkew, women whose partners aren't supportive during the pregnancy are "more likely to view their pregnancy as unwanted." Finally, your being involved now makes it more likely that your partner will breastfeed your baby (we'll talk about why that's so important later on).

For you, being an involved dad will reduce the chance that you'll engage in risky behavior. You'll probably start taking better care of yourself, you'll be happier in your relationship with your partner, and you'll even perform better at work.

WHAT'S NEW IN THIS EDITION

In the years since the first edition of *The Expectant Father* was published, I've received literally thousands of letters (yes, people still do send letters) and emails from readers offering comments and suggestions on how to make this book better. I've incorporated many of them into this edition, and I know that the book is greatly improved as a result. Let me give you a quick rundown:

- **ADOPTIVE FATHERS.** Although your partner may not actually be carrying a baby, the two of you are still very much "psychologically pregnant." There's a lot of research, in fact, that suggests that in the months leading up to the adoption of their child, expectant adoptive fathers deal with many of the same emotional and psychological issues that biologically expectant fathers do.
- **MULTIPLES.** We've expanded the sections geared toward expectant fathers of twins, triplets, and so forth.
- **OVERCOMING INFERTILITY.** As the average age of new parents increases, more and more couples are experiencing infertility. So we've included a whole

chapter on infertility in the Appendix as well as information on what you can do to increase the chances that you and your partner will conceive.

- **THE ART OF FATHERHOOD.** An increasing number of couples are conceiving through the use of ART (assisted reproductive technology), which includes IVF (in vitro fertilization), artificial insemination, donor sperm, donor eggs, and gestational carriers (who used to be referred to as surrogates). We've included a number of sections that deal with the fascinating issues facing ART dads and their partners.

- **GI DADS.** Every year, a huge number of men (and women) from all branches of the service spend at least part of their partner's pregnancy thousands of miles away. Many of them come home to a child who was born while they were deployed. As a Marine myself (I got out long ago, but as we all know, there's no such thing as an "ex-Marine"), I knew I needed to do as much as I could to help our service members. For that reason we've included several sections in this book designed to help expectant military dads stay involved before, during, and after the pregnancy so that they can hit the ground running when they get back home. I go into these issues in much more detail in my book *The Military Father: A Hands-on Guide for Deployed Dads*.

WE NEED YOUR HELP

I'd love to hear your experiences, feelings, comments, and suggestions, and I'll try to incorporate them into future editions of this book. You can email me at armin@MrDad.com. And as long as you're online, please visit my website (mrdad.com). Info on how to connect with me via social media is in the Resources appendix of the book, on page 300.

Now, close your eyes, take a deep breath, and let's get you started on this new and wonderful stage of your life!

First Decisions

Among the first major questions you and your partner will face after learning she's pregnant are: *Where are we going to have the baby? Who's going to help us deliver it? How much is it all going to cost?* To a certain extent, the answers will be dictated by your health insurer, but there are still a range of options to consider. As you weigh all your choices, give your partner at least 51 percent of the vote. After all, the ultimate decision really affects her more than it does you.

WHERE AND HOW

Hospitals

For most couples—especially first-time parents—the hospital is the most common place to give birth. It's also, in many people's view, the safest. In the unlikely event that complications arise, most hospitals have specialists on staff twenty-four hours a day and are equipped with all the necessary life-saving equipment and medications. And in those first hectic hours or days after the birth, the on-staff nurses monitor the baby and mother and help both new parents with the dozens of questions that are likely to come up. They also run interference for you and help fend off unwanted intrusions. If you have a choice among several hospitals in your area, be sure to take a tour of each one before making your decision.

Most of the time, you'll end up going with the hospital where your partner's doctor or midwife has privileges (or where your insurance plan says you can go). Some people do it the other way around: they select the hospital first and then find a practitioner who's associated with that hospital.

Many hospitals now have birthing rooms (or entire birthing centers) that are carefully decorated to look less sterile and medical and more like a bedroom at home, although the effect is really more like a nice motel suite or a quaint bed-and-breakfast. The cozy decor is supposed to make you and your partner feel more comfortable. But with the wood furniture cleverly concealing sophisticated monitoring equipment, the cabinets full of sterile supplies, and nurses dropping by every hour or so to give your partner a pelvic exam, it's going to be hard to forget where you are. Keep in mind that at some hospitals, birthing rooms are assigned on a first-come-first-served basis, so don't count on getting one—unless you can convince your partner to go into labor before anyone else does that day. In other hospitals, *all* the labor rooms are also birthing rooms, so this won't be an issue.

Hospitals, by their nature, are pretty busy places, and they have all sorts of rules and policies that may or may not make sense to you. Giving birth in a hospital generally involves less privacy for you and your partner, and more routine (and sometimes intrusive) procedures for her and the baby.

That said, if your partner is considered "high risk" (meaning she's carrying twins or more, is over thirty-five, has had any complications during a previous delivery, had complications during this pregnancy, has any medical risk factors, or was told as much by her practitioner), a hospital birth will—and should—be your only choice.

Freestanding Birthing Centers

Of the 1–2 percent of births that take place outside a hospital, about 30 percent happen in private birthing centers. Usually staffed by certified nurse-midwives (CNMs), these facilities tend to offer a more personal approach to the birthing process. They look and feel a lot like home—nice wallpaper, hot tubs, and sometimes even a kitchen. They're generally less rigid than hospitals and more willing to accommodate any special requests your partner or you might have. For example, there are fewer routine medical interventions, your partner may be allowed to eat during labor (a big no-no at most hospitals), and she'll be able to wear her own clothes—none of those unflattering hospital gowns unless she really wants one. The staff will also try to make sure your partner and baby are never separated. One downside is that you and your newly expanded family may need to check out as soon as six to ten hours after the birth.

Private birthing centers are designed to deal with uncomplicated, low-risk pregnancies and births, so expect to be prescreened. And don't worry: if something doesn't go exactly as planned, birthing centers are always affiliated with a doctor and are usually either attached to a hospital or only a short ambulance ride away.

If you're interested in exploring this option, start by getting a recommendation from your partner's practitioner or friends and family. Or, contact the American Association of Birth Centers at www.birthcenters.org.

Home Birth

With all their high-tech efficiency and stark, impersonal, antiseptic conditions, hospitals are not for everyone. As a result, some couples (less than 1 percent) decide to have their baby at home. Home birth has been around forever (before 1920, that's where most births happened) but has been out of favor in this country for a long time. It is, however, making something of a comeback as more and more people (most of whom aren't even hippies) decide to give it a try.

My wife and I thought about a home birth for our second baby but ultimately decided against it. While I don't consider myself particularly squeamish, I just couldn't imagine how we'd avoid making a mess all over the bedroom carpet. What really clinched it for us, though, was that our first child had been an emergency Cesarean section. Fearing that we might run into problems again, we opted to be near the doctors.

If you're thinking about a home birth, be prepared. Having a baby at home is quite a bit different from the way it's made out to be in those old westerns. You'll need to assume much more responsibility for the whole process than if you were using a hospital. It takes a lot of research and preparation. At the very least, you're going to need a lot more than clean towels and boiling water.

Making the decision to give birth at home does *not* mean that your partner can skip getting prenatal care or that the two of you should plan on delivering your baby alone. You'll still need to be in close contact with a medical professional to ensure that the pregnancy is progressing normally, and you should make sure to have someone present at the birth who has plenty of experience with childbirth (no, not your sister or your mother-in-law, unless they happen to be qualified). So if you're planning on going this route, start working on selecting a midwife right now.

Statistically, it's pretty unlikely that you'll go this route. But in case you're considering it, I want to take you through some of the reasons people commonly give for wanting to have their baby at home, and some situations that would make a home birth unnecessarily risky.

Natural vs. Medicated Birth

In recent years giving birth "naturally"—without drugs, pain medication, or any medical intervention—has become all the rage. But just because it's popular doesn't mean it's for everybody. Labor and delivery are going to be a painful experience—for both of you, although in different ways—and many couples elect to

15

take advantage of the advances medical science has made in relieving the pain and discomfort of childbirth. Whichever way you go, make sure the decision is your partner's. Proponents of some childbirth methods (see pages 159–63) are almost religiously committed to the idea of a drug-free delivery, to the extent that they often make women who opt for any pain medication feel as though they're failures. Besides making a lot of new parents feel bad about themselves when they should be celebrating the birth of their baby, that militant attitude is simply out of touch with reality. Nationwide, about half of women give birth using an epidural (which is the most common method of pain relief), and in some big-city hospitals that rate is north of 85 percent.

There are advantages and disadvantages to both medicated and unmedicated births, and we'll talk about them when we get closer to your baby's due date. But for now, the most important thing is to be flexible and not let your friends, relatives, or anyone else pressure you into doing something you don't want to do.

You and your partner may be planning a natural childbirth, but conditions could develop that necessitate intervention or the use of medication (see pages 60-62). On the other hand, you may be planning a medicated delivery but could find yourself snowed in someplace far from your hospital and any pain medication, or the anesthesiologist may be at an emergency on the other side of town.

WHO'S GOING TO HELP?

At first glance, it may seem that your partner should be picking a medical practitioner alone—after all, she's the one who's going to be poked and prodded as the pregnancy develops. But considering that more than 90 percent of today's expectant fathers are present during the delivery of their children, and that the vast majority of them have been involved in some significant way during the rest of the pregnancy, you're probably going to be spending a lot of time with the practitioner as well. So if at all possible, you should feel comfortable with the final choice, too. Here are the main players.

Private Obstetrician

If your partner is over twenty, she's probably been seeing a gynecologist for a few years. And since many gynecologists also do obstetrics, it should come as no surprise that most couples elect to have the woman's regular obstetrician/gynecologist (OB/GYN) deliver the baby.

Private OB/GYNs are generally the most expensive way to go, but your insurance company will probably pick up a good part of the bill. Most private OBs, however, aren't strictly private; they usually have a number of partners, which

WHY TO HAVE THE BABY AT HOME

- The surroundings are more familiar, comfortable, and private.
- You don't like—or are afraid of—hospitals and doctors. Or you had a negative experience with a previous birth.
- You've already had one or more uncomplicated hospital births.
- You can surround yourselves with anyone you pick.
- The birth is more likely to go exactly as you want than it might anywhere else. And your partner will be treated less like a patient than she would be in a hospital.
- You can pay attention to the spiritual aspects of the delivery, an intimate matter that you might be discouraged from, or feel embarrassed about, in the hospital.
- Hospitals are full of sick people and it's best to stay far away from them.
- It's cheaper.

WHY NOT TO HAVE THE BABY AT HOME

- Your partner is over 35 or has been told by her doctor that she's "high risk."
- She's carrying twins (or more) or you find out that the baby is breech (feet down instead of head down).
- She goes into labor prematurely.
- She developed preeclampsia, a condition that affects about 10 percent of pregnant women and that can have very serious complications if it's not detected and treated early (see pages 61–62 for more on this).
- She has diabetes or a heart or kidney condition, has had hemorrhaging in a previous labor, has had a previous Cesarean section, or smokes cigarettes.
- No insurance coverage.

means that the doctor you see for your prenatal appointments might not be the one in attendance at the birth. So make sure that you're aware of and comfortable with the backup arrangements—just in case your baby decides to show up on a day when your regular doctor isn't on call. Labor and delivery are going to be stressful enough without having to deal with a doctor you've never met before.

Researcher Sandra Howell-White found that women who view childbirth as risky, or who want to have a say in managing their pain or the length of their labor, tend to opt for obstetricians.

Family Physician (FP)

Although many FPs provide obstetrical care, not all do, so check with yours to see whether he or she does. If not, he or she will refer your partner to someone else for the pregnancy and birth. One of the big advantages of going with your family doctor is that after the birth, he or she often can see your partner and baby on the same visit. The time saved running around from doctor to doctor will be welcome.

Like most doctors, FPs are frequently in group practices, and there's no guarantee that the doctor you know will be on call the day the baby comes. So, if you can, try to meet with the other doctors in the practice, as well as any OB/GYNs your family doctor might work with. (Most FPs can't do C-sections or assisted deliveries, and will need OB/GYN backup. In addition, since malpractice insurance covering maternity care and childbirth is very expensive, many FPs will refer pregnant patients to an OB who already has that coverage. Make sure you're comfortable with this person, since he or she may be doing the delivery if things get complicated.)

Midwife

Although midwives are not as common in the United States as they are in Europe and other parts of the world, they're becoming increasingly popular. And you might want to consider bringing one into the process, even if your partner has a regular OB.

In Howell-White's study, women who expect their partners to be actively involved in labor and delivery and who place a high value on getting information on the birth process are more likely to opt for a midwife. Interestingly, so are women who have no religious affiliation.

Certified nurse-midwives (CNMs) are licensed nurses who have taken a minimum of two or three years of additional training in obstetrics and passed special certification exams. They can deliver babies in hospitals, birthing centers, or at home. But because their training is usually in uncomplicated, low-risk births, CNMs have to work under a physician, just in case something comes up.

Some states have created a new designation, certified midwife (CM), which allows practitioners who aren't nurses, but who go through the same training and take the same exams as CNMs, to work as midwives.

Many standard OB/GYN practices, recognizing that some of their patients might want to have a midwife in attendance at the birth, now have a CNM (or in some cases a CM) on staff. Officially, then, your partner is still under the care of a physician—whose services can be paid for by insurance—but she'll still get the more personalized care she wants. Keep in mind, though, that because midwives aren't MDs, they can't perform surgery and they're able to handle only low-risk cases.

If you're considering using a CNM or a CM and need some help with your search, the American College of Nurse-Midwives (midwife.org) can put you in touch with one in your area and fill you in on any applicable regulations. If you've already found a midwife but want to be sure she's properly certified, visit the American Midwifery Certification Board (www.amcbmidwife.org).

There are also plenty of midwives out there who are neither certified nor licensed. Lay midwives have a lot of experience working with pregnant women and may even have a lot of specialized training. But they're not regulated and may not have passed any specific midwife exams, which means that in most cases they can work in home settings but not in hospitals or birthing centers.

Like CNMs or CMs, lay midwives must work with a physician, in case of an emergency. The Midwives Alliance of North America (MANA.org) can help you find out more about lay midwives and make contact with one near you.

Doula

Although it sounds like it should mean "a little duel," *doula* is actually a Greek word that means "a woman caregiver of another woman." Many doulas have had children of their own, and all of them go through an intensive training period in which they are taught how to give the laboring woman *and* her partner emotional and physical support throughout labor, and information about the delivery. Doulas have become increasingly popular over the years, and we'll talk a lot more about them on pages 165–67. For now, though, as you're just beginning the process, there's one very important thing to think about.

Doulas are *not* medical professionals, they're generally not regulated, and they may not be particularly welcome in hospitals. Here's how childbirth educator Sarah McMoyler and I described, in our book *The Best Birth*, the sometimes combative relationships that can develop. "The problem is that some doulas have an agenda and see their role as protecting mom and baby from what they believe are unnecessary interventions. Sometimes they take that agenda a couple steps too far and start playing doctor, inserting their non-medical opinion into a science-based hospital arena. As you can imagine, this can create tension and confusion, and is, frankly, completely inappropriate." Because this kind of attitude can interfere with the medical team's ability to do its job, a number of OB/GYN practices and hospitals around the country have banned doulas from their delivery rooms. That said, several studies have shown that having a doula can reduce the length of labor. But before you plunk down a deposit, check with your OB.

What to Ask Your Prospective Practitioner

Besides a medical school degree, OB/GYNs may have little else in common. Each will have a slightly different philosophy and approach to pregnancy and birth. The same (except for the medical school part) can be said for midwives. So before making a final decision about who's going to deliver your baby, you should get satisfactory answers to the following questions and any others you can think of. (If at all possible, make a separate appointment to do this. You'll never be able to get everything in a fifteen-minute appointment. And no, there are no stupid questions—we're talking about your partner and baby here.)

ESPECIALLY FOR OB/GYNS

- How do you feel about the father being there for prenatal exams and attending the delivery? Are you enthusiastic about it or just tolerant?
- Do you recommend any particular childbirth preparation method (Lamaze, Bradley, and so on)?
- At which hospital(s) do you deliver your babies?
- Are you board certified? Do you have any specialties or special training?
- How many partners do you have and how often are they on rotation?
- What percent of your patients' babies do you deliver? What are your backup arrangements if you can't be there?
- Where do you stand on the natural-vs.-medicated debate?
- What's your philosophy about Cesareans, labor inductions, and episiotomies?
- What's your C-section rate, and how do you make the decision to proceed with the surgery?
- Do you permit fathers to attend Cesarean sections? If so, where do they stand (up by the woman's shoulders or down at the "business end")?
- What is your definition of a "high-risk" pregnancy?
- What kind of monitoring do you recommend? Require?
- How do you feel about the mother lifting the baby out herself if she wishes?
- How do you feel about the father assisting at the birth?
- Do you routinely suction the baby or use forceps during delivery?
- Do you usually hand the naked baby straight to the mother?
- Do you allow the mother or father to cut the umbilical cord?

ESPECIALLY FOR MIDWIVES

- Are you licensed or certified? By which organization?
- How many babies have you delivered?
- Which physicians and hospitals are you associated with?
- How often does a physician get involved in the care of your patients?
- What is the role of the physician in your practice?
- What position do most of the women you work with adopt for the second stage of labor?
- How do you make the decision to transfer the patient to a hospital or the care of a physician? How often does that happen?

FOR BOTH OB/GYNS AND MIDWIVES

- Do you have an advice line we can call when we panic about something?
- What are your rates and payment plans?
- What insurance, if any, do you take?
- What percentage of your patients had natural, unmedicated births in the past year?
- What's your definition of "high risk"?
- If labor starts when you're not on call, will you come in anyway?
- What and who (besides you, Dad) is allowed in the delivery room (friends, relatives, doulas, cameras, webcams, etc.)?
- Are you willing to wait until the umbilical cord has stopped pulsating before you clamp it?
- What prenatal tests do you suggest getting? Which ones do you require?
- Which tests do you usually order for women like your partner (her age, race, medical history, and risk factors)?
- How many sonograms (ultrasounds) do you routinely recommend?
- Are women free to walk, move, and take a shower throughout the early stages of labor? Can the baby be put to the breast immediately after delivery?
- Are you willing to dim the lights when the baby is born?
- How much experience have you had with twins or more? (This is a very important question if you and/or your partner have a family history of multiple births or if you suspect that your partner is carrying more than one baby.)

BILLS

Having a baby isn't cheap. Exactly how much you have to come up with will depend on how and where your baby is born, and which of the infinite combinations of deductible, coinsurance, copays, and out-of-pocket maximums you have. According to the Agency for Healthcare Research and Quality, a part of the U.S. Department of Health and Human Services, the average charge for a vaginal delivery is just under $9,000—nearly triple what it was in 1993. And the average charge for a Cesarean is almost $16,000—2.5 times higher than in 1993. Private insurance covered an average of 80 percent of prenatal care charges and 88 percent of delivery charges. But even if you have good insurance, that 12–20 percent can still add up in a hurry. Do keep in mind, though, that what the practitioner receives will almost always be quite a bit less than the sticker price.

In the sections that follow, you'll get an idea of how the costs for a typical—and a not-so-typical—pregnancy and childbirth experience might break down. It's a good idea to look over your insurance policy, find out how much it will be picking up, and start figuring out now how you're going to pay for the rest of it. Oh, and all of this is in addition to anything you might have paid for fertility diagnosis and treatment. What we're talking about here are just the costs that come up after your partner gets pregnant. Putting together a budget can be important even if you're adopting. In many cases, adoptive parents are in close contact with the birth mother throughout her pregnancy and delivery. You and your partner might go with her to the doctor's appointments, see the ultrasound, hear the baby's heartbeat, and pick up the bills—most of which won't be reimbursed by your insurance company—for everything. If you're doing an international adoption, you won't have to worry about covering the birth mother's medical expenses, but you'll probably need to budget in the cost of several overseas trips. In addition, you'll need to take into account the many other adoption-related expenses you're likely to incur, including agency fees, attorney's fees, and the home study you'll have to go through.

Pregnancy and Childbirth

Most doctors charge a flat fee for your partner's care during the entire pregnancy. This generally covers monthly visits during the first two trimesters, biweekly visits for the next month or so, and then weekly visits until delivery. But don't make the mistake of thinking that that's all you'll pay. Bills for blood and urine tests, ultrasounds, hospital fees, and other procedures will work their way into your mailbox at least once a month. Here's what you can expect to pay (before your insurance pays its part) for having your baby:

OB/GYN

Expect to pay $2,500–6,500 for general prenatal care and a problem-free, vaginal delivery. Add a few thousand more for a C-section. Most doctors will meet with you to discuss their rates and the services they provide. For a list of important questions to ask, see pages 20–21. In addition, be sure to discuss which insurance plans, if any, they participate in (it might actually be easier to start with the doctors your insurance covers and choose from there). You should also ask whether they'll bill your insurance company directly or will want you to make a deposit (most will want to collect about 25 percent of the anticipated bill up front); whether you can make your payments in installments; and whether they expect their fee to be paid in full before the delivery.

MIDWIFE

The average cost of a delivery by a midwife is $2,000–4,000, but it can vary greatly depending on where you live and whether you expect her to be with you throughout labor or just the part that's right before the birth. If you're delivering at home, you'll also need to add the cost of the supplies the midwife thinks you'll need for the birth (sterile pads, bandages, and so on).

Lab and Other Expenses

- Blood: Over the course of the pregnancy, you can expect to be billed anywhere from $200 to $1,500 for various blood tests.
- Ultrasound: At least $250 each. In an ordinary pregnancy, you'll have between none and three.

Prenatal Testing

If you and/or your practitioner decide that you're a candidate for amniocentesis or any other prenatal diagnostic test, you can expect to pay $1,000–1,500. In most cases genetic counseling is required beforehand, and that costs an additional $400–600. If you're having any prenatal testing done just because you'd like to find out the sex of the baby or want reassurance of its well-being (and not because you're in a high-risk group), your insurance company may not pay for it. But if your partner is thirty-five or older, they probably will pay for testing.

At the Hospital

- If you're paying for it yourself, a problem-free vaginal delivery and a twenty-four-hour stay in a hospital will run anywhere from $4,500 to $9,000, depending on where you live. Add $5,000–7,000 for a Cesarean.

- If you're planning to spend the night in the hospital with your partner, add about $250 per day.
- Anesthesiologists usually charge from $1,000 to $1,500, depending on what they do and the time spent doing it.
- Although a lot of people worry about preterm delivery, there's also the issue of late delivery. If your baby decides to stay inside any more than seven to ten days past his due date, your partner may need to have labor induced. If that happens, add another $1,000–3,000.
- If your partner does deliver early (by more than a couple of weeks) and your baby needs to spend time in intensive care, the bills—most of which you will hopefully never see—can go into the hundreds of thousands.

If Your Partner Needs a Cesarean Section

If your partner ends up having a C-section (which happens more than 30 percent of the time—up from 21 percent in 1993), all bets are off. Even though it's routinely done, it's still considered major surgery, and is expensive. The operation, which your OB/GYN will perform, is not included in his or her flat fee, and you'll have to pay for at least two other doctors to assist, plus a nurse, who must be in attendance to care for the baby. In addition, a C-section entails a longer recovery period in the hospital—usually four to five days—as well as extra nursing care, pain medication, bandages, and other supplies. If the baby is in good health, you can probably take him home while your partner stays in the hospital, but chances are you'll want the baby to stay with your partner, especially if she is breastfeeding. The baby's additional time in the nursery costs more too.

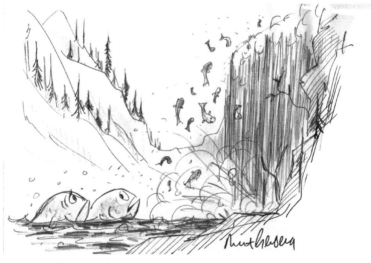

"Listen, are you absolutely sure you want to have kids?"

An Important (and Possibly Profitable) Word of Advice

Make sure that you and your partner check your birth-related bills very carefully. Hospitals can make mistakes—in fact, a study by credit giant Equifax found that nine out of ten hospital bills contain errors, and they're rarely in your favor. After we'd recovered from the shock of the C-section bills for the birth of our first child (which started off at about $17,000), we asked a doctor friend to go over them with us. He found that we'd been charged for a variety of things that hadn't happened and overcharged for a lot of the things that had. For example, we'd been billed $25 for a tube of ointment that the hospital's own pharmacy was selling for $1.25. We (actually, mostly our insurance company) ended up paying closer to $15,000. And for the second pregnancy, our nitpicking review of the bills cut about 20 percent off the total.

Look for double billings, services you never received (say, a private room when you were actually in a shared one, or brand-name drugs when you really got generics), and any kind of suspicious jargon. A wonderful exposé done by ABC News found that people had been billed hundreds of dollars for a "disposable mucus recovery system" (a 79-cent box of tissues) and "thermal therapy" (ice cubes in a bag). Also keep an eye out for procedures that never happened. I've heard stories about new parents being billed for their baby's circumcision. That would have been fine, except that they had a girl.

While some of these things may seem silly, they can really add up—especially if you're footing a big portion of the bill. In the Equifax study, the average error was more than $1,300. And according to a joint study done by Harvard's Medical and Law Schools, "[n]early half of all Americans who file for bankruptcy do so because of medical expenses." About 10 percent of those are childbirth related.

Even if all the bills are being paid by your insurance, reviewing those bills can still be profitable. Although most insurance companies have their own internal auditors, all they'll be able to catch are charges that are above the "usual and customary" and/or procedures that simply aren't covered. They won't know about most of the things mentioned above and will be ecstatic if your review ends up saving them money. In fact, some insurers are so thrilled that they'll actually give you a percentage (sometimes as much as half) of the money they save. Naturally, though, you'll have to ask for your reward. So, read your policy carefully and, if you still have questions, talk to your agent or one of the company's underwriters.

And while you're reading your insurance policy, here are a few other things to look out for:

- How long before the birth does the insurer need to be notified about the pregnancy and estimated due date? Not complying with the carrier's instructions could mean a reduction in the amount they'll pay for pregnancy and birth-related expenses.

- When can the baby be added to the policy? Until the baby is born, all pregnancy- and birth-related expenses will be charged to your partner.

After the birth, however, your partner and the new baby get separate bills (all baby-related expenses, such as medication, pediatrician's exams, diapers, blankets, and various other hospital charges, will be charged to the baby). Some carriers require you to add the baby to your (or your partner's) policy as far in advance as thirty days before the birth; most give you until thirty days after. Again, failing to follow the insurer's instructions could result in a reduction of coverage.

LOW-COST ALTERNATIVES

Obstetrical Clinics

If you live in a city where there is a large teaching hospital, your partner may be able to get prenatal care at its obstetrical clinic. If so, you'll spend a lot less than you would for a private physician. The one drawback is that your baby will probably be delivered by an inexperienced—yet closely supervised—doctor or a medical student. This isn't to say that you won't be getting top-quality care. Clinics are often equipped with state-of-the-art facilities, and the young professionals who staff them are being taught all the latest methods by some of the best teachers in the country.

Your Rights to Free and Subsidized Medical Care

If worse comes to worst, hospital emergency rooms are required by federal law to give your partner an initial assessment—and any required emergency care—even if you can't afford to pay. But that's no substitute for the kind of ongoing prenatal care that will ensure a healthy pregnancy, healthy baby, and healthy mom.

So if you're uninsured or underinsured—according to the American Pregnancy Association (americanpregnancy.org/), that's the case for 13 percent of pregnant women—or just need some help paying for that prenatal care your partner needs, your first step should be to find out what Medicaid benefits she's eligible for. (If you're in this category, don't feel bad. Nearly half of all births in the U.S. are financed by Medicaid.) Since benefits vary by state, you should also make contact with your state's health department as well. You'll be able to get most of your questions answered at the Medicaid website (medicaid.gov).

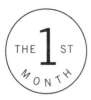

Salad Days

WHAT'S GOING ON WITH YOUR PARTNER

Physically

- Morning sickness (nausea, heartburn, vomiting)
- Food cravings or aversions
- Dizziness, irritability, headaches
- Fatigue
- Breast changes: tenderness, enlargement

Emotionally

- Thrilled, stunned, a little frightened, or even completely bummed out (not all pregnancies are planned) that she's pregnant. Sometimes all of these at the same time.
- A heightened feeling of closeness to you
- Apprehension about the nine months ahead
- Mood swings and sudden, unexplained crying

WHAT'S GOING ON WITH THE BABY

It's going to be a busy first month. About two hours after you had sex, one very lucky sperm will have fertilized the egg, and, voilà, you've got yourself a *zygote*. By the end of the day, the zygote will divide into two cells and is now, technically, an *embryo*. Your tiny bundle of cells will continue to divide, and four to seven days after conception it will implant itself comfortably into the wall of your partner's uterus, where it'll stay until birth. By the end of this month, your little embryo will be about one quarter-inch long—10,000 times bigger than when it was just a zygote—and will have a heart (but no brain), and tiny arm and leg buds.

WHAT'S GOING ON WITH YOU

Thrills

I still have the white bathrobe I was wearing the morning my wife and I found out we were expecting for the first time. I remember standing nervously in the kitchen, the countertop cluttered with vials of colored powders and liquids, droppers, and the small container filled with my wife's "first morning urine." (Fortunately, do-it-yourself pregnancy detection kits are a lot less complicated today than they used to be, but I'm not sure they're anywhere near as much fun.) Feeling like a Nobel Prize–winning chemist on the edge of making a discovery that would alter the course of the entire world, I carefully dropped several drops of the urine into one of the vials of powder. I stirred the mixture with the specially provided swizzle stick, rinsed it, and slowly added the contents of the other vial.

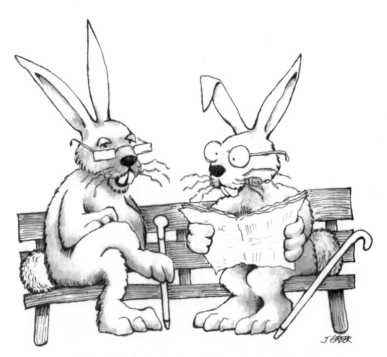

"Young kids today don't know how good they have it. . . .
I remember the old days before home pregnancy tests."

Fresh or Frozen

Whether your baby was conceived in a lab or a bed, your future child will develop in the same way. A few days after conception, the embryo—now about eight cells—may be implanted in your partner's uterus. Some clinics wait a few more days, until the embryo develops into a *blastocyst*. The reason is that in the wild, fertilization usually takes place in the fallopian tubes and the embryo travels for a few days until arriving in the uterus, where it implants in the wall. Not all embryos, however, develop into blastocysts, so waiting until they do gives your fertility doc a better shot at implanting something that has a strong chance of survival.

If you're doing IVF, the eggs you use will come either from your partner or another woman. And you can order them in one of two ways: fresh or frozen. Fresh embryos result in somewhat more pregnancies and live births than frozen ones. However, fresh isn't always a possibility (the eggs may have been fertilized before you or your partner went through a medical procedure—like chemotherapy—that could potentially have damaged either her eggs or your sperm. Or the eggs may have been retrieved from a faraway donor). Interestingly, fresh may not always be better. In independent studies, researchers in Finland, the U.S., and Australia all found that while defrosted embryos result in fewer pregnancies, the babies that are produced that way are less likely to be born prematurely, be born underweight, or die soon after birth. No one has any idea why that is.

In all honesty, the results we got twenty minutes later weren't a complete surprise. But that didn't make it any less thrilling. I'd always wanted to have children, and suddenly it seemed that all my dreams were finally going to come true. It was like hitting the million-dollar jackpot on the nickel slots.

Relief . . . and Pride

The pregnancy test's positive result filled me with an incredible feeling of relief. Secretly, I'd always been afraid that I was sterile and that I'd have to be satisfied with taking someone else's kids to the circus or the baseball game. I also felt a surge of pride. After all, I was a man, a fully functional man—all right, a stud, even. And by getting my wife pregnant, I'd somehow lived up to my highest potential.

If you're not the biological father of your child (your partner conceived using donor sperm), you probably won't have these feelings. But that in no way means

Morning Sickness

Somewhere between half and 90 percent of all pregnant women experience "morning sickness." Despite the catchy name, the nausea, heartburn, and vomiting can strike at any hour of the day. No one's quite sure what causes morning sickness. Some suggest that it's the pregnant woman's reaction to changing hormone levels, in particular *human chorionic gonadotropin* (hCG), which is produced by the placenta and is the same stuff that's picked up by home pregnancy kits. Others, such as researchers Margie Profet, Samuel Flaxman, and Paul Sherman, contend that morning sickness is the body's natural way of protecting the growing fetus from *teratogens* (toxins that cause birth defects) and *abortifacients* (toxins that induce miscarriage). Morning sickness seems to go hand in hand with food aversions, which a lot of pregnant women also have. The most common aversions are to meat, fish, poultry, and eggs—all foods that can spoil quickly and can carry disease.

Whatever the cause, for most women, morning sickness typically starts four to six weeks after conception and disappears by fourteen to fifteen weeks. Until then, here are a few things you can do to help your partner cope:

- Give her some good news. It turns out morning sickness may actually be a good thing. Women who don't have nausea or vomit are three times more likely to miscarry than those who do have those symptoms, according to researcher Gideon Koren. And women over thirty-five (whose risk of miscarriage is higher) benefited the most. In addition, women with morning sickness are less likely to deliver too early, have very low-birth-weight babies, or have babies with birth defects. Oh, and those babies do have higher IQs. Knowing this probably won't make your partner feel any better, but it might give her something to smile about as she's leaning over the toilet bowl.
- Encourage her to drink a lot of fluids (although some women with morning sickness have trouble tolerating milk). You might also want to keep a large water bottle next to the bed. She should avoid caffeine, which tends to be dehydrating, and she might want to start the day with a small amount of

that you're any less manly—or that you're going to be any less of a dad—than the rest of us.

Many expectant ART dads feel a different kind of relief: all those months and years of infertility treatment—the emotional ups and downs, the optimism and disappointment—are now a thing of the past. Other dads take longer to get to this point, and some never completely shake the infertility mentality.

nonacidic juice, such as apple or grape, or flat soda; the sweet flavor will probably encourage her to drink a little more than she might otherwise.

- Be sensitive to the sights and smells that make her queasy—and keep them away from her. Fatty or spicy foods are frequent offenders.
- Encourage her to eat a lot of small meals throughout the day—every two or three hours, if possible—and to eat before she starts feeling nauseated. Low blood sugar can make the nausea worse. A high-protein, high-carbohydrate diet may help. And basic, bland foods like rice and yogurt are particularly good because they're less likely to cause nausea than greasy foods.
- Go for a walk. Some women find that exercise reduces nausea.
- Make sure she takes her prenatal vitamins—with food—if her doctor says to do so. He may also suggest that she take some additional vitamin B and K. For some women, the prenatal vitamins may actually be making the morning sickness worse. OB Lissa Rankin often switches her patients to a chewable vitamin. If that doesn't work, she takes them off the vitamins altogether for a few months. "It's more important to stay hydrated and take in some nutrients than to take a vitamin," she says.
- Put some pretzels, crackers, or rice cakes by the bed—she'll need something to start and end the day with, and these are low in fat and calories and easy to digest.
- Explore alternative treatments. Acupressure bands that press on the inside of the wrist have reduced symptoms in some women, and so has eating or drinking ginger or taking vitamin B6 supplements. In addition, some research indicates that sniffing peppermint oil and isopropyl alcohol (the stuff they rub on your arm before giving you a shot) can shorten the duration of symptoms. But be sure to check with her practitioner before she starts sniffing or eating or pressing on anything.
- Be aware that she needs plenty of rest and encourage her to get it.

Irrational Fears

At some point after the initial excitement passes, a surprising number of men find themselves experiencing an irrational fear that the child their partner is carrying is not theirs. Psychologist Jerrold Lee Shapiro interviewed more than two hundred men whose partners were pregnant, and found that 60 percent "acknowledged fleeting thoughts, fantasies, or nagging doubts that they might not really be the biological father of the child." The majority of these men don't actually believe their partners are having affairs. Rather, Shapiro writes, these feelings are symptoms of a common type of insecurity: the fear many men have that they simply aren't capable of doing anything as incredible as creating life, and that someone more potent must have done the job. Most guys get over these feelings pretty quickly.

Dads whose baby was conceived using donor sperm and aren't biologically connected have their own kind of irrational fears. A lot of guys worry that they won't be able to bond with their baby or that sperm samples have been switched and that they'll end up with a child of a different race. Actually, the issue isn't so much race as physical similarity. Most IVF couples don't feel the need to make the circumstances of the pregnancy public. And, like any other dads, they hope their children will look like them—at least enough so that they won't have to deal with the inevitable "Gee, the baby doesn't look anything like you" comments. They may choose to tell the kids the true story of their birth later on. But that's a topic we'll tackle in the sequel to this book, *The New Father: A Dad's Guide to the First Year*.

STAYING INVOLVED

Exercise

If your partner was already working out regularly before the pregnancy, she probably won't need any extra encouragement to exercise. And if her doctor approves, she can continue her regular fitness routine, and do pretty much any kind of working out she wants to (see "Workout No-Nos" on page 34 for some exceptions). Be aware, though, that some health clubs—out of fear of getting sued—may ask a pregnant woman to provide a letter from her doctor. If your partner wasn't physically active before pregnancy, this isn't the time for her to take up rock climbing or start training for a marathon. That doesn't mean, however, that she should spend the entire pregnancy on the sofa. Getting exercise is critical (the Centers for Disease Control and Prevention—CDC—recommends thirty minutes per day of moderate exercise). It will help improve her circulation and keep her energy level high.

Exercising during pregnancy may also help your partner keep her weight gain steady and reasonable, help her sleep better, improve her mood, and reduce some of the normal pregnancy-related discomforts. Plus, it will improve her strength and endurance, both of which will come in very handy during labor and delivery. Researchers James Clapp and Elizabeth Noble found that women who exercise during the pregnancy have shorter labors and give birth to healthier babies. Others, including Bradley Price, have found that exercise may even lessen the chance

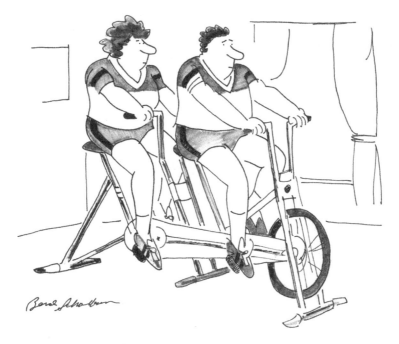

that your partner will deliver prematurely, have complications during labor, or need a Cesarean section.

Finally, there's Canadian neuroscientist Dave Ellemberg, who found that compared to couch-potato expectant moms, pregnant women who did twenty minutes of moderate exercise (leading to slight shortness of breath by the end) three times per week had babies with "more mature cerebral activation." Translation: their brains developed more quickly. Ellemberg believes that those babies could "acquire speech more rapidly" and reach developmental milestones sooner.

But because pregnancy can make even the buffest woman feel a little run down, she may not always feel like working out. One way to help motivate her to get the exercise she needs is to work out with her. (See below for a list of good activities you can do together.) The most important thing is to start easy and not push her if you see she's feeling tired or winded. If your budget doesn't permit joining a gym or a health club, you can always buy pregnancy workout DVDs or even download pregnancy exercise apps to your phone.

Whatever you do, remember that you and your partner will get the greatest benefit and least chance of injury if you exercise regularly—thirty minutes on as many days as you can—rather than sporadically. Here are some great ways of exercising together:

- Walking—doesn't matter whether it's fast or slow, through your neighborhood, on a trail, or on a treadmill.

Workout No-Nos

- High-impact sports. I've spoken with dozens of OB/GYNs over the years and have yet to find one who seriously believes that it's possible to induce a miscarriage by ordinary falling—especially in the first trimester. Severe, sudden impacts such as car crashes can sometimes cause a miscarriage, though. Same with sudden starts and stops, such as might occur on a roller coaster. That said, it's a good idea to limit or avoid high-contact sports, like boxing, hockey, or roller derby.
- Any sport that might cause her to take a hard fall. This includes horseback riding, in-line skating, ice skating, and, starting in about the seventh month, bicycling. For a nonpregnant person, taking a tumble doing one of these sports could be dangerous. For someone who's having balance issues, the risks are even greater.
- Downhill skiing. Unless you're an expert, don't, and even then take it easy. My wife skied when she was seven months pregnant but avoided the most challenging runs, where she'd have risked a serious fall. Unless your partner's doctor prohibits it, cross-country skiing should be fine.
- Scuba diving. The fetus can't decompress like adults can.
- Heavy lifting. This can put unnecessary pressure on internal organs.
- Overdoing it. If she can't carry on a normal conversation while exercising, she's working too hard.
- Overheating. Your partner shouldn't overdress, and she should keep her workouts moderate. Remind her to take plenty of breaks and drink lots of water before, during, and after the workout.
- Hot tubs / steam baths / saunas. During the first six to eight weeks of the pregnancy, it's best to stay away from anything that could raise your partner's body temperature above 102°F (39°C). To cool itself, the body moves blood away from the internal organs—including the uterus and the fetus that's inhabiting it—and toward the skin. After eight weeks, she should be okay. But even then, if she does decide to slip into the hot tub, make sure she drinks plenty of water.

One final word of advice: *Do not panic* if your partner did any of these things before you found out she was pregnant. First of all, there's nothing you can do about it now, and torturing yourselves won't undo it. Second, the chances are slim that anything she did will have an impact on the baby in any significant way. Just be careful from here on out.

- Running—but do yourselves and your knees a favor: get good shoes and run on a soft surface.
- Low-impact aerobics and low-impact exercise machines such as stair-steppers, treadmills, and bicycles.
- Swimming, water aerobics, or snorkeling.
- Cycling—stationary or street is fine, but you should probably skip those bumpy dirt-bike rides.
- Tennis or golf.
- Light weight-lifting.
- Yoga—but avoid extreme stretches; this can cause damage to your partner's connective tissues, which are somewhat weakened during pregnancy.

Before starting any kind of workout program, discuss the details with your provider and get his or her approval. If you're doing anything that will work up a sweat, be sure to get enough fluids. Both of you should drink a glass or so of water an hour before starting and another four to eight ounces every fifteen to twenty minutes while you're working out.

Nutrition

Although the names keep changing (once upon a time it was the Four Basic Food Groups, then came the Food Guide Pyramid, then MyPyramid, then MyPlate), the principles of good nutrition haven't changed all that much since you learned about them back in sixth grade. And a healthy pregnancy diet looks pretty much like a healthy nonpregnancy diet: eat plenty of fruits and veggies, whole grains, and lean protein, limit fats and salt, and drink a lot of water. There are a few differences, though. Now that your partner is pregnant, she'll need more calcium, folate, iron, and protein (we'll talk about this in detail below). Overall, after the first trimester, she should get about 300 more calories a day than before (more if she's carrying twins or better). Of course, if she was underweight before the pregnancy or is pregnant with multiples, she might need a little more than that. Defer to her doctor on this one.

If she was overweight before getting pregnant, this is not the time to go on a diet. At the same time, the fact that she's "eating for two" is not a license to eat anything she wants. In fact, a growing body of solid research is finding that what a woman eats while she's pregnant can directly—and permanently—affect the baby's long-tern health and risk of developing diabetes, heart disease, obesity, and other diseases. Her practitioner will undoubtedly suggest a diet for her to follow, but here are a few important nutritional basics to keep in mind:

CALCIUM

Calcium is critical to the manufacture of the baby's bones. And because so much of your partner's calcium intake goes directly to the baby, she needs to make sure there's enough left over for herself—1,200–1,500 mg per day. If not, the growing fetus will leach it from your partner's bones, potentially increasing her risk of developing osteoporosis later in life. The best sources of calcium are milk and other dairy products. But if your partner is allergic to milk or is lactose intolerant (a condition that affects as many as fifty million Americans), many doctors will advise her to stay away from it—especially if she's planning to breastfeed (her milk allergy could be passed to the baby). Good alternate sources of calcium include pink salmon (canned, with soft bones, is okay), tofu, broccoli, calcium-fortified orange juice, eggs, and oyster-shell calcium tablets.

FOLATE

Folate (or folic acid) is a B vitamin that plays an important role in preventing neural tube defects, which are major defects of the brain and/or spine. These defects happen in the first few weeks of pregnancy—often before a woman knows she's pregnant. Since about half of all pregnancies are unplanned, experts recommend that every woman of childbearing age take a folate supplement, just in case. Your partner should get around 600 micrograms per day during the pregnancy. Some docs bump that to 800 micrograms per day for the first trimester. Folate is so important that many grain products, including some flours, pastas, and cereals, are fortified with it. Additional good sources of folate include asparagus, avocados, bananas, beans, beets, broccoli, citrus fruits, dark green veggies, eggs, lentils, seeds and nuts, and yogurt.

IRON

Your pregnant partner needs 27 mg of iron per day—nearly twice as much as before. If she doesn't get enough, she may become anemic and begin to feel exhausted. She should try to get three servings of iron-rich foods per day. Spinach, dried fruits, lean beef or poultry, fortified cereals, and legumes are all good sources, but since a lot of your partner's iron intake is being used to manufacture the fetus's blood, she may need still more than she can possibly get from food alone. If so, her doctor will prescribe some over-the-counter supplements, but probably not until sometime after the third month. If possible, your partner should take the tablets with a glass of orange juice—it (along with other sources of vitamin C) will help her body absorb the iron. One warning: iron supplements frequently cause constipation.

PROTEIN

The average woman needs 45 grams of protein a day, but your pregnant partner should take in about 70 grams per day. If she's pregnant with twins, however, she'll need to up her protein intake by another 20–25 grams a day, but not until she's in the fourth or fifth month. When the fetus is eight weeks old, it has about 125,000 brain-cell neurons. But then production goes into hyperdrive—one thousand new neurons every *second*—so by the end of the nineteenth week, there are more than twenty-five billion, the most your child will *ever* have.

Many nutritionists believe that a high-protein diet—especially during the first nineteen weeks of pregnancy—supports this surge in brain-cell growth in the baby. Fortunately, most women already eat plenty of protein, so your partner won't need any encouragement to eat more. But if you feel you need to be involved, lean proteins are always the best bet.

Low-fat milk is one of the easiest sources of protein: one glass has about 8 grams. Drinking milk may have other benefits as well. Dr. Fariba Mirzaei of the Harvard School of Public Health found that daughters of mothers who drank four glasses of milk per day while pregnant were 56 percent less likely to develop multiple sclerosis than daughters of women who drank less than three glass per month. Other researchers have found a positive connection between an expectant mother's milk drinking and her children's height (they're taller) and IQ (they're smarter). If your partner can't drink milk, high doses of vitamin D produced similar results. But check with her practitioner before she takes any supplements. Other good sources are skinless chicken, lean meats, low-fat cheese, tofu, peanut butter, and cooked fish (but be careful with fish; see "Nutritional and Chemical No-Nos" on pages 40–43). Eggs (cooked, not raw) are another excellent choice; hard-boiled, they travel well and make a handy between-meal snack.

FRUITS AND VEGGIES

Eat a rainbow. Well, not really. But your partner (and you, for that matter) should try to eat fruits and vegetables in as wide a variety of colors as you can. Besides helping form red blood cells, green and yellow vegetables (which, strangely enough, include cantaloupe and mango) are excellent sources of iron and vitamins A and B, which will help your partner's body absorb all that extra protein she'll be eating. Vitamin A may also help prevent bladder and kidney infections. In addition, these vegetables are an excellent source of folic acid, which we discussed above. The darker the green, the better it is for your partner.

When it comes to fruit, the more-colorful-the-better rule holds true. Fruits are bursting with all sorts of vitamins and minerals, including antioxidants, which can protect against a variety of diseases and illnesses. Vitamin C is critical to the body's manufacture of collagen, the stuff that holds tissue together. It also helps ensure the baby's bone and tooth development. Vitamin D is involved in an amazing number of body functions and not getting enough of it can cause all sorts of problems, including increasing the likelihood that your partner will give birth early, have a C-section, develop gestational diabetes or preeclampsia, or give birth to a baby with skeletal problems. One of the best sources of Vitamin D is sunlight, but talk to her OB about whether she needs a supplement.

Overall, your partner should have a total of at least seven servings a day of fruits and vegetables.

CARBS

Grains (including breads and cereals) are basically fuel for your partner's body, and she should have at least four servings a day. Since her body will burn the fuel first, if she doesn't get enough there may not be enough for the baby. Grains are generally low in calories and high in zinc, selenium, chromium, and magnesium—all essential nutrients. They're also high in fiber, which will help your partner combat the constipating effect of iron supplements. Good sources include whole-grain breads (keep her away from white bread and white rice for a few months if you can), brown rice, fresh potatoes, peas, dried beans, and quinoa.

Going Organic

Grocery store shelves are filled with organic everything. But how much of this craze is hype, just another excuse to raise prices? Well, there's no way to give you an exact statistic, but it seems to make sense that we should try to minimize the amount of pesticides, hormones, antibiotics, and other nasty-sounding gunk that shows up in our food. The Environmental Working Group has a complete list (ewg.org/foodnews/list.php) of the produce items that you and your partner might want to avoid, as well as the ones that pose little or no danger (meaning there's no sense paying extra for organic). Generally speaking, foods with peels you don't eat are okay—and the harder the peel, the better. I've included a dozen of the worst and the best below. If you can't stay away from the bad ones, at least wash them very, very carefully.

NO NEED TO BUY ORGANIC		DEFINITELY BUY ORGANIC	
Avocado	Asparagus	Apples	Bell peppers
Sweet Corn	Mango	Strawberries	Nectarines
Pineapple	Papaya	Grapes	Cucumbers
Cabbage	Kiwi	Celery	Cherry tomatoes
Onions	Eggplant	Peaches	Snap peas
Sweet Peas	Cantaloupe	Spinach	Potatoes

WATER

As if she doesn't have enough to do already, your partner should try to drink at least eight 8-ounce glasses of water (or unsweetened, noncaffeinated fluids) a day—more if she's doing a lot of exercise or if she's pregnant during the summer. This will help her to replace the water she loses when she perspires (which she'll do more during pregnancy) and to carry away waste products. Keep in mind that at any given moment, about half of the population is walking around somewhat dehydrated, which puts them at increased risk of developing a variety of problems, including kidney stones and urinary tract cancers.

FATS

Despite all the hype about low- or no-fat diets, the fact is that your partner, like everyone else in the world, needs to consume at least some fat. She'll probably be getting most of what she needs in the other things she's eating during the day.

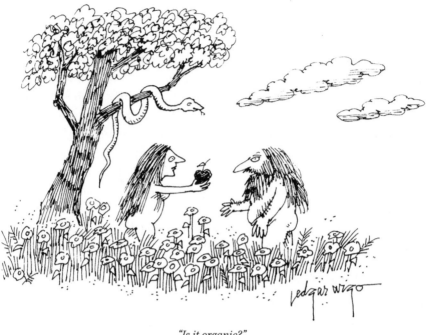

"Is it organic?"

But no more than 30 percent of her total caloric intake should come from fat. A diet too rich in fatty foods isn't good for her or your growing baby-to-be. Monounsaturated fats (avocado, peanuts, almonds, olive oil, canola oil) are best, followed by polyunsaturated fats (margarine, mayonnaise, walnuts). The worst kinds are saturated fats (bacon, lard, butter) and trans fats—basically anything that has the words *partially hydrogenated* or *hydrogenated* on the ingredients panel.

NUTRITIONAL AND CHEMICAL NO-NOS

Here's the deal. Generally speaking, if your partner eats it, drinks it, breathes it, or smells it, so does your growing baby.

- Cigarettes. When a mother-to-be inhales cigarette smoke, her womb fills with carbon monoxide, nicotine, tar, and resins that inhibit oxygen and nutrient delivery to the baby. Maternal cigarette smoking increases the risk of low-birthweight babies and miscarriage. There's also some evidence that paternal smoking (exposing your partner and your baby to secondhand smoke) is just as bad. If you think the baby is somehow protected from your smoke by being inside your partner, or if you think that smoking doesn't matter this early in the pregnancy, you're dangerously wrong. Bottom line: if you're a smoker, quit now. If she is, encourage her to quit and help her any way you can. Interestingly, a lot of men put off quitting—or asking their partners to quit—out of fear that withdrawal might lead to some marital tension. Bad choice. The potential danger to your baby far outweighs the danger to your relationship. Oh, and if you're thinking of e-cigarettes (and why not? Everything else in our lives seems to have an "e" or an "i" in front of it), think again. While they're less toxic than tobacco cigarettes, and they cut down on second-hand smoke, they're hardly safe. Most e-cigs use liquid nicotine, which, besides being addictive, can cause high blood pressure and other heart-related issues in your wife, and can reduce blood flow to the placenta, potentially doing permanent damage to your baby. E-cigs may also contain propylene glycol, which, when heated, can turn into a powerful carcinogen. They also produce nanoparticles, which can irritate the lungs and aggravate asthma and other lung issues.

Here's a great example of what happens when people get something only half right. Remember what I said about smoking causing low-birth-weight babies? Well, in Great Britain, smoking during pregnancy—especially among teen girls—is disturbingly common. These young girls somehow got the idea into their head that having a smaller baby would make labor and delivery less painful. What they didn't understand was that low birth weight is only the beginning. Smoking also increases the odds of miscarriage, birth defects, stillbirth, and premature birth. Babies born too soon have a higher risk of all sorts of problems later in life: respiratory illness, cerebral palsy, mental retardation, and heart problems, just to name a few. And they often go through nicotine withdrawal right after birth, just like crack babies. It also affects the mom, by increasing her risk of developing *placental previa* (where the placenta covers the opening to the uterus) and *placenta abruption* (where the placenta separates from the wall of the uterus before delivery), as well as of going into labor prematurely. Am I scaring you? I sure as hell hope so.

- Alcohol. Complete abstinence is the safest choice (although your partner's practitioner may sanction a glass of wine once in a while to induce relaxation). Regular, high-dose alcohol consumption can cause Fetal Alcohol Syndrome, a set of irreversible mental and physical impairments and abnormalities. Even moderate social drinking has been linked to low-birth-weight babies, learning impairments, and miscarriages in the early stages of pregnancy. "[I]f you have a glass of chardonnay here and there, you do so at your own risk," writes OB Lissa Rankin in her book, *What's Up Down There? Questions You'd Only Ask Your Gynecologist If She Was Your Best Friend.* "It's probably just fine to enjoy the occasional glass of wine. There's a big difference between being reckless (a definite no-no) and having one drink at dinner. But there's just no data to help us make safe recommendations." If you're worried about any drinking your partner may have done before you found out you were pregnant, talk to her practitioner about it.

- Fasting. Unless she has a doctor's approval, your partner should never, ever go twenty-four hours without eating. This is especially important in the first nineteen weeks of pregnancy, when the baby's brain is developing.

- Over-the-counter or prescription drugs. Your partner should talk with her doctor before taking any medication, including aspirin, ibuprofen, and cold medicines—especially anything that contains alcohol or codeine. Antidepressants in particular have come under a lot of scrutiny lately. Several recent studies have linked one class of antidepressants, SSRIs (which include Prozac, Zoloft, Celexa, and Paxil), with increased risk of several fetal abnormalities. Others haven't found any connection. But as you might expect, untreated depression can cause plenty of problems too. So if your partner has struggled with depression, talk with her doctor about whether the risks of taking antidepressants are outweighed by the risks of not taking them.

- Caffeine. Avoiding an excessive amount of caffeine is especially important in the early months. Some studies have shown that pregnant women who drink more than three or four good-sized cups of coffee per day have a greater risk of having a miscarriage, delivering prematurely, or having a low-birth-weight baby than women who can walk by a Starbucks and keep their wallet in their purse. Most studies seem to indicate that a cup or two a day is okay, but check with her practitioner to get the final word.

- Recreational drugs. Abstain during pregnancy—unborn children can be born addicted.

- Certain foods. Raw meats and fish may contain _Toxoplasma gondii_, which can blind the fetus or damage its nervous system. Unpasteurized milk and soft cheeses such as Brie may contain _Listeria_, another dangerous bacterium. Raw eggs and chicken may contain salmonella. Practitioners do disagree, however, on the magnitude of the risk involved. My wife's first OB/GYN was Japanese and had absolutely no problem with her eating sushi. Some fish you do need to watch out for, though. The FDA recommends that pregnant women stay away from shark, swordfish, mackerel, and tilefish, all of which contain high levels of mercury. Limit albacore tuna to a serving or two per week. If she wants fish or seafood, salmon, pollock, and shrimp are low-mercury choices.

- Cat feces. Okay, cat feces don't have much to do with nutrition, but they do contain high quantities of the same parasite found in some raw meats. So if you have a cat and you want to be chivalrous, take over the duty of cleaning the litter box for the duration of the pregnancy. Actually, litter boxes don't pose much of a problem for most women. She's got a much better chance of coming into contact with cat poop when she's outside, digging in the garden (which, in many cats' view, is nothing more than a giant litter box anyway).

- Insecticides, weed killers, and the like. As long as you're taking over the gardening, put on your gloves and take a load of chemical fertilizer and pesticides to the nearest toxic waste disposal place (your regular trash company won't take it if they know it's there). Prolonged and repeated exposure to those toxic substances has been linked to birth defects. If you really need pesticides and fertilizers, now's the time to switch to organics. Also, keep your partner far away from other potential chemical contaminants, such as diazinon (a common cockroach killer), as well as no-pest strips, flea sprays and collars, and pesticide bombs. Two chemicals in particular—PCBS and DDE (an insecticide byproduct)—can have some very negative effects. Kids exposed to those chemicals in utero tend to be taller (about two inches) and weigh more (an average of eleven to fifteen pounds) as teens than kids who weren't exposed, and they often enter puberty too early.

- Hair dyes. Long-term use of hair dyes by adults has been linked to increased risk of several types of cancer. But could hair dye be absorbed through a pregnant woman's scalp, enter her bloodstream, and harm her unborn baby? The jury's out on that one. The American Pregnancy Association says that hair dyes (and other chemical-intensive products) are fine during pregnancy. After all, your partner isn't planning to drink the stuff—she's putting it in her hair, right? Other experts in reproductive health, including Joanne Perron, point to research that indicates that using hair dye may affect a growing fetus on the cellular level and could increase a child's risk of developmental and reproductive disorders. May. Could. Big words. But why take the risk? The easiest solution is for your partner to avoid dyeing her hair while she's pregnant—at the very least, during the first three months, when the baby's organs and nervous system are forming. If you can't convince her that her hair looks wonderful just the way it is, Google "nontoxic hair dye."

A WORD ABOUT A VEGETARIAN DIET

If your partner is a vegetarian, there's no reason why she and the baby can't get the nutrition they need—especially if she eats eggs and milk. But if she's a strict vegan, she'll need to be especially sure that she's getting enough protein and other nutrients. Check with her doctor or a good nutritionist for special guidance.

A FINAL NOTE ON NUTRITION

Helping your partner eat right is one of the best things you can do to ensure that you'll have a healthy, happy baby (and a healthy, happy partner). But don't be too hard on her. Being pregnant is tough enough without having someone standing over her shoulder criticizing every choice she makes. While she'd undoubtedly be better off eating nothing but healthy foods all the time, an occasional order of fries or a candy bar isn't going to do any long-term damage. In fact, there's some evidence that eating dark chocolate may actually be good for her. Several studies have found a correlation between dark chocolate and reduced heart attack risk, weight management, and stress relief. In one study, pregnant women who had five or more servings of chocolate every week (in the third trimester) were 40 percent less likely to develop preeclampsia (a very dangerous blood pressure condition; see pages 63–64 for more).

Finally, be supportive. This means that you should try to eat as healthily as she does. If you absolutely must have a banana split and you're not planning to share, do it on your own time (and don't brag about it).

The Hunger Campaign

One of the things I constantly underestimated while my wife was pregnant was how incredibly hungry she would get, and how quickly it would happen. Even though she might have had a snack before leaving the office, by the time she got home she'd be ravenous again.

If you've been doing most of the cooking at your house, things probably won't change much during the pregnancy. But if your partner has been making the meals, there are a few things you can do to simplify her life significantly:

- Learn to cook simple, quick meals. There are plenty of cookbooks specializing in meals that can be made in less than thirty (or twenty or ten!) minutes. Easier yet, there are quite a few blogs and websites that can help. I like realfoodby-dad.com, www.stayatstovedad.com, cookingfordads.net, and dadcooksdinner.com. You can also stock up on healthy microwavable dinners or order take-out meals, but that can get expensive pretty fast.
- Do some meal planning. This means you'll have to spend some time reading cookbooks or surfing websites, looking for things that sound good. As you're reading, be sure to write down the ingredients you'll need. Although meal

A Special Note for Adoptive and ART Dads

If you're one of the many expectant adoptive parents who has met your future baby's birth mother, or you've hired a surrogate, do whatever you can to support her pregnancy without being annoying. Encourage her to exercise, stop smoking, eat right, take her prenatal vitamins, go to her regularly scheduled medical appointments, and so on.

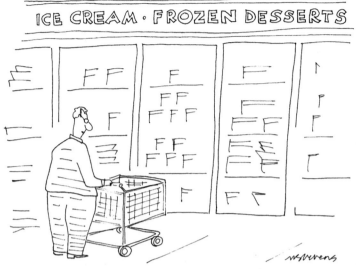

"Why have you brought me here?"

planning doesn't sound all that difficult, it's time-consuming—especially when you add in the extra time you'll have to spend at the grocery store.

- Do the shopping. Even if your partner still plans the meals and makes out the shopping lists, your going to the store will spare her an hour or so a week of walking around on floors that are tough even on nonpregnant people's feet. In addition, many women who have severe morning sickness find that being in a grocery store, surrounded by so much food, is just too much to stomach. If your partner did the shopping before the pregnancy, ask her to make a *detailed* list of the items she usually bought.
- Make her a nutritious breakfast shake. Let her spend a few more precious minutes relaxing in bed in the morning (see below for a good recipe).
- Keep some snacks in the glove compartment when you're out together. Her energy can crash at any time, and a handful of nuts, some raisins, or a granola bar can really help.

RECIPES

Power Shake

½ cup skim milk   12 strawberries
1 banana   juice of 2 oranges

Combine ingredients in a blender or food processor and serve over crushed ice or straight up chilled.

Stocking Up

If you keep the following items on hand, you or your partner should be able to throw together a healthy meal or snack anytime.

- Unsweetened cereals
- Whole-wheat pasta
- Tomato or vegetable juice
- Whole-grain bread
- Skim milk
- Nonfat cottage cheese
- Low-fat, naturally sweetened yogurt
- Fresh eggs (and some hard-boiled ones too)
- Natural peanut butter
- Pure fruit jams
- Bottled water
- Crackers
- Fresh vegetables that can be eaten raw, including carrots, cucumbers, celery, and tomatoes
- Fresh fruit
- Frozen berries and grapes
- Raisins and other dried fruits
- Doughnuts (okay, not very often, but you've got to give yourselves a break once in a while)

Basic Quick Snacks

- Peel and slice carrots and celery the night before for your partner to take to work for lunch.
- Boil eggs: put a few eggs in a pot with enough water to cover them, cover the pot, bring to a boil. As soon as the water boils, turn off the heat and let the eggs sit in the pot for 20 minutes. Then rinse with cold water and shell.
- Mix up some GORP (dried fruits, nuts, raisins, sunflower seeds).

Chocolate Banana Pancakes

½ cup white flour
½ cup whole-wheat flour
2 teaspoons baking powder
¼ teaspoon cinnamon
    pinch salt
½ tablespoon white sugar
½ tablespoon brown sugar (if you're missing either kind of sugar, just use a whole tablespoon of the one you have)

1 egg
1 teaspoon vanilla extract (optional, but great)
1 tablespoon vegetable oil
    a bit less than 1 cup milk
½ cup chocolate chips
1 tablespoon butter or margarine
3 bananas, sliced

Mix the dry ingredients in a large bowl. Add the egg, vanilla, oil, and milk. Mix into a smooth batter. Add the chocolate chips and mix again. Melt the butter on a heated griddle. Pour the batter onto the griddle in large spoonfuls. Then quickly place several banana slices on each pancake. When the bubbles that form on the surface of the pancakes pop, flip them over. Cook until the second side is as brown as the first, and remove from griddle.

Open-Face Mexican Omelet

3 eggs

1 teaspoon cilantro, finely chopped

1 small tomato, chopped

¼ cup green and/or red pepper, chopped

¼ cup red onion, diced

black pepper to taste

If eating the egg yolks aggravates your partner's morning sickness, use only the whites. Whisk eggs in a bowl or measuring cup and pour into a medium nonstick frying pan. Turn heat on low. As eggs begin to cook, add all other ingredients. Simmer until egg becomes firm, and slide omelet onto plate for serving.

Microwave Oatmeal

⅓ cup oats (you can use 1-minute, 5-minute, quick, or regular)

⅔ cup water

½ banana, sliced

dash cinnamon

⅛ teaspoon vanilla extract

milk

1 tablespoon wheat germ

Put the oats in a 1-quart microwave-safe bowl. Stir in the water, banana, cinnamon, and vanilla. Microwave on high for 2 to 3 minutes, or until the concoction starts steaming or bubbling. Take out and stir again. Add milk to taste. Sprinkle with wheat germ for extra vitamins and protein.

Any of the following salads can be served as a main course for lunch or as a side dish for dinner.

Tomato and Basil Salad

The combination of these two ingredients makes a refreshing salad. When available, use fresh basil and local tomatoes for the best flavor.

2 vine-ripened tomatoes

6–8 basil leaves

4 tablespoons balsamic vinegar

4 tablespoons extra virgin olive oil

freshly ground black pepper to taste

Slice tomatoes and arrange on a serving plate. Shred basil leaves and sprinkle over tomatoes. Cover with the vinegar and oil. Add freshly ground pepper. Cover and refrigerate for at least 1 hour. Remove from refrigerator a half hour before serving.

Reading the Small Print

Getting healthy food isn't always as easy as it might seem, and even though labeling requirements are getting more stringent, most food manufacturers aren't about to do you any favors. So as you're pushing your cart around the grocery store, be sure to read the labels carefully. In particular, watch out for the following:

- Ingredients. The first ingredient on the list is always the one there's the most of—no matter what you're buying. So, if that healthy ingredient (oat bran!!!) splashed all over the front of the box turns out to be at the bottom of the list, try something else.
- Sugar—and all the synonyms. Watch out for fructose, corn syrup, corn sweeteners, sucrose, dextrose, cane syrup, malt syrup, honey, and many more. They're just fancy ways of saying "sugar."
- Words like "drink," "flavored," or "cocktail." Despite the healthy-looking label, most fruit "drinks" or fruit-"flavored" drinks contain less actual juice than you might guess—often as little as 10 percent, with the rest usually water and…wait for it…sugar.
- Servings. This is one of the most potentially deceptive areas in food labeling. In most cases, the number of calories, grams of fat and protein, and other nutritional information is given per serving. That's all very nice, except that

Mixed Green Salad with Balsamic Vinaigrette

Combining different types of greens, such as Boston lettuce, red leaf lettuce, radicchio, arugula, and endive, makes a green salad more interesting. Raw cucumbers, snow peas, French beans, shredded carrots, and cooked beets also add to the flavor, color, and nutrition of a mixed salad. Stay away from croutons, which are high in calories and low in nutrition.

Thoroughly wash and dry greens, place each serving on a plate, and arrange whatever selection of vegetables you like on top. Just before serving, pour about three tablespoons of balsamic vinaigrette dressing (see recipe below) over each salad.

BALSAMIC VINAIGRETTE

2 cloves garlic, crushed

⅔ cup balsamic vinegar

1 teaspoon Dijon mustard

½ teaspoon parsley, chopped

manufacturers don't all use the same serving size. For example, I recently saw an eight-ounce package of fairly healthy frozen lasagna. The calories, protein, and fat all seemed okay—until I noticed that the serving size was actually only six ounces. This means that since one person would eat the entire eight ounces (I would, anyway), there was really 33 percent more fat and calories than expected.

- Percentage of calories from fat. Most nutritionists agree that pregnant women should limit their percentage of calories from fat to about 30 percent. Manufacturers are now required by law to make this calculation for you, so pay careful attention to the "nutrition facts" you'll find on any packaged food.
- A word about additives. When it comes to ingredients, my rule of thumb has always been that if you can't pronounce it, don't eat it. In addition, even some easy-to-pronounce items don't belong in your partner's stomach. So while she's pregnant, keep her away from artificial sweeteners (aspartame, Splenda, Saccharin, Truvia, and others), nitrates and nitrites (preservatives commonly found in lunch meats, hot dogs, and bacon), and monosodium glutamate (MSG, a flavor enhancer especially popular in Asian food and, for some odd reason, gefilte fish). All of these may have negative effects on your unborn child.

½ teaspoon chives, chopped	⅔ cup oil
½ teaspoon basil, chopped	salt and pepper

Mix garlic, vinegar, mustard, and herbs together. Whisk oil into the vinegar mixture. Add salt and pepper to taste.

Cucumber Salad

2 large cucumbers, sliced	½ cup nonfat plain yogurt
1 medium Bermuda onion, diced	1 teaspoon fresh dill, chopped
1 cup cider vinegar	

If the cucumbers are not waxy, leave the skin on. Slice the cucumbers thinly (a food processor does the job best). Combine the diced onion with the cucumber slices in a large bowl that can be refrigerated. Pour the vinegar and yogurt over the mixture, cover, and leave in the refrigerator overnight. Serve cold as a side dish, garnished with the dill.

Low-Calorie Pizza

Create your own combination of toppings, including artichokes, olives, and squash, and use an assortment of cheeses, such as blue, cheddar, Swiss, and even low-fat cottage cheese.

- 4 soft tortillas (found in grocery freezer)
- 2 fresh plum tomatoes, sliced
- 3 cloves garlic, minced or crushed
- 1 cup mushrooms, sliced and sautéed
- 1 medium onion, chopped and sautéed
- 6 teaspoons fresh herbs (oregano, thyme, and basil), minced (or 2 teaspoons dried)
- ½ cup shredded cheese or low-fat cottage cheese

Preheat oven to 350°F. Place tortillas on a lightly greased cookie sheet. Cover with tomatoes, garlic, mushrooms, onions, and herbs. Add cheese. Bake for 20 minutes or until tortilla is crisp. Serve hot.

Quick and Easy Vegetarian Spaghetti Sauce

- 2 large onions, chopped
- 4 tablespoons olive oil
- ½ pound mushrooms, thinly sliced
- 2 16-ounce jars meatless spaghetti sauce
- 2 14.5-ounce cans stewed tomatoes
- 1 4-ounce can tomato paste
- 1 pound tofu, diced into ½-inch cubes
- 1½ teaspoons dried basil
- a generous pinch of cayenne pepper
- 1 bay leaf
- salt and pepper to taste
- 1 teaspoon sugar
- ½ teaspoon garlic powder
- 1 tablespoon rice vinegar

In a saucepan, sauté onions in the olive oil over medium heat until they're translucent. Add mushrooms, and sauté for 5 more minutes (until the mushrooms begin to release their liquid). Add all the other ingredients and simmer for 40 minutes. If sauce won't be used immediately, let cool, pour into two serving containers, and store in freezer. Defrost as needed.

Low-Calorie Cream of Zucchini Soup

This recipe can be varied by substituting carrots, potatoes, or celery for zucchini.

- 3 medium-size zucchini, seeded and cut into ¼-inch slices
- 1 medium white onion, diced
- 1 small chicken bouillon cube (optional; bouillon cubes usually contain MSG)
- 1 cup nonfat plain yogurt
- 1 tablespoon fresh dill
- salt and pepper

Put zucchini, onion, and bouillon cube in a saucepan. Add just enough water to cover. Bring to a boil and cook until soft (about 10 minutes). Let cool. Transfer to a blender or food processor, add yogurt and dill, and blend until smooth. Add salt and pepper to taste.

Spa Potato Chips

3 baking potatoes, peeled and thinly sliced

nonstick cooking spray
paprika to taste

Preheat oven to 350°F. Slice potatoes as thinly as possible (a food processor is best). Spray a cookie sheet with nonstick cooking spray. Spread out potatoes evenly in pan. Sprinkle with paprika and bake for about 15 minutes, or until crisp.

Spicy Peanut Butter Pasta

1 pound angel-hair pasta
1 tablespoon sesame oil
4 tablespoons peanut or safflower oil
6 cloves garlic, minced
1 generous pinch (⅛ teaspoon) red pepper flakes
10 scallions, thinly sliced

½ cup creamy peanut butter
6 tablespoons rice wine vinegar
6 tablespoons soy sauce
4 teaspoons white sugar
1 cucumber, peeled, seeded, and diced (optional)
cilantro to taste (optional)

Cook pasta according to directions on package. Drain and drizzle with the sesame oil. Set aside. Sauté garlic and pepper flakes in the peanut or safflower oil in a large frying pan. Add scallions. Turn heat to high and stir for one minute. Remove from heat. Add remaining ingredients and use a wire whisk to thoroughly mix into a thick sauce. Pour over pasta while sauce is still warm. Garnish with cucumber and/or cilantro, if desired.

Garlic Roasted Chicken

1 roasting chicken (3 to 4 pounds)
5 garlic cloves
1 carrot, sliced
2 celery stalks, sliced
4 small white onions

2 teaspoons olive oil
½ cup white wine (optional)
¼ cup water
salt and pepper to taste

Preheat oven to 450°F. Clean chicken and rinse thoroughly with water. Pat dry. Sprinkle inside and out with salt and pepper. Using fingers, make pockets under skin and stuff with garlic cloves. Place chicken in a deep baking dish. Stuff cavity of chicken with carrot and celery slices and onions. Drizzle olive oil on top of chicken. Pour wine and water over chicken. Bake chicken at 450°F for ten minutes to sear. Then reduce heat to 350°F and cook for 30 to 40 minutes, or until the juices run clear when the thigh is pierced with a fork.

Rack of Lamb

A festive, delicious dish that is easy to prepare.

¼ cup bread crumbs

3 cloves garlic, crushed

2 teaspoons parsley flakes

salt and pepper to taste

1 rack of lamb (ask the butcher to crack the rack, remove excess fat, and French-cut the ribs)

5 teaspoons Dijon mustard

Preheat oven to 450°F. In a small bowl, mix the bread crumbs, garlic, parsley, and salt and pepper. Place rack of lamb in a baking pan, meat side up. Spread mustard on top and bake for 10 minutes. Remove from oven. Using a fork, press the bread-crumb mixture into mustard, reduce heat to 350°F, and cook for about 20 more minutes, or until medium rare.

Fruit Salad with Creamy Yogurt Dressing

A refreshing, low-calorie dish for breakfast, lunch, or dessert. As a side dish or dessert, this recipe serves four. As a main course for lunch, it serves two.

1 green apple, cored and diced

1 banana, sliced

juice of 1 lime

1 small bunch of red or green seedless grapes

5 strawberries, halved

2 kiwis, peeled and sliced

1 seedless navel orange (or other citrus fruit), sectioned

1 cup low-fat vanilla yogurt (or nonfat plain yogurt)

1 teaspoon cinnamon

½ cup shredded coconut (optional)

4–8 fresh mint leaves (optional)

In a large mixing bowl, combine banana and apple, pour lime juice over them, and mix. Add remaining fruit and mix again. In a separate bowl combine yogurt and cinnamon. Just before serving, mix the yogurt dressing and coconut into the fruit. If fresh mint is available, garnish each serving with one or two leaves.

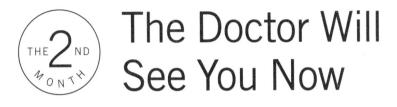

The Doctor Will See You Now

THE 2ND MONTH

WHAT'S GOING ON WITH YOUR PARTNER

Physically

- Continuing fatigue
- Continuing morning sickness
- Frequent urination
- Tingly fingers
- Breast tenderness and darkening nipples

Emotionally

- Continued elation and at the same time some ambivalence about being pregnant
- Inability to keep her mind on her work
- Fear you won't find her attractive anymore
- Continuing moodiness
- Fear of an early miscarriage, especially if you used ART

WHAT'S GOING ON WITH THE BABY

During this month, the baby will officially change from an embryo to a fetus. By the end of the month, he or she (it's way too early to tell which by looking) will be about the size of an almond and will have stubby little arms (with wrists but no fingers yet), sealed-shut eyes on the side of the face, ears, and a tiny, beating heart (on the outside of the body). If you bumped into a six-foot-tall version of your baby in a dark alley, you'd run the other way.

WHAT'S GOING ON WITH YOU

The Struggle to Connect

Just about every study that's ever been done on the subject has shown that women generally connect with their pregnancies sooner than men do. Although they can't feel the baby kicking inside them yet, the physical changes they're experiencing make the pregnancy more real for them. For most men, however, pregnancy at two months is still a pretty abstract concept. For me—as excited as I was—the idea that we were really expecting was so hard to grasp that I actually forgot about it for several days at a time.

Excitement vs. Fear

But when I remembered we were about to become parents, I found myself in the midst of a real conflict—one that would plague me for months. On the one hand, I was still so elated that I could barely contain myself; I had visions of walking with my child on the beach, playing catch, reading, helping him or her with homework, and I wanted to stop strangers on the street and tell them I was going to be a father. On the other hand, I made a conscious effort to stifle my fantasies and excitement and to keep myself from getting attached to the idea. That way, if we had a miscarriage or something else went wrong, I wouldn't be devastated.

Dads who have been through a miscarriage on a previous pregnancy or done several unsuccessful ART cycles are especially susceptible to this kind of self-protective (and completely understandable) denial.

Increased or Decreased Sexual Desire

It was during the times when I let myself get excited about becoming a father that I noticed that my wife's and my sex life was changing. Perhaps it was because I was still reveling in the recent confirmation of my masculinity, or perhaps it was because I felt a newer, closer connection to my wife. It may even have been the sense of freedom resulting from not having to worry about birth control. Whatever the reason, sex in the early months of the pregnancy became wilder and more passionate than before. But not all men experience an increase in sexual desire during pregnancy. Some are turned off by their partner's changing figure; others are afraid of hurting the baby (a nearly impossible task at this stage of the game). Still others may feel that there's no sense in having sex now that they're pregnant.

Whatever your feelings—about sex or anything else for that matter—try to talk them over with your partner. Chances are she's experiencing—or soon will be—very similar feelings. One thing you may *not* want to discuss with your partner is your dreams. According to Berkeley, California (where else?), psychologist

Alan Siegel, a lot of expectant dads experience an increase in dreams about having sex—with their partner, old girlfriends, and even prostitutes. For some guys, these dreams are an expression of their concern that the pregnancy will mess with their sex life. The brain is probably saying to itself, "Well, big guy, if you can't get any in the flesh, you can still have some pretty wild fantasies..." For other guys, sexual dreams are a way of reassuring themselves that fatherhood—and all those mushy, protective feelings that go with it—in no way detracts from their masculinity.

STAYING INVOLVED

Going to the OB/GYN Appointments

The general rule that women connect with the pregnancy sooner than men has an exception: men who get involved early on and stay involved until the end have been shown to be as connected with the baby as their partners. And at this stage, the best way to get involved is to go to as many of your partner's OB/GYN appointments as possible.

Although I always love being told that I'm healthy as a horse, I've never really looked forward to going to the doctor. And going to someone else's doctor is even less attractive. But over the course of three pregnancies, I think I missed only two OB medical appointments. Admittedly, some of the time I was bored out of my mind, but overall it was a great opportunity to have my questions answered and to satisfy my curiosity about just what was going on inside my wife's womb.

There's no doubt that you can get at least some basic questions answered by reading a couple of the hundreds of pregnancy and childbirth books written for women. But there are a number of other, more important reasons to go to the appointments:

- You will become more of a participant in the pregnancy and less of a spectator. In other words, it will help make the pregnancy "yours."
- It will demystify the process and make it more tangible. Hearing the baby's heartbeat for the first time (in about the third month) and seeing his or her tiny body squirm on an ultrasound screen (in about the fifth month) bring home the reality of the pregnancy in a way that words on a page just can't do.
- As the pregnancy progresses, your partner is going to be feeling more and more dependent on you, and she'll need more signs that you'll always be there for her. While going to her doctor appointments may not seem quite as romantic as a moonlit cruise or a dozen roses, there are very few better ways to remind her that you love her and reassure her that she's not in this thing alone.
- The more you're around, the more seriously the doctor and his or her staff

Looking for Validation

If you're adopting, the time between your decision to adopt and the actual arrival of your child could be considered a "psychological pregnancy." Unlike a biological pregnancy, you won't, in most cases, know exactly how long it's going to take from beginning to end. But what's interesting is that most expectant adoptive parents go through an emotional progression similar to that of expectant biological parents, says adoption educator Carol Hallenbeck. The first step is what Hallenbeck calls "adoption validation," which basically means coming to terms with the idea that you're going to become a parent through adoption instead of through "normal" means. During their psychological pregnancy, adoptive parents often experience the same kind of denial that I described above, not letting themselves get too excited out of fear that the adoption could take far longer than they expected or that it will fall apart completely.

If you and your partner have hired a surrogate, there's a good chance that you'll be going through a psychological pregnancy as well. Unlike an adoptive couple, you have a much better idea of when your baby will be born, but you may still go through what might be called "surrogacy validation."

This may seem straightforward, but it's usually not. For many parents, according to researcher Rachel Levy-Shiff, adoption (or surrogacy) is a second choice, a decision reached only after years of unsuccessfully trying to conceive on their own and after seemingly endless disappointments and intrusive, expensive medical procedures. Infertility can make you question your self-image, undermine your sense of masculinity (how can I be a man if I can't get my partner pregnant?), force you to confront your shattered dreams, and can take a terrible toll on your relationship. If you're having trouble accepting the fact that you won't be having biologically related children, I urge you to talk to some other people about what you're feeling. Your partner certainly has a right to know—and she might be feeling a lot of similar things. In addition, the adoption agency you're working with will probably have a list of support resources for adoptive fathers. Give them a try.

will take you and the more involved they'll let you be (see pages 75–76 for more on this).

If you're planning to go to your partner's checkups, you'd better get your calendar out. Here's what a typical schedule looks like:

MONTH	IF YOU'RE EXPECTING ONE BABY	IF YOU'RE EXPECTING MULTIPLES
1–5	Monthly	Monthly
6	Monthly	Every other week
7	Every other week	Every other week
8	Every other week	Weekly
9	Weekly	Weekly

Of course, taking time off from work for all these appointments may not be realistic. But before you write the whole thing off, check with the doctor—many offer early-morning or evening appointments.

Screening and Testing

Besides being a time of great emotional closeness between you and your partner, pregnancy is also a time for your partner to be poked and prodded. Most of the tests she'll have to take, such as the monthly urine tests for blood sugar and the quarterly blood tests for other problems, are purely routine. Others, though, are less routine and sometimes can be scary.

The scariest of all are the ones to detect birth defects, most commonly Down syndrome and other chromosomal abnormalities. One of the things you can expect your partner's doctor to do is take a detailed medical history—from both of you. These medical histories will help the practitioner assess your risk of having a child with severe—or not so severe—problems (see pages 59–60 for more on this). If you're in one of the high-risk categories, your doctor may suggest some additional prenatal screening.

The words *screening* and *testing* are often used interchangeably, but there's actually a big difference between them. Noninvasive procedures such as ultrasounds and blood tests are used to assess potential risks. If the risk is high enough, the doctor may order a *test* to confirm a diagnosis. Those tests are usually invasive (to your partner and your baby) and involve some risk. The OB will be able to help you decide whether the benefits of taking the test (knowing whether your baby is healthy) outweigh the potential risks (causing a miscarriage).

If you did ART and PGD (preimplantation genetic diagnosis; see pages 298–99), you and your partner may not have to be tested at all—the lab was able to test the embryo itself for more than a hundred diseases and abnormalities. If any were found, that particular embryo wouldn't have been implanted. However, because there is a small risk of getting a false negative on the PGD, many fertility doctors will recommend additional testing once the pregnancy is underway.

NONINVASIVE PROCEDURES

ULTRASOUND (SONOGRAM)

This noninvasive test is painless to the mother, safe for the baby, and can be performed any time after the fifth week of pregnancy. By bouncing sound waves around the uterus and off the fetus, ultrasounds produce a picture of the baby and the placenta. To the untrained eye, standard, 2-D images look remarkably like Mr. Potato Head, without the glasses and mustache. 3-D ultrasounds generate a more complete image of the fetus. And 4-D ultrasounds (sometimes called dynamic 3-D) actually let you see your future baby in action, sucking his thumb, napping, swimming, and doing whatever else fetuses do to pass the time.

In the first trimester, your doctor will probably recommend an ultrasound only if there's something going on that's a little out of the ordinary. The most common reason is that the size of the uterus doesn't correspond to the age of the fetus when measured from your partner's last period. The doc may also order an ultrasound if your partner has experienced any bleeding, if there's any doubt as to the number of fetuses, or if he or she suspects an ectopic pregnancy (a pregnancy that takes place outside the uterus). At this stage, the ultrasound can confirm that there's a heartbeat and can measure the baby (starting with the charmingly named Crown-Rump Length, which will give you a better due date estimate).

Depending on your partner's risk, her doctor may offer or recommend a *nuchal translucency ultrasound* (NT scan), a special type of ultrasound that measures fluid in the nuchal fold, a spot at the base of your baby's head. Excess fluid in that area is often associated with chromosomal abnormalities and some heart conditions. The test needs to be done between 11 and 14 weeks and is usually part of what's called the combined first trimester screening, which includes a blood test measuring your partner's levels of *pregnancy associated plasma protein* A (PAPP-A) and a hormone called hCG. The combined test is about 85 percent accurate and has a false-positive rate of 5 percent.

There's also an *integrated screening*, which uses the results of the combined screening and adds in the Quad test I describe below, which is done between 15 and 20 weeks. Taken together, this increases the detection rate and reduces the false-positive rate to about 1 percent.

Second-trimester ultrasounds are usually the ones that low-risk couples see first. They're used to determine the sex of the baby (this one is optional), to get a more accurate estimate of the due date, or just because you're curious about what the baby looks like. If this is the first ultrasound, your practitioner will want to confirm the number of residents in the uterus, see how well they're moving around, and make sure all the body parts and organs are the right size and in the right place. The test may also be used to firm up the due date and to confirm anything that may have come up in other prenatal testing, including the Triple or Quad Screen, amniocentesis, and CVS (see pages 61–62).

During the last part of the pregnancy—and especially if the baby is overdue—your partner's doctor may order additional ultrasounds to determine the baby's position, to make sure the placenta is still functioning, or to confirm that there's still enough amniotic fluid left to support the baby.

TRIPLE OR QUADRUPLE SCREENS

The Triple Screen measures three chemicals that may show up in your partner's blood: AFP (Alpha-Fetoprotein), hCG (human chorionic gonadotropin), and estriol. The Quad adds one more substance, Inhibin A, to the screen, and there's actually a Penta, which includes yet another substance, ITA (Invasive Trophoblast Antigen). Together they're used to flag potential abdominal wall abnormalities and a variety of neural-tube defects (defects relating to the brain or spinal column), the most common of which are spina bifida and anencephaly (a completely or partially missing brain). Whether you have the Triple, the Quad, or the Penta (is this is sounding like Olympic gymnastics judging, or is it just me?) will depend on what your doctor orders. Theoretically, the more things you test for, the lower the false-positive rate.

These simple blood tests are conducted when your partner is 15–20 weeks pregnant, and the results are usually available within a week, sometimes even the next day. It's important to understand that a "positive" result is not necessarily an indication of the presence of an abnormality, just that there *might* be a problem. Most turn out perfectly fine, but if your partner does get a positive result, she'll be asked to take additional tests, such as an ultrasound and amniocentesis, which should clear up any doubts you have. Since these screens are really designed to let your partner know whether she needs additional testing, she may not want to bother if she's planning to have an amnio or an in-depth ultrasound test.

TESTS *YOU* MAY HAVE TO TAKE

No, you're not pregnant, but there are still a few times when you may need to give a little blood to make sure all is well with your baby. A variety of genetically transmitted birth defects, for example, affect some ethnic groups more than others. So, based on your family histories, your partner's doctor may order one or both of you to get additional blood tests. OB Saul Weinreb told me that "every person in the world is estimated to carry thousands of potentially harmful genetic mutations, which means that every couple has an approximately equal chance of having a baby with a random genetic disease they had no idea they carried." The good news is that science has been able to identify certain diseases that occur more commonly in certain ethnic groups. So rather than think of these groups as somehow genetically worse off than others, think of them as being lucky that there are tests for conditions that may affect them. New tests are being developed every day. Among the most commonly identifiable conditions are:

- Sickle-cell anemia. If you're African American or if your family came from the Caribbean, Italy, Sardinia, or India, you may want to be tested whether your practitioner suggests it or not. If your partner knows she's negative, though, ask the doctor whether you should bother.
- Tay-Sachs and Canavan Disease. If either you or your partner is of Ashkenazi (Eastern European) descent, get tested. Tay-Sachs is also found in some non-Jewish French Canadians. Interestingly, once your partner is pregnant, it is more accurate to test you for these conditions than to test her. If your results come back positive, she'll need to be tested, though.
- Cystic fibrosis. The American College of Obstetricians and Gynecologists now recommends that OBs offer cystic fibrosis testing routinely.
- Thalassemia. Affects mainly families of Asian, Southeast Asian, African, Middle Eastern, Greek, or Italian origins.

You may also have to be tested if your partner has a negative Rh (for rhesus, like the monkey) factor in her blood. If you're positive (and most of us are), your baby might be positive as well. If this is the case, your partner's immune system might think the Rh-positive baby is some kind of intruder and try to fight it. This can lead to fetal brain damage or even death. Fortunately, this problem is preventable: your partner will have to get some anti-Rh injections, starting around the 28th week of the pregnancy.

INVASIVE PROCEDURES

AMNIOCENTESIS

This extremely accurate test is usually performed at 15–18 weeks, and can identify nearly every possible chromosomal disorder, including Down syndrome. It can't, however, detect deformities such as cleft palate. If your baby is at risk of any other genetic conditions, your partner's doctor can order additional testing (but these tests are not done routinely). Amnio is also sometimes used in the third trimester of pregnancy to help doctors determine whether the fetus's lungs are mature enough to survive an emergency premature delivery, if they're worried about that. The test involves inserting a needle through the abdominal wall into the amniotic sac, where about an ounce of fluid is collected and analyzed. Results are usually available in one to three weeks. Unless your partner is considered at high risk (see page 61), or either of you needs to be reassured that your baby is healthy, there's

Reasons Your Partner (or You) Might Consider Genetic Testing

- One of you has a family history of birth defects, or you know you're a carrier for a genetic disorder such as cystic fibrosis, muscular dystrophy, or hemophilia.
- One of you is a member of a high-risk ethnic group, such as African Americans, Native Americans, Jews of Eastern European descent, Greeks, Italians, and others (see "Tests *You* May Have to Take," pages 59–60).
- Your partner is thirty-five or older.
- Your partner has had several miscarriages.
- Your partner had a positive Triple (or Quad or Penta) Screen (see page 59).
- One of you might be a carrier of specific genes that have been linked with birth defects.

Other Reasons for Prenatal Testing

Prenatal testing is also available to people who, while not considered at risk, have other reasons for wanting it done. Some of the most common reasons include:

- Peace of mind. Having an amniocentesis or a Chorionic Villi Sampling (CVS) test can remove most doubts about the chromosomal health of your child. For some people, this reassurance can make the pregnancy a much more enjoyable—and less stressful—experience. If the tests do reveal problems, you and your partner will have more time to prepare yourselves for the tough decisions ahead (for more on this, see pages 71–72).
- To find out the sex of the baby (or, in some cases, to determine who the biological father is).

no real reason to have this test. The chances that a twenty-five-year-old woman will give birth to a baby with a defect that an amnio can detect are about 1 in 500. The chances that the procedure will cause a miscarriage, however, are 1 in 200. For women over thirty-five, though, amnio begins to make statistical sense: the chances she'll have a baby with chromosomal abnormalities are roughly 1 in 190 and rise steadily as she ages. At forty, they're about 1 in 65; at forty-five, 1 in 20.

CHORIONIC VILLI SAMPLING (CVS)

Generally this test is performed at 9–12 weeks to detect chromosomal abnormalities and genetically inherited diseases. The test can be done by inserting a needle

Cell-Free Fetal DNA

One of the most exciting developments in prenatal testing is Cell-Free Fetal DNA (also called cfDNA or cffDNA) testing, which has the potential to eliminate the need for the vast majority of invasive diagnostics. Cell-Free Fetal DNA testing, which can be done as early as 10 weeks, analyzes tiny bits of the fetus's DNA that are running around in the mom-to-be's blood. According to Diana Bianchi, a pediatric geneticist at Tufts Medical Center, the results are ten times more accurate in predicting Down syndrome, and five times more accurate in predicting several other genetic conditions. The CffDNA test is nearly 100 percent accurate in ruling *out* problems, meaning that a negative result should relieve your anxieties. But it does produce some false positives, so a positive diagnosis would still need to be confirmed by amnio, CVS, or PUBS. Still, according to Bianchi, "Nine out of 10 women who are currently being referred for further testing would not need invasive tests." The test is expensive, isn't available everywhere, and may not be covered by insurance, so if you're interested, check with your partner's doc.

through the abdominal wall or by threading a catheter through the vagina and cervix into the uterus. Either way, small pieces of the chorion—a membrane with genetic makeup identical to that of the fetus—are snipped off or suctioned into a syringe and analyzed. The risks are about the same as for amnio, and the two tests can identify pretty much the same potential abnormalities. The main advantage to CVS is that it can be done a lot earlier in the pregnancy, giving you and your partner more time to consider the alternatives. That's why the number of amnios is falling, while CVSs are rising.

PERCUTANEOUS UMBILICAL BLOOD SAMPLING (PUBS)

No, PUBS has nothing to do with bars, although you may need one after thinking about all this. The PUBS test is usually conducted at 17–36 weeks and is sometimes ordered to confirm possible genetic and blood disorders detected through amnio or CVS. The procedure is virtually the same as an amnio, except that the needle is inserted into a blood vessel in the umbilical cord; some practitioners believe this makes the test more accurate. Later in the pregnancy, PUBS may be used to determine whether the fetus has chicken pox, *Toxoplasma gondii* (see page 42), or other dangerous infections. Preliminary results are available within about three days. In addition to the risk of complications or miscarriage resulting from the procedure, PUBS may also slightly increase the likelihood of premature labor or clotting of the umbilical cord, and because it can't be performed any earlier than 17 weeks, it's not nearly as popular as amnio or CVS.

Dealing with the Unexpected

For me, pregnancy was the proverbial emotional roller-coaster ride. One minute I'd find myself wildly excited and dreaming about the new baby, and the next I was filled with feelings of impending doom. I knew I wanted our babies, but I also knew that if I got too emotionally attached and anything unexpected happened—like an ectopic pregnancy, a miscarriage, or a birth defect—I'd be crushed. So, instead of allowing myself to enjoy the pregnancy fully, I ended up spending a lot of time torturing myself by reading and worrying about the bad things that could happen.

ECTOPIC PREGNANCY

About 1–2 percent of all embryos don't embed in the uterus but begin to grow outside the womb, usually in the fallopian tube, which is unable to expand sufficiently to accommodate the growing fetus. Undiagnosed, an ectopic pregnancy would eventually cause the fallopian tube to burst, resulting in severe bleeding. Fortunately, the vast majority of ectopic pregnancies are caught and removed by the eighth week of pregnancy—long before they become dangerous. Unfortunately, there is no way to transplant the embryo from the fallopian tube into the uterus, so there's no choice but to terminate the pregnancy. As quickly as technology is advancing, though, I'm sure transplantation will be possible in the not-too-distant future.

PREECLAMPSIA

This is one of the most common pregnancy complications—about 10 percent of pregnant women, most between the ages of eighteen and thirty, suffer from it, although the highest risk groups are very young teens and women in their forties. Preeclampsia is sometimes referred to as toxemia or PIH—protein-induced hypertension—because one of the symptoms is high protein in the urine. Basically, it's an increase in the mother's blood pressure late in the pregnancy. This can deprive the fetus of blood and other nutrients and put the mother at risk of a stroke or seizure. Women who have a history of high blood pressure or blood vessel abnormalities are especially prone, as are daughters of women who had preeclampsia when they were pregnant. And Norwegian researchers Rolv Skjærven and Lars J. Vatten found that "men born after a preeclampsia-complicated pregnancy had a moderately increased risk of fathering a preeclamptic pregnancy." But most of the time it comes as an unpleasant surprise to everyone.

In its early stages there usually aren't any symptoms, but it can be detected by a routine blood pressure check. If the condition worsens, the woman may develop headaches, water retention, vomiting, pain in the abdomen, blurred vision, and seizures. Interestingly, researchers now suspect that preeclampsia is actually a disorder in which the mother's immune system rejects some of the father's genes that are in the fetus's cells. They suspect that women may be able to "immunize" themselves *before* getting pregnant if they build up a tolerance by exposing themselves to their partner's semen as often as possible. This explains why preeclampsia is far more common during first pregnancies, or at least the first pregnancy with a new partner. It also explains why fewer women over thirty develop this condition. (Still, it can happen to older moms or those who have multiple children.)

There's no guaranteed way to prevent preeclampsia, but there are a few things that could reduce the risk. Staying well hydrated, cutting back on salt, and getting enough exercise may help your partner keep her blood pressure under control. So can increasing her fiber intake. One study found that women who ate over 25 grams of fiber every day cut their risk by 50 percent. And in one of the greatest pieces of good news for pregnant women, Elizabeth Triche and her colleagues found that "women who had five or more servings of chocolate each week in their third trimester were 40 percent less likely to develop preeclampsia than those who ate chocolate less than once a week." Apparently, there's a chemical in chocolate, theobromine, that dilates blood vessels and reduces blood pressure. But do you really think your partner needs an excuse to eat more chocolate?

MISCARRIAGES

The sad fact—especially for pessimists like me—is that miscarriages happen fairly frequently. Some experts estimate that between a fifth and a third of all pregnancies end in miscarriage (sometimes also called "spontaneous abortion"). In fact, almost every sexually active woman not on birth control will have one at some point in her life. (In most cases the miscarriage occurs before the woman ever knows she's pregnant—whatever there was of the tiny embryo is swept away with her regular menstrual flow.)

Before you start to panic, there are a few things to remember: First, over 90 percent of couples who experience a single miscarriage get pregnant and have a healthy baby later. Second, many people believe that miscarriages—most of which happen within the first three months of the pregnancy—are a kind of Darwinian natural selection. Some have even called them "a blessing in disguise." In the vast majority of cases, the embryo or fetus had some kind of catastrophic defect that would have made it incompatible with life. Still, if you and your partner have a miscarriage, you probably won't find any of this particularly reassuring. And it won't make it hurt any less.

Until very recently, miscarriage, like the pregnancy it ends, had been considered the exclusive emotional domain of women. Truth is, it isn't. While men don't have to endure the physical pain or discomfort of a miscarriage, their emotional pain can be just as severe as their partner's. They still have the same hopes and dreams about their unborn children, and they still feel a profound sense of grief when those hopes and dreams are dashed. And many men, just like their partners, feel tremendous guilt and inadequacy when a pregnancy ends prematurely.

Some good friends of mine, Philip and Elaine, had a miscarriage several years ago, after about twelve weeks of pregnancy. For both of them, the experience was devastating, and for months after the miscarriage they were besieged by sympathetic friends and relatives, many of whom had found out about the pregnancy only after it had so abruptly ended. They asked how Elaine was feeling, offered to visit her, expressed their sympathy, and often shared their own miscarriage stories. But no one—not even his wife—ever asked Philip what he was feeling, expressed any sympathy for what he was going through, or offered him a shoulder to cry on.

Psychologists and sociologists have conducted many studies on how people grieve at the loss of a fetus. But the vast majority of them have dealt only with women's reactions. The ones that have included fathers' feelings generally

If You're Expecting Twins

If your partner was carrying twins (or more), miscarrying one "does not seem to have negative implications regarding the health or genetic integrity of the surviving fetus," say doctors Connie Agnew and Alan Klein. Miscarrying a twin may, however, put your partner at a slightly higher risk of going into preterm labor.

If your partner is carrying three or more fetuses, you may have to deal with the question of "selective reduction." Basically, the more fetuses in the uterus, the greater the risk of premature birth, low birth weight, and other potential health hazards. Simply—and gruesomely—put, all these risks can be reduced by reducing the number of fetuses. It's an agonizing decision that only you and your partner can make. Since 1980, the number of twin births has doubled, and the number of unplanned triplets, quads, and so on has more than quadrupled. Fortunately, as ART methods improve, that trend has been slowly declining, which means that fewer and fewer couples will be faced with this heartrending decision.

conclude that men and women grieve in different ways. Dr. Kristen Goldbach found that "women are more likely to express their grief openly, while men tend to be much less expressive, frequently coping with their grief in a more stoical manner." This doesn't mean that men don't express their grief at all, or that they feel any less grief than women. Instead, it simply highlights the fact that in our society men, like my friend Philip, have virtually no opportunity to express their feelings—at least not in the "traditional" way. Many men respond to their grief by doing everything they can to get life back to normal. That often means going back to work and putting in extra-long hours. It's a way of getting away from the self-blame and feeling of helplessness at not knowing how to comfort their partner. It's a way of avoiding the barrage of baby images that was probably always there but now seems much more pervasive. It's a way of coping with their grief and, unfortunately, of ignoring it.

Trying Again

If you've suffered a miscarriage and have decided to try to get pregnant again, your goal is to prepare a healthy environment for the baby to swim around in, and to prevent birth defects or other complications.

One of the most crucial times of the pregnancy is between 17 and 56 days after conception. That's when the organs start developing. But because this stage happens so early on, it's entirely possible that your partner might not know she's pregnant. And by the time she finds out, she may have already done all sorts of things that could affect the baby—things she'll wish she hadn't done.

For that reason, it's important to prepare yourselves for the next pregnancy as far in advance as you can. From six to nine months would be great, but even a month or two can make a big difference.

Preconception

The rest of this book is devoted to how to have a healthy, safe pregnancy and a healthy mom and baby. But right now, we're talking about steps you can take *before* your partner conceives again that can boost your chances of getting pregnant, make for a less eventful pregnancy, and potentially help you reduce or avoid the expense and emotional ups and downs of fertility treatments.

You never know when your partner is going to burst out of the bathroom waving a little white stick and announce, "Honey, I'm pregnant!" So before the two of you hop in the sack, there are a few things that she should do, you should do, and the two of you should do together to get ready.

Pregnancy after a Miscarriage

Getting pregnant after having lost a baby can bring up a jumble of feelings for both you and your partner. For example, you'll probably be feeling incredibly happy that you're expecting again. But you may also be worried that this pregnancy will end the same way the last one did. That could keep you from allowing yourself to become truly engaged in and enjoy the pregnancy—at least until after you're past the point when the miscarriage happened last time. If your partner is feeling this, she may deliberately keep herself from bonding with the baby, trying to save herself the grief if the worst happens again. If it's been a while since the miscarriage, you might be angry—in an abstract sort of way—that you're still expecting, when by all rights you should be holding a baby in your arms right now. But if your partner got pregnant right away, you might be feeling guilty at not having let an appropriate (whatever that means) amount of time pass.

Everyone deals with post-miscarriage pregnancy differently, but there are a few things that may make it a little easier:

- Try not to worry. It may have happened before, but chances are it won't happen again. Only 1 in about 200 women are what are called "recurrent miscarriers," meaning that they have had three miscarriages and have never delivered a child.
- Don't pay attention to other people's horror stories (you'd be amazed at how insensitive some people can be).
- Don't tell anyone about the pregnancy until you're absolutely ready to, and then tell only people you'd want to support you if something bad were to happen (see pages 82–83 for more on this).
- Get some more ultrasounds or listen to the heartbeat—this might help to reassure you that all is well.
- Get some support. If your partner can help you, great, but she may be preoccupied with her own thoughts. Otherwise, find someone else who's been there and tell him or her how you're feeling.
- Support your partner. Encourage her to talk about what she's feeling and don't make any judgments about what she says. And try to keep her calm. As the pregnancy progresses, for example, and she can feel the baby's movements, she may become fixated on counting them—worried that there are either too many or too few. Just so you know, anywhere from 50 to 1,000 a day is normal.

WHAT SHE SHOULD DO

- Make an appointment with her health-care provider for a preconception physical. The doctor will:
  - Evaluate any and all medications your partner is taking to see whether they're safe during pregnancy.
  - Probably prescribe prenatal vitamins and possibly folic acid supplements (folic acid lowers the risk of some birth defects of the brain and spinal cord).
  - Address any medical conditions, such as diabetes, asthma, high blood pressure, depression, epilepsy, obesity, or any problems with previous pregnancies. All of these reduce her ability to get pregnant, and if she does conceive, can increase pregnancy complications and the risk of miscarriage, preterm delivery, and birth defects.
  - Make sure her immunizations are up-to-date, in particular chicken pox (varicella), German measles (rubella), and hepatitis B.
  - Screen her for sexually transmitted diseases.
  - Discuss the birth control methods she's been using. If she's been on the pill, she may need to go through a couple of pill-free months before trying to conceive.
- Get healthy. According to the Centers for Disease Control (CDC), 11 percent of women smoke during pregnancy, and 10 percent consume alcohol. Of women who could get pregnant, 69 percent don't take folic acid supplements, 31 percent are obese, and about 3 percent take prescription or over-the-counter drugs that are known teratogens (substances that can interfere with fetal development or cause birth defects). Getting healthy means:
  - Limit caffeine. Some studies show that caffeine can decrease a woman's fertility and increase the risk of miscarriage or other problems. Other studies find no connection. Just to be safe, though, it's probably best if she cuts back to no more than two or three cups of coffee per day or switches to decaf.
  - Exercise. It's much better for a pregnant woman to continue an exercise routine she already has in place than to start a new one. If your partner hasn't been working out regularly, add this to the list of things to talk about with her health-care provider.
  - Watch her weight. If she's overweight (her doctor will tell her whether it's a problem or not), now's the time to start slimming down. She definitely doesn't want to be dieting during the pregnancy. According to the CDC, "reaching a healthy weight before pregnancy reduces the risks of neural tube defects, preterm delivery, diabetes, Cesarean section," and other conditions associated with obesity.

- Pay attention to diet and nutrition. What your partner eats immediately before conception and in the first days and weeks of the pregnancy can have a big impact on fetal development and the baby's long-term health. See pages 35–44 for details on her diet and nutritional needs.
- Quit smoking and drinking. Both decrease fertility and increase the chances of a premature or low-birth-weight birth, or pregnancy loss.
- Stay out of hot tubs. A recent study by health-care giant Kaiser Permanente found that women who used a hot tub after conception were twice as likely to miscarry as women who didn't. Other studies haven't found much of a connection, but Kaiser's lead researcher, De-Kun Li, recommends that "women in the early stages of pregnancy—and those who may have conceived but aren't sure—might want to play it safe for the first few months and avoid hot tubs" as a way of reducing "unnecessary risk of miscarriage."

WHAT YOU SHOULD DO

- Talk to your doctor. Give him your medical history and tell him about your plans to do the dad thing. You want to find out whether there are any issues that you need to address before you start planning those romantic, candlelit, birth-control-free evenings. One especially important topic you'll want to discuss is how to make sure your sperm is healthy. Here are some ways to do that:
  - Keep your balls cool. Sperm is very sensitive to heat, which is why your testicles—where those little swimmers of yours live—hang outside your body, where it's a few degrees cooler. Heating them up by a couple of degrees (say, by spending any more than five minutes in a hot tub or hot bath, sitting with your legs crossed for extended periods of time, or wearing tight underwear that keeps your testicles up against your body) could reduce sperm production or cause abnormalities. We all know that women have fertility cycles, but were you aware that we do too? Turns out that sperm are on a ninety-day cycle, meaning that whatever happens to them today won't show up for three months or so.
  - Call in the vice squad. Smoking, using illegal drugs (or misusing legal ones), and drinking alcohol have all been linked to lowered fertility, miscarriage, and birth defects.
  - Watch the toxins. Hazardous chemicals, pesticides, and even noxious fumes could damage sperm and, if you inadvertently bring them home (for example, on your clothes), they could hurt your partner too.
  - Lose some weight. Dr. A. Ghiyath Shayeb, from the University of Aberdeen, Scotland, found that obese men produce lower volumes of seminal fluid

(the liquid that carries the sperm) and have a higher proportion of abnormal sperm. "[M]en who are trying for a baby with their partners should first try to achieve an ideal body weight," writes Shayeb.

- Have a little more fun. Traditional thinking has it that if you want to improve your chances of getting your partner pregnant, you should not ejaculate for at least a couple of days before trying. But Australian OB David Greening disagrees. Greening studied men with DNA-damaged sperm. After seven days of ejaculating daily (no, it didn't matter how), the percentage of damaged sperm dropped significantly. And motility—a measure of how straight and how quickly sperm swim toward those ever-elusive eggs—increased.
- Hang out with some dads. Talk to other guys about what it's like to be a dad, the challenges they've faced, and how they overcame them. Ask a ton of questions.

WHAT BOTH OF YOU SHOULD DO

- Make sure you've discussed any possible medical issues with a qualified health-care provider. If you haven't already, talk over any and all pregnancy-related risk factors. These include:
  - Her age. Getting pregnant at thirty-five or older increases the risk of certain genetic abnormalities, such as Down syndrome.
  - Your age. (See pages 296–97 for more).
  - Family history. Could either of you be a carrier of any genetic disorders, birth defects, or conditions such as cystic fibrosis or hemophilia?
  - Belonging to a high-risk ethnic group. African Americans may want to be tested for sickle-cell anemia. Individuals of African or Mediterranean descent may want to be tested for thalassemia; Jews of Ashkenazi (Eastern European) descent may want to be tested for Tay-Sachs and/or Canavan disease.
- Take a quick look at your HR manual and investigate your family leave options. We'll talk about this more on pages 136–42. But the more time you have to prepare yourself and your employer, the better.
- Look at your finances. How are you going to pay for all this? Do you have insurance? If so, check your deductibles and copays—and whether you have maternity coverage at all. If you or she just started a job, does the policy have a waiting period before benefits kick in? If you don't have insurance, what are your options? Could you qualify for Medicaid?
- Sit down with your partner and have some serious discussions about your plans. Hopefully she'll get pregnant at the perfect time. But if that doesn't happen, how do you feel about fertility treatments? Would you consider artificial

insemination using your sperm? Would you consider using donor sperm? How about in vitro (test tube) fertilization? What about using donor eggs? And if you do use any kind of technology, are you prepared to parent twins or more? Don't try to resolve anything in a single conversation.

Birth Defects

If one of the tests discussed earlier in this chapter indicates that your baby will be born deformed or with any kind of serious disorder, you and your partner have some serious discussions ahead of you. There are two basic options for dealing with birth defects in an unborn child: keep the baby or terminate the pregnancy. Fortunately, you and your partner won't have to make this decision on your own; every hospital that administers diagnostic tests has specially trained genetic counselors who will help you sort through the options.

There's no question that the availability of genetic testing has changed the landscape with regard to birth defects. Two recent studies analyzed birth data from a fifteen- to twenty-year period. One found a slight increase in the number of Down syndrome births, the other a slight decrease. As we've discussed, more and more women are putting off childbirth. And since women over thirty-five are about five times more likely than those in their twenties to have a Down syndrome baby, researchers would have expected the number of births to double. The reason that didn't happen is quite simple: with genetic testing able to identify Down syndrome babies very early in the pregnancy, many couples are choosing abortion. If you're considering terminating the pregnancy for genetic reasons, remember that communicating clearly and effectively with your partner is probably the most important thing you can do during this stressful time. The decision you make should not be taken lightly—it's a choice that will last a lifetime—and you and your partner must fully agree before proceeding with either option. But ultimately, your partner should make the final decision.

Coping with Your Grief

If you and your partner choose to terminate your pregnancy or reduce the number of fetuses, or if the pregnancy ends in miscarriage, the emotional toll can be devastating. That's why it's critical for the two of you to seek out the emotional support you're entitled to as soon as possible. While there's nothing that can be done to prepare for or prevent a miscarriage, telling your partner how you feel—either alone or with a member of the clergy, a therapist, or a close friend—is very important. And don't just sit back and wait for her to tell you what *she's* feeling. Take the initiative: be supportive and ask a lot of questions.

Avoid the temptation to try to "fix" things. You can't. And don't try to console your wife with statements like, "We can always have another one." Your intentions are good, but it won't go over well.

You and your partner do not have to handle your grief by yourselves: counseling and support are available to both women and men who have lost a fetus through miscarriage, genetic termination, or selective reduction. Going to a support group can be a particularly important experience for men—especially those who aren't getting the support they need from their friends and family. Many men who attend support groups report that until they joined the group, no one had ever asked how they felt about their loss. The group setting can also give men the chance to escape the loneliness and isolation and stop being strong for their partners for a few minutes and grieve for themselves. If you'd like to find a support group, your doctor or the genetic counselors can refer you to the closest one—or the one that might be most sympathetic to men's concerns.

Some men, however, are not at all interested in getting together with a large group of people who have little in common but tragedy. If you feel this way, be sure to explain your feelings tactfully to your partner—she may feel quite strongly that you should be there with her and might feel rejected if you aren't. If you ultimately decide not to join a support group, don't try to handle things alone; talk to your partner, your doctor, your cleric, or a sympathetic friend, or read—and maybe contribute to—some of the blogs that deal with grief from the dad's perspective. Keeping your grief bottled up will only hinder the healing process.

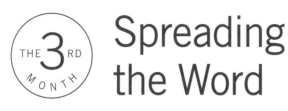

THE 3RD MONTH

Spreading the Word

WHAT'S GOING ON WITH YOUR PARTNER

Physically

- Fatigue, morning sickness, breast tenderness, and other early pregnancy symptoms are beginning to disappear
- Continuing moodiness
- She doesn't look pregnant yet, but she's having trouble fitting into her clothes anyway

Emotionally

- Heightened sense of reality about the pregnancy from hearing the baby's heartbeat
- Continuing ambivalence about the pregnancy and wondering how she's ever going to get through the next six months
- Frustration and/or excitement over her thickening waistline
- Turning inward—beginning to focus on what's happening inside her
- Beginning to bond with the baby

WHAT'S GOING ON WITH THE BABY

By now, the little fetus looks pretty much like a real person—except that he or she (even a really sharp ultrasound technician would be hard pressed to tell you which) is only about two or three inches long, weighs less than an ounce, and has translucent skin and a gigantic head (although "gigantic" is a relative term—it's roughly the size of a grape now). All the internal organs are there. Teeth, fingernails, toenails, and hair are developing nicely, and the brain is not far behind. By the end of this month, the baby will be breathing amniotic fluid and will be able to curl its toes, turn its head, open and close its mouth, and even frown.

WHAT'S GOING ON WITH YOU

A Heightened Sense of Reality

During the third month, the pregnancy begins to feel a little more tangible. By far the biggest reality booster for me was hearing the baby's heartbeat, even though it didn't sound anything like a real heart at all (more like a fast hoosh-hoosh-hoosh). Somehow, having the doctor tell us that what we were hearing was really a heartbeat—and a healthy one at that—was mighty reassuring.

Ambivalence

Most expectant dads have moments—or weeks or months—when they're less than completely excited about the pregnancy. Some are petrified that something terrible will happen to their partner or the baby, or that they'll be stuck in traffic on the way to the hospital and they'll have to deliver the baby all by themselves on the side of the road. Some see the whole thing as an inconvenience, or a never-ending suck of time and money. Others don't like the idea that they might lose their sex life, their youth, their independence, their friends, their savings, and that coveted spot at the center of their partner's universe. A lot of times these feelings of ambivalence or lack of interest are followed by guilt—for not being more supportive or not being a better spouse—or fear that these less-than-warm-and-fuzzy feelings are a surefire sign that you'll be a lousy dad. Give yourself a break, will you?

There are a number of factors that can increase or decrease these feelings of ambivalence:

- Is your partner the woman of your dreams, or were you pressured into your relationship? Similarly, is this the relationship of a lifetime, or do you have a feeling that it's not going to last?
- Are you totally ready to be a dad, or do you feel that you were pressured into the pregnancy? Have you accomplished everything you wanted to accomplish at this stage of your life, or are you sitting on a bunch of unfulfilled dreams?
- Are you financially ready (whatever that means to you) for fatherhood, or are you worried about money?

As you can probably guess, the more ambivalence you feel, the less you'll be involved during the rest of the pregnancy and after your baby is born.

Feeling Left Out

While becoming more aware of the reality of the pregnancy is certainly a good thing, it's not the only thing that you'll be feeling around this point. Toward the end of this first trimester, your partner will probably begin to spend a lot of time concentrating on what's happening inside her body, wondering whether she'll be a good enough mother, and establishing a bond with the baby. She may be worried about the baby's health or concerned that every little ache and pain she feels is a sign of some horrible disease. She's probably internalizing her feelings about all this and may become a little self-absorbed. And if she has a close relationship with her mother, the two of them may develop a deeper bond as your partner tries to find good role models.

Everything she's going through at this point is completely normal. The danger, however, is that while your partner is turning inward, spending more time with her girlfriends, or bonding with her own mother and the baby, you may end up feeling left out, rejected, or even pushed out of the way. This can be particularly painful. But no matter how much it hurts, resist the urge to "retaliate" by withdrawing from her. Be as comforting as you can be, and let her know—in a nonconfrontational way—how you're feeling (see the "Your Relationship" section, pages 86–90). Fortunately, this period of turning inward won't last forever.

Excluded—or Welcomed—by Your Partner's Practitioners

For some men—especially those who are feeling emotionally left out by their partners—the joy they experience at the increasing reality of the pregnancy can be outweighed by the bitterness they feel at the way they're treated by their partner's doctors. Pamela Jordan, a nurse and a pregnancy expert, found that most men feel that their presence at prenatal visits is perceived as "cute" or "novel." I frequently hear from expectant dads that medical professionals have a tendency to treat them as if they're mere onlookers or intruders, and consider their partners the only ones worth interacting with. If they were talked to at all during visits, it was only to discuss how to support their partners. The fact that an expectant dad might have very specific, unique, and important needs and concerns didn't seem to occur to anyone.

If you *are* interested in being involved and your partner's practitioner isn't as welcoming as you'd like, I can just about guarantee that your experience of the whole pregnancy will be tainted. Whether you realize it or not, you probably have some pretty clear ideas about how you'd like the pregnancy and birth to go. If you're reduced to the role of spectator, you're not going to get what you want, and you're going to feel stressed and resentful. That will influence your level of involvement throughout the rest of the pregnancy and will make it a lot harder to adjust to all the changes that new fatherhood will bring.

I don't mean to suggest that this kind of thing happens everywhere, or that the fault always lies entirely with the medical staff. A lot of guys feel a little squeamish around (or are just plain put off by) gynecological stuff, and they hide in the corner to avoid having to deal with it. And if your partner has a male OB, it can also be a little odd to be in the room while another guy has his hands in places you thought were off-limits to everyone but you. (Yes, pelvic exams are standard medical procedures, and if you go to enough appointments, you'll get used to them, but still ...)

Fortunately, more and more medical professionals (but not nearly enough) are welcoming dads into the fold. In my case, over the course of three pregnancies, all of the OBs went out of their way to include me in the process. They made a special point of looking at me when talking about what was happening with my wife and the baby. They encouraged me to ask questions, and answered them thoroughly.

Part of the reason for this was that from the very beginning I made it clear that I *wanted* to be involved and I peppered them with questions, so it was pretty much impossible for them to ignore me. I suggest that you do the same, especially if you have even the slightest suspicion that your partner's practitioner is ignoring you or not taking you seriously.

Our first OB even invited me to take a look at my wife's cervix. I was a little put off by the idea, but getting to see the cervix—through which our baby would emerge just six months later—somehow made the pregnancy seem less mysterious and made me feel much more a part of the whole thing. (At the same time, I've got to admit that the experience was a little odd.) If your OB doesn't offer you a look, ask for one—but expect some raised eyebrows. Be sure to ask your partner first, though. She might feel that it's more than a bit intrusive—especially since it's a part of her body that she may never see. Plus, she may simply not want anyone but her practitioner looking at her in such a clinical way. Can't blame her for that one.

Physical Symptoms: Couvade

Although most of what you'll be going through during your pregnancy will be psychological, don't be surprised if you start developing some physical symptoms as well. Various studies estimate that as many as 90 percent of American expectant fathers experience *couvade* syndrome (from the French word meaning "to hatch"), or "sympathetic pregnancy." Couvade symptoms are typically the same as those traditionally associated with pregnant women—weight gain, nausea, mood swings, food cravings—as well as some not necessarily associated with pregnant women: headaches, toothaches, itching, diarrhea, even cysts. Symptoms—if you're going to have them at all—usually appear in about the third month of pregnancy, decrease for a few months, then pick up again in the month or two before the baby is born. In almost every case, though, the symptoms "mysteriously" disappear at the birth. Here are some of the most common reasons an expectant father might develop couvade symptoms:

SYMPATHY OR FEELINGS OF GUILT FOR WHAT THE WOMAN IS GOING THROUGH

Men have traditionally been socialized to bite the bullet when it comes to pain and discomfort. When our loved ones are suffering and we can't do anything to stop it, our natural (and slightly irrational) instinct is to try to take their pain away—to make it ours instead of theirs. This is especially true if we have even the slightest feeling—no matter how crazy—that we're responsible for the pain in the first place. If your partner has been suffering from morning sickness or has had any other pregnancy-related difficulties, you (and she) may feel that it's your fault. And if her symptoms have been particularly rough, she might even reinforce your subconscious guilt by reminding you that you're the one who "got her into all this" in the first place.

JEALOUSY

There's no question that your partner is going to be getting a lot more attention during the pregnancy than you are. And some men who develop couvade symptoms undoubtedly do so in a subconscious attempt to shift the focus of the pregnancy to themselves. It's as if they're saying, "Hey, she's not the only one around here who's tossing her cookies," or "Excuse me, but my pants aren't fitting so well anymore either." My father, who was pacing the waiting room while my mother was in labor with me, suddenly got a gushing nosebleed. Within seconds the delivery room was empty—except for my mother—as three nurses and two doctors raced out to take care of my poor, bleeding father. I'm sure he didn't do it on purpose, but for one brief moment during the delivery, Dad was the complete center of attention. Similarly, physical symptoms could be a kind of public way of asserting paternity.

Although it's not exactly a couvade symptom, a lot of expectant dads take up hobbies or begin projects that allow them to create something new, just like their partner.

YOUR HORMONES COULD BE RAGING

No, I haven't got that backward. While she's pregnant, several of your partner's hormone levels gradually rise. These include *prolactin*, which helps get her breasts ready to lactate (produce milk), and *cortisol*, which appears to be associated with parent-child bonding. It used to be that everyone thought these hormone changes were triggered by the developing fetus. But in several fascinating studies, researcher Anne Storey and her colleagues found something that may change a few minds. Storey took blood samples from expectant mothers and fathers at various points during the pregnancy and found that expectant dads' levels of cortisol and prolactin (which you wouldn't think guys would even have) paralleled their partners'. "The differences for mums were much more drastic, but the patterns were similar," said Dr. Storey, who's Canadian—hence the cute "mums."

Some guys seem to be more susceptible to this kind of thing than others. In talking with the men in her study, Storey found that those who had experienced tiredness, weight gain, changes in appetite, or any other physical couvade symptoms had higher-than-average levels of prolactin and lower-than-average levels of testosterone compared to expectant dads who didn't have these symptoms. Fortunately, this doesn't mean that you'll be developing breasts anytime soon. Like your partner's, your hormone levels will return to normal not long after your baby is born, and your manliness will remain intact.

These hormone changes could also contribute to an extremely common, non-physical type of couvade symptom. Most expectant dads find themselves somewhat more interested in children than before the pregnancy. Is it simply curiosity, or is it the body's way of preparing the expectant dad for his changing responsibilities? Hard to say. But studies have shown that the stronger an expectant dad's couvade symptoms, the better he'll care for his newborn. Maybe there's something about sharing (sort of) the physical part of pregnancy that helps develop the dad-baby bond. If any of this is hitting home, though, you may want to think twice before you let your partner read this page—especially if you've been making fun of *her* out-of-control hormones. If none of this is hitting home, that's fine too. There are no rules about how you're supposed to be feeling.

GOOD OLD-FASHIONED STRESS

Researcher Robert Rodriguez cites evidence that men with unplanned pregnancies seem to have more symptoms than others, and that working-class men (who, presumably, are more likely to worry about money) have more frequent symptoms than middle-class dads.

YOU MAY BE SENDING MESSAGES TO YOUR PARTNER

Generally speaking, women are more vulnerable during pregnancy and parenthood than men; you can always take off, she can't. (At the risk of sounding politically incorrect, a number of researchers have speculated that this is precisely why women have traditionally looked for men who will be "good providers.") As a result, expectant mothers are often particularly concerned about whether their partners are going to be there for them and whether they're really committed to being fathers. On one level, you can reassure your partner by telling her you love her, by going to all the prenatal doctor appointments, and by educating yourself and staying as involved as you possibly can. But words aren't always enough.

Some evolutionary psychologists have speculated recently that on a far more subconscious level, expectant dads' physical couvade symptoms could be a chemically driven way of showing their partners just how committed they truly are. After all, you could be lying when you tell her you love her and that you're excited about being a dad. But it's a lot harder to fake a nosebleed or a backache or weight gain. In short, your physical symptoms may be nature's way of giving your partner a way to evaluate your true feelings about her and the baby, as well as your reliability as a partner and fellow parent.

A LITTLE HISTORY

Most researchers today agree that in Western societies, couvade symptoms appear unconsciously in those expectant fathers who experience them. But as far back as 60 B.C.E. (and continuing today in many non-Western societies), couvade has been used deliberately in rituals designed to keep fathers involved in the experience of pregnancy and childbirth. Not all of these rituals, however, have been particularly friendly to women. W. R. Dawson writes that in the first century C.E. mothers were routinely ignored during childbirth, while their husbands were waited on in bed. And more recently, in Spain and elsewhere, mothers frequently gave birth in the fields where they worked. They then returned home to care for the baby's father.

But in some other cultures, men tried to do the same thing they try to do today: take their partner's pain away by attracting it to themselves. In France and Germany, for example, pregnant women were given their husband's clothes during labor in the belief that doing so would transfer the wives' pains to their husbands. Perhaps the most bizarre couvade ritual I've come across is one that enabled dads-to-be to literally share the pain of childbirth. Apparently, the Huichol people of Mexico used to position the dad in a tree or on the roof above his laboring wife. Ropes were tied around his testicles and with each contraction she could yank on the ropes and give her husband a taste of what she was going through. Seems a little much to me, but I'm sure there are plenty of women who would disagree.

Perhaps the most interesting aspect of ritual couvade is the importance attached to the supernatural bond between the father and the unborn child. Whatever the fathers did during the pregnancy was believed to have a direct impact on the unborn child. In Borneo expectant fathers ate nothing but rice and salt—a diet said to keep a new baby's stomach from swelling. In other countries a man who hammered a nail while his wife was pregnant was thought to be dooming her to a long, painful labor, and if he split wood, he would surely have a child with a cleft lip. Afraid of making his own child blind, an expectant father wouldn't eat meat from an animal that gives birth to blind young. He also avoided turtles—so that his child would not be born deaf, with deformed limbs (flippers), and anencephalic (with a cone-shaped head).

While it's pretty doubtful that couvade rituals actually reduced any woman's childbirth pains or prevented any deformities, they do illustrate an important point: men have been trying to get—and stay—involved in pregnancy and childbirth for thousands of years. As Bronislav Malinowski noted in his 1927 book, *Sex and Repression in Savage Society*:

> Even the apparently absurd idea of couvade presents to us a deep meaning and a necessary function. It is of high biological value for the human family to consist of both father and mother; if the traditional customs and rules are there to establish a social situation of close moral proximity between father and child, if all such customs aim at drawing a man's attention to his offspring, then the couvade which makes man simulate the birth-pangs and illness of maternity is of great value and provides the necessary stimulus and expression for paternal tendencies. The couvade and all the customs of its type serve to accentuate the principle of legitimacy, the child's need of a father.

Couvade for Adoptive and ART Dads Too? Yep.

Given that couvade symptoms seem to be an expression of fathers' desires to get some confirmation of their special status in their children's lives, it shouldn't come as much of a surprise that adoptive fathers often experience them as well. In fact, according to adoption educator Patricia Irwin Johnson, "sympathetic symptoms of pregnancy" are fairly common. "One or both partners may experience repeated, and even predictably scheduled, episodes of nausea," says Johnson. "Food cravings and significant weight gain are not unusual. One or both may complain of sleep disturbances or emotional peaks and valleys."

Men who are becoming fathers thanks to IVF or some other ART procedure aren't immune to couvade symptoms either. In fact, some research suggests that fathers who have (or whose partner has) experienced infertility may actually be *more* susceptible than dads who conceived naturally. The same may also be true for expectant dads who were adopted as babies.

STAYING INVOLVED

Spilling the Beans

Another thing (this month anyway) that will make the pregnancy seem more real is telling other people about it. By the end of the third month, I'd pretty well gotten over my fears of miscarriage or other pregnancy disasters, and we'd decided it was safe to put the word out to our family and close friends. Somehow just saying "My wife's pregnant" (I switched to "We're expecting" a while later) helped me realize it was true.

The decision about when to let other people in on your pregnancy is a big one. Some people are superstitious and opt to put off making the announcement for as long as possible. Others rush to the phone or start emailing, texting, tweeting, and updating their Facebook pages before the urine is even dry on the pregnancy test stick. Even if you're in the first category, sooner or later you're going to have to start spreading the word—and the end of the third month is a pretty good time.

There are, of course, advantages and disadvantages to making either an early or a late announcement. For example, if you tell people early, you'll probably get a lot of support, reassurance, referrals, and hand-me-downs. But after a while you may start looking around for an off switch. If you tell early and something does go wrong, that support will be there for you. On the other hand, retracting good news is not an easy thing to do.

If you decide to tell people later, you'll have complete control over the information flow. You'll keep from drowning in advice, but some of that advice might have been good. And if something were to go wrong, you wouldn't have to worry about retracting the good news, but you wouldn't have as much of a support network to lean on either.

Ultimately, whom you decide to tell, and in what order, is your own business. But here are a few ideas you might want to keep in mind.

FAMILY

Unless you have some compelling reason not to, you should probably tell your family first. Your close friends will forgive you if they hear about the pregnancy from your Aunt Ida; if it happens the other way around, Aunt Ida may take real offense. There are a few cases, however, when telling your family first might not be a great idea. One couple we knew kept their pregnancy a secret from their friends for five months—and from their family for longer—hoping that the husband's brother and sister-in-law, who had been trying to get pregnant for years, would succeed in the interim.

FRIENDS

If you do decide to tell your friends first, don't count on your secret staying a secret for very long—good news travels a lot faster than you might think, and nothing travels faster—or further—than a tweet or a Facebook status update. As in the case of relatives, be considerate of friends who have been trying but who haven't been as successful as you.

THE OFFICE

You'll probably want to tell your coworkers and your boss (if you have one) at about the same time as you tell your friends. But remember that society has some pretty rigid work/family rules for men, so be prepared for a less-than-enthusiastic response from some people (see the "Work and Family" section, pages 136–42, for a complete discussion). Whatever you do, though, don't wait until the last minute to tell the folks at work—especially if you're planning to take some time off or make any work schedule changes after the birth.

YOUR OTHER CHILDREN

If you have other children, give them plenty of time to adjust to the news. But don't tell them until after you want everyone else to know. Until they're over six, kids don't understand the concept of "keeping a secret." When she was four, one of my oldest daughter's big thrills in life was to gleefully whisper in people's ears things that were supposed to be secrets. In her mind, whispering something didn't actually count as saying it.

Make a special effort to include your other children as much as possible in the pregnancy experience. Our oldest daughter came with us to most of the doctor appointments and got to hold the Doppler (the thing you hear the fetus's heartbeat through) and help the doctor measure my wife's growing belly.

Finally, keep in mind that it's perfectly normal for expectant siblings to insist that they, too, are pregnant—just like Mommy. Insisting that they're not may make them feel excluded and resentful of the new baby. This is especially true for little boys.

A FEW SPECIAL CIRCUMSTANCES

If your partner had a miscarriage and you're expecting again, the rules (to the extent that there are any) for telling family and friends change somewhat. You might want to tell selected people immediately—you may be craving your family's or friends' support, or you may just need someone to be happy for you. Most people, though, want to put it off as long as possible (although in another month or so it'll be pretty obvious). Here are some common reasons why:

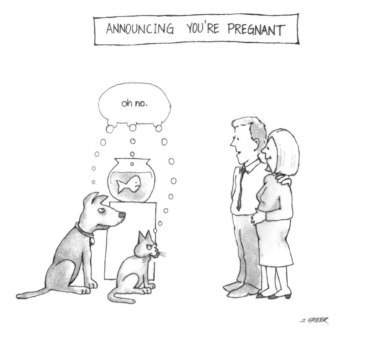

ANNOUNCING YOU'RE PREGNANT

- You may be worried that there could be another miscarriage and don't want to put yourself through the pain of calling everyone to give them bad news. This is especially true if your partner has had more than one.
- If your partner got pregnant right after a miscarriage, you may worry that other people will think you're being disrespectful by not grieving longer.
- You may want to wait until you're over the hump—past the point when the miscarriage happened last time. If you have other kids who know about the previous miscarriage, it's a good idea to wait until the pregnancy is pretty far along. They may worry about your partner or the new baby, and they might even be afraid that something they did caused the first miscarriage. If you have even the slightest inkling that this is the case, spend some time gently explaining to your other children that they are not responsible at all, that sometimes things happen that we just can't explain.

Telling friends and family that you've decided to adopt, that you're doing ART, or that you're using a gestational carrier can also be surprisingly tricky. Some couples are perfectly fine with the idea. But for most, it's a lot more complicated. To start with, you or your partner might be ashamed at what you might consider the inadequacy of not being able to get pregnant naturally. And then there's the grief one or both of you may feel. Depending on which options you're considering, you may have to come to terms with the loss of your dreams of having a biologically related child and keeping your genetic line alive. Or the disappointment at being deprived of the opportunity to go through a pregnancy and birth.

Although you'd think that everyone would be overjoyed at your decision to adopt (or, if you're using donor sperm or eggs, to tell people about it), that's not always the case. Some people—especially relatives—might not be too happy that you're bringing an "outsider" into your family. You have every right to expect your family to respect your decision and treat you and your partner with respect. At the same time, as Patricia Irwin Johnson points out, your family has the right to expect certain things from you:

- Information. They can't be sensitive about something they don't understand. You might want to recommend that they read some books on adoption (see Selected Bibliography).
- Sensitivity. You must acknowledge that your decision to adopt might cause some people some pain. Your parents, for example, might be disappointed that they're not going to become grandparents the "right" way or that a genetic family link has been broken. Like you, they may need some time to mourn the loss of their hopes and dreams.
- Patience. Even if they do have information and a good understanding of adoption, they're still lagging behind you and your partner in terms of knowledge. So give them some time to catch up and don't expect instant support and understanding. If someone makes a dumb or insensitive remark about adoption or donor sperm, or anything else, resist the urge to bite her head off. Instead, take her aside and point out the mistake as nicely as you can.

What If You're Not Married?

Even in the twenty-first century, when it's the norm for couples to live together before getting married, having a child out of wedlock still raises a lot of eyebrows in some circles. Your most liberal-minded friends and relatives might surprise you by suggesting that you "make an honest woman of her" before the baby comes. Try to keep your sense of humor about these things. You and your partner are grown-ups and capable of making the decisions you think best. And anyway, most unmarried parents-to-be find that their relatives' joy at the prospect of a new little niece, nephew, or grandchild frequently overshadows those same relatives' disappointment over your lack of a marriage certificate.

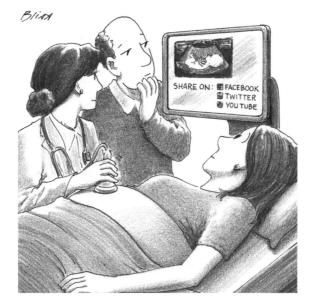

No matter how or when you do it, telling people you're expecting will open a floodgate of congratulations and advice; after a few weeks, you may wonder what anyone used to talk about at parties before. Just about everyone has something to say about what you should and shouldn't do now that you're expecting. You'll hear delightful stories, horror stories, and just plain boring stories about pregnancy and childbirth. You'll probably also have to endure endless "jokes" about your masculinity, speculation about who the "real" father is, and questions about what the mailman or the milkman looks like—mostly, unfortunately, from other men. With attitudes like these, is it any wonder that 60 percent of men have at least fleeting doubts as to the true paternity of their children?

Immediately after breaking the news to our friends and family, my wife and I began to feel some slight changes in our relationship with them. What had once been our private secret was now public knowledge, and just about everyone wanted to share it with us. People would drop in unannounced, usually bearing either gifts or advice—just to see how things were going—and the phone never stopped ringing.

After a few days, you and your partner may start to feel a little claustrophobic. If this happens, don't hesitate to establish some ground rules. For example, you might want to ask your friends and families to call before coming over, or you might set up—and let everyone know about—specific visiting hours. You should also prepare yourself for the possibility that you may feel a little left out. Most people are going to be asking how your partner is feeling, what she's going through, and so on. Few, if any, will ask you the same questions.

Trying to Keep the Secret

Despite your attempts to control the flow of information, if you're not careful about what you do, people—especially your close friends—are going to guess. If you're serious about not wanting anyone to know, here are a couple of things to keep in mind:

- Stay away from expressions like "in her condition" or "I think she really needs to rest." That's exactly how I inadvertently leaked the news to a friend who had asked how we liked working out on the Stairmaster machine at the gym.
- Be unobtrusive if you change your habits. If your partner used to drink or smoke before she got pregnant, you might want to think a little about how your friends and family will react to her new, vice-free lifestyle (but that's no excuse not to quit smoking and drinking). When my wife was pregnant with our second daughter, we agreed to meet some good friends at a bar one Saturday night. No one really noticed that my wife was drinking mineral water instead of her usual beer. But when she ordered an ice-cold glass of milk, the jig was up.

If you start feeling that you're being treated more like a spectator than a participant in the pregnancy, there are three basic solutions. First, you can just ignore the whole thing—no one's deliberately trying to exclude you; it just doesn't occur to most people that pregnancy, at least at this stage, affects men all that much. Second, you can sulk. This (although sometimes satisfying) will probably not get you the kind of attention you're craving. Third, you can take a proactive role and volunteer information about how the pregnancy is affecting you. Tell people about how excited you are, how much weight you've put on, and how bad those stomachaches you've been having hurt. Confide your hopes and fears to your friends—especially those who already have kids and can offer advice. If you're lucky, they'll then start asking you for updates.

Your Relationship

WITH EACH OTHER

Pregnancy is not only a time of great joy and anticipation, it's also a time of great stress. And even though you and your partner are both pregnant at the same time, you're not experiencing the pregnancy in exactly the same way or at the same pace. This can lead to an increasing number of misunderstandings and conflicts.

As Jerrold Shapiro writes, when a couple becomes a family, "generally all the things that are good get better, and all the things that are bad get worse." As your pregnancy continues, then, it's critical to learn to talk—and listen—to each other, and to find ways to help each other through this marvelous, but emotionally bumpy, experience.

As men, we've been conditioned to try to protect our partners from harm. And when our partners are pregnant, protecting them may include trying to minimize the levels of stress in their lives. One way we try to do this is by not talking about our own concerns. Somewhere along the line, we got this idea that being strong for our partner means not ever acknowledging how much the pregnancy—and the whole transition to fatherhood—is affecting us.

Researchers Carolyn and Philip Cowan found that this overprotective, macho attitude has some very negative side effects. First, because we never give ourselves the chance to talk about our fears and concerns, we never learn that what we're going through is normal and healthy. Second, our partners never get the chance to find out that we understand and share their feelings. As a result, instead of decreasing stress around the house, we end up increasing it—for her and for ourselves.

There's also some evidence that there are other benefits to talking about how you're feeling—and getting your partner's support for those feelings. Researcher Geraldine Deimer found that men who receive their partners' emotional support during pregnancy have better physical and emotional health and are better able to maintain good relationships with their spouses than men who don't get that kind of support.

DANGEROUS ASSUMPTIONS

When I was in the Marines, one of my drill instructor's favorite comments was: "Never assume anything. Assuming makes an ass out of u and me." The sergeant's spelling problems notwithstanding (he also thought habitual thieves were called hypochondriacs and Italians ate bisgetti), he was right about the dangers of making assumptions.

Here are a few important things you may have assumed were no problem but could end up biting you in the butt. Not all these issues are important to everybody, but if you haven't discussed them already, do it now. A lot of couples avoid bringing up these issues because they're afraid it'll lead to a fight—and no one wants to upset a pregnant woman, right? Well, in my view it's better to talk about these things now, a little at a time, than to seethe about them for the next six months and then have some kind of explosion. Because these issues are so important, give yourself partial credit toward your fifteen-minutes-a-day homework assignment outlined on page 89.

- Your involvement in the pregnancy. Dr. Katharyn Antle May has found that there are three basic styles of father involvement during pregnancy. The *Observer Father* maintains a certain emotional distance and sees himself largely as a bystander; the *Expressive Father* is emotionally very involved and sees himself as a full partner; the *Instrumental Father* sees himself as the manager of the pregnancy and may feel a need to plan every medical appointment, every meal, and every trip to the gym. Whatever your style is, make sure to talk it over with your partner. After all, she's pregnant too. Be aware that there's a direct correlation between your level of involvement in the pregnancy (as perceived by your partner) and her satisfaction with your relationship, according to Susanne Biehle, a social psychologist at DePauw University. Also be aware that her definition of involvement may not be the same as yours. For example, you may consider providing financially for your growing family as involvement, while she may not.
- Your involvement in family tasks. How much child care are you planning to do when the baby comes? How much is your partner expecting you to do? How much are you expecting her to do? This is going to sound harsh, but the reality is that you'll be as involved with your children as your partner will let you be. If she wants you to take an active role in child care, chances are you'll want the same thing. But if she wants to keep these activities to herself, you'll probably be less involved. In addition, the Cowans have found that men who take a more active role in running their households and rearing their children "tend to feel better about themselves and about their family relationships than men who are less involved in family work."
- Religion. Both you and your partner may never have given a thought to the religious education—if any—you plan to give your child. If you have thought

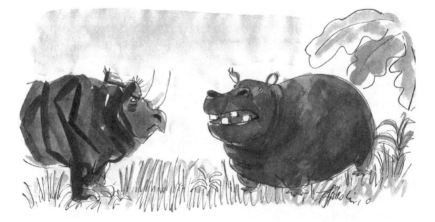

"You're entirely too touchy. My saving grace is my ability to laugh at myself."

An Important Homework Assignment

In the first year after the birth of their baby, 90 percent of couples in researcher Jay Belsky's studies experienced a tremendous drop-off in the quality and quantity of their communication. Half the time it was permanent.

If you think about this, it makes perfectly good sense. Right now, besides being in a relationship together, you and your partner have your own individual lives, hobbies, friends, jobs, and interests. You're both growing and developing as people—as individuals and as a couple. That's what has made you the lovable guy you are and the lovable woman she is. But once your baby shows up, you're going to be making an abrupt change to the all-baby-all-the-time channel, constantly thinking about, talking about, and doing things with your baby. All that personal growth stuff is going out the window, at least for a while.

The cure for this is to set aside fifteen minutes every day to talk about something, anything, other than the baby. I know this sounds awfully simple, but if you get into the habit now, while your life is still relatively calm, you'll be taking a huge step toward keeping your relationship fresh. It really does work, and making a commitment to doing it every day is absolutely critical. The more satisfied you feel in your relationship *before* you have children, according to researchers Chih-Yuan Lee and William Doherty, the more time you'll spend with your child during the first year of his or her life.

about it, make sure you're both still thinking along the same lines. If you haven't, this might be a good time to start.

- Discipline styles. How do you feel about spanking your children? Never? Sometimes? How does she feel about it? How you were raised and whether your parents spanked you will have a great deal to do with how you'll raise your own children.
- Sleeping arrangements. It's never too early to give some thought to where you want the baby to sleep: In your bed? In a bassinet next to you? In a separate room? Be prepared, though: things have a way of changing after the baby shows up.
- Work and child-care expectations. Is your partner planning to take some time off after the birth before going back to work? How long? Would you like to be able to take some more time off? How long? What types of child-care arrangements do you and she envision?

• Finances. Do you need two paychecks to pay the mortgage? If you can get by on one, whose will it be?

And throughout the pregnancy, don't forget your feelings—good, bad, or indifferent. Talk about your excitement about having a child, your dreams, your plans for the future, your fears, worries, and ambivalence, and how satisfied you are with your level of involvement during the pregnancy. Don't forget to ask your partner what she's feeling about the same things. Have these discussions regularly—what the two of you are thinking and feeling in the third month may be completely different from what you'll be thinking and feeling in the fourth, sixth, or ninth month. As difficult as it may seem, learning to communicate with each other now will help you for years to come.

Getting Time Alone

There may be times when you find the pressures of the pregnancy so overwhelming that you need just to get away from it for a while. If so, take advantage of the fact that you don't have a baby inside you, and give yourself some time off. Go someplace quiet where you can collect your thoughts or do something that will give you a break from the endless conversations about pregnant women and babies. Before you go, though, be sure to let your partner know where you're headed. And whatever you do, don't rub it in; she'd probably give anything to be able to take a breather from the pregnancy—even for a couple of hours. Here are a few things you might want to do with your free time:

• Hang out with some childless friends.
• See a movie or a play.
• Read.
• Start a blog about what you're feeling and thinking during the pregnancy. If you're writing stuff that you'd rather not have your partner know about, you might want to make your posts private.
• Go to the batting cages and let off a little steam.
• Go for a long drive or for a walk on the beach or in the woods.
• Be a kid for a while and spend a couple of hours playing video games. If you haven't got a PlayStation, Xbox, or Wii of your own, download a few from your favorite gaming site or grab some quarters and head for the nearest arcade.
• Sleep (good luck with that).
• If you feel guilty that you're getting a break when your partner isn't, use the time to do something for the family, like updating your blog or building a Facebook fan page and posting all those cute ultrasound pictures.

THE 4TH MONTH

Money, Money, Money

WHAT'S GOING ON WITH YOUR PARTNER

Physically

- Nipples darkening; freckles and moles might get darker and more obvious (a normal side effect of her increasing skin pigmentation)
- As her morning sickness begins to wane, she'll start to recover her appetite—for food and for sex
- Clumsy—dropping and spilling things
- She may be able to feel some slight movements (although she probably won't associate them with the baby unless she's already had a child)
- She may notice some strange changes in her vision; if she wears contacts, they may be bothering her
- She may get gingivitis (swollen, bleeding gums)—60 to 75 percent of pregnant women do
- She may be starting to show; most people won't be able to say for sure, but if she's a celebrity and ends up on the cover of *People* magazine or *Us Weekly*, there would be a big arrow pointing to her "bump"

Emotionally

- Great excitement when she sees the sonogram
- Worries about miscarriage are beginning to fade
- Concerned about what it really means to be a mother
- Continuing forgetfulness and mood swings
- Increasingly dependent on you—needs to know you'll be there for her, that you still love her

- She may get very depressed when her regular clothes stop fitting her and may become nearly obsessed with her appearance

What's Going On with the Baby

During this month, the baby will grow to about four or five inches long and tip the scales at about four ounces. His heart will finish developing and will start pounding away at 120–160 beats per minute—about twice as fast as yours—and his whole body is covered with smooth hair called *lanugo*. The fetus can—and often does—kick, swallow, and suck his thumb. He can also tell when your partner is eating sweet things or sour things and reacts accordingly (swallowing more for sweet, less for sour). He can also respond to light and dark—if you shine a strong light on your partner's abdomen, the baby will turn away.

WHAT'S GOING ON WITH YOU

Increasing Sense of the Pregnancy's Reality

By the time the fourth month rolls around, most men are still in what Katharyn May calls the "moratorium phase" of pregnancy—intellectually we know that she's pregnant, but we still don't have any "real" confirmation. Oh, sure, there was the pregnancy test, the blood test, the doctor's pelvic exams, her swelling belly and breasts, the food cravings, and hearing the baby's heartbeat a month before. Even with all that, I had the lingering suspicion that the whole thing was an elaborate, *Mission: Impossible*-style fake. Or maybe she was making the whole thing up as an excuse to get out of doing the laundry. Hmmm.

But the day my wife and I went in for the ultrasound, everything began to change. Somehow, seeing the baby's tiny heart pumping and watching those bandy little arms and legs squirm convinced me that we might really be expecting after all.

If you're expecting twins (or more), you may want to pay extra attention to the ultrasound (you may also want to see if you can schedule a couple of extras over the next few months) because the way the fetuses behave in utero may give you some insight into what you can expect after they're born. Each twin has its own temperament from the very early stages of development, and each set of twins establishes a characteristic pattern of behavior, according to researcher Alessandra Piontelli. Both the temperament and the way the twins interact continue for at least the first year after birth. Even odder (assuming that's possible), one group of researchers found that with triplets, two of the fetuses may interact with each other while ignoring the third. After the birth, that dynamic continued for a year or so, with the third baby isolated by his siblings.

Of course, seeing the ultrasound is only one of a number of things you can do to make the pregnancy seem more real. That's a good thing, because the more real it is, the more significance it will have to you—and the more you'll get involved. And as we've discussed earlier, involvement *now* leads directly to involvement *later.*

So, besides the ultrasound, what are some other activities you can do now to up the reality factor? Researchers Jacinta Bronte-Tinkew and Allison Horowitz identified five:

- Discussing the pregnancy with the mother. Check (hopefully you've been doing that for a while now).
- Listening to the baby's heartbeat. Check.
- Feeling the baby move. Coming soon to a belly near you.

Commissioning Connection

For most expectant mothers, it doesn't take much imagination for the pregnancy to feel real—all they have to do is pay attention to what's going on with their own bodies. Expectant dads can connect by being around the pregnant woman and doing all the things listed in this section. But what if you've outsourced the pregnancy and someone else is carrying your baby? Connecting with *that* pregnancy will present some challenges.

British researchers Fiona MacCallum and Emma Lycett studied relationships between commissioning couples and surrogate mothers. They found that whether the surrogate mother is a friend, relative, or someone completely unknown to the commissioning couple, the three players have to establish some kind of bond (which some have referred to as a "forced friendship").

In MacCallum's and Lycett's study, 98 percent of commissioning mothers and 90 percent of fathers rated their relationship with the surrogate mother as "harmonious." Sure, there were a few issues here and there—some couples thought the surrogate was overexerting herself, others found the relationship a little chilly—but just about everyone was satisfied with how things went.

Seventy-nine percent of the commissioning mothers saw the surrogate mother at least once a month, often going to all the OB visits. Only 55 percent of the men did this, but in many of these cases, the surrogate requested that the dad not be there. Eighty-one percent of the moms were there for the birth, but only 31 percent of the dads. Again, this was in large part at the request of the surrogate.

- Attending a childbirth prep class. Give it another couple of months.
- Buying something for the child. An ongoing effort.

To give you a hint as to where all this is leading, "Men who participated in more of these prenatal activities," write Bronte-Tinkew and Horowitz, "were more likely to exhibit positive engagement in cognitively stimulating activities (e.g., reading to the child), warmth (e.g., hugging the child), nurturing activities (e.g., soothing an upset child), physical care (e.g., changing diapers), and caregiving activities (e.g., bathing the child)."

Can We Really Afford This?

Besides being fun, seeing the ultrasound filled me with a wonderful sense of relief. After counting all the fingers and toes (not an easy task, considering how small they were and how fast they were moving), I felt I could finally stop worrying about whether our baby would be all right.

But my newfound sense of ease didn't last long. I suddenly became possessed by the idea that we couldn't possibly afford to have a baby—not an uncommon thought among expectant fathers. Not surprisingly, though, expectant fathers in their early and mid-twenties feel more financial pressures than dads-to-be who are over thirty-two. These "older" fathers tend to be more settled in their careers and make more money than the young bucks.

Even well into the twenty-first century, American society still values men's financial contribution to their families much more than it does their emotional contribution. And expressing strong feelings, anxiety, or even fear is not what men are expected to do—especially when their wives are pregnant. So, as the pregnancy progresses, most expectant fathers fall back on the more traditionally masculine way of expressing their concern for the well-being of their wives and little fetuses: they worry about money.

Some men express their financial worries by becoming obsessed with their jobs, their salaries, the size of their homes, even the rise and fall of interest rates. Expectant fathers frequently work overtime or take on a second job; others may become tempted by lottery tickets or get-rich-quick schemes. Clearly, a new baby (and the associated decrease in household income while the mother is off work) can have a significant impact on the family's finances. But as real as they are, write Libby Lee and Arthur D. Colman (authors of *Pregnancy: The Psychological Experience*), men's financial worries "often get out of proportion to the actual needs of the family. They become the focus because they are something the man can be expected to handle. The activity may hide deeper worry about competence and security." In other words, calm down.

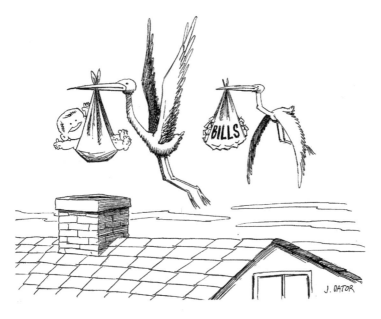

In some ways, work and fatherhood are inseparable. But very few people (except the dads themselves) see providing for the family as involvement. Shawn Christiansen and pioneering fatherhood researcher Rob Palkovitz have come up with four explanations for this selective blindness:

- There's an assumption that men should provide. Because we're *supposed* to do it, all the financial support dads contribute gets taken for granted.
- Providing is invisible. This is partly because work generally takes place away from the family. "When family members do not see fathers in the act of providing," write Christiansen and Palkovitz, "they may not be as acutely aware of the energy, sacrifice, and labor extended in order to provide."
- There are some negative connotations associated with the traditional provider role. The more time dads spend at work, the less time they can spend at home. So people often see them as uninvolved, or uncaring, or emotionally distant.
- People don't think the right way about providing. We have a tendency to set up a dynamic of work vs. family (see pages 136–44 for more on this), as though it's one or the other. But men see providing for their family as just one component of what it takes to be a good father.

Safety—Your Partner's and the Baby's

As if worrying about finances weren't enough, many expectant fathers find themselves preoccupied with the physical health and safety of the other members of their growing family (but not their own—studies have shown that men go to the

Ways to Show Her You Care

Here are nearly a hundred ideas—in no particular order—that will make you popular around the house (and make your wife the envy of all of her friends—pregnant and otherwise). If you come up with one that's not on this list, email us. We'll include it in the next edition.

- Offer to give her back rubs and foot massages.
- Get her a gift certificate for a real, professional massage. Many spas have prenatal packages designed to comfort pregnant women.
- Suggest activities that might be harder to do when the baby comes, like going to movies or concerts.
- Bring home roses for no reason at all.
- Write a bunch of little love notes and hide them in her purse or around the house so she can find them.
- Vacuum the house—even under the bed—without being asked.
- Give your wife lots of hugs; research shows that the more she's hugged, the more she'll hug the baby after he comes.
- Go to the store and buy her a package of the most girly, moisturizing bubble bath you can find.
- If you're traveling on business, arrange to have a friend take her to dinner.
- Kiss her. Hard, long. Then do it again.
- Read to the baby (see pages 115, 118–22 for more on this).
- Offer to pick up a pizza on your way home from work—and surprise her with a pint of her favorite frozen yogurt too. Two pints, if you're planning on having any.
- Buy her a maternity pillow.
- Run errands (pick up dry cleaning, shop, go to the drugstore, and so forth). Better yet, do them before she asks you to.
- Treat her to a manicure or pedicure. Extra points for both. Even more extra points if you go along with her and get your nails done too.
- Dry her tears when she has an unexplained meltdown.
- Do a little house cleaning. If you don't have time, hire a housekeeper.
- Do the laundry before it piles up. Then fold it and put it away.
- Tell her you think she's going to be a great mother.
- Apologize for something—even if you didn't do anything wrong.
- Frame your first ultrasound pic of the baby. If you've made the pregnancy public, maybe post it on Instagram.
- Hold her hand while you're out walking.

- If she arrives home after you, have a candlelight dinner on the table, complete with sparkling cider.
- Listen attentively when she wants to tell you about what a miserable day she had—even if yours was worse.
- Hand over the TV remote and watch what she wants.
- Load and unload the dishwasher.
- Write her a love letter and send it to her in the mail.
- Plan a romantic, predelivery babymoon weekend (together, of course). This could be the last time for quite a while.
- Buy a toy or outfit for the baby, have it gift-wrapped, and let her unwrap it.
- Thank her for making you the happiest guy in the world.
- Indulge her cravings.
- Buy her a pretty maternity dress. Don't even think about the words *circus tent.*
- Go on a long walk with her.
- Slow dance in your living room.
- Arrange for some of her girlfriends to pick her up and take her out for an evening (nonalcoholic, of course) on the town.
- Plan a baby-naming ceremony.
- Start putting together a list of all the local take-out restaurants.
- Learn baby CPR.
- Offer to give her a back rub—again.
- If you smoke, stop.
- Stream a chick flick, make some popcorn, and curl up to watch it together. Force yourself.
- Tell her she's beautiful. Then tell her again a few hours later.
- Pay extra attention to making sure she has enough to eat—pack some snacks for her before the two of you go out for an evening or for a hike.
- Organize a surprise baby shower for her.
- Keep a list of your favorite names or buy her an interesting name book.
- Paint a picture for or write a letter to your unborn baby.
- Set up some interviews with potential child-care people.
- Buy her a Mother's Day or Valentine's Day gift—even if it's November.
- Go to her prenatal appointments.
- Keep a journal (either written or recorded) of what you're thinking and feeling during the pregnancy.

Ways to Show Her You Care *continued*

- Do something with her that she knows you absolutely hate to do.
- Schedule a tour of the hospital where your baby will be born.
- Sign the two of you up for a childbirth prep class.
- Help her address envelopes for the birth announcements.
- Get your social media ducks lined up so you can let everyone know as soon as the baby arrives.
- Learn to prepare a few easy recipes (see pages 45–52).
- Smile and nod agreeably when she says, "You have no idea what it's like to be pregnant." She's right, you know.
- If you already have children, take them to the park and let your partner have time alone to relax or run an errand she's been putting off.
- Surprise her with breakfast in bed on a lazy Sunday. Or, on a workday, get up five minutes earlier and surprise her with a power shake.
- Let her win your next argument. And the fifteen or twenty after that.
- Take the day off from work and hang around the house with her.
- Give other expectant mothers seats on trains and buses.
- Make a donation to a local children's hospital or school.
- Don't tell her she looks tired or needs a rest.
- Discuss your fears with your partner. Listen to hers, too, but don't make fun of them—no matter how insignificant they may seem to you.
- Tell her about some of the cool things you're reading about in this book. She really wants to know that you're interested in the pregnancy.
- Paint or wallpaper the baby's room.
- Chocolates and flowers. It's mathematically impossible to overdo either one. Or jewelry, for that matter.
- Help put together the changing table and crib. Or do it yourself.

doctor much less frequently than usual when their partners are pregnant). In some cases, men's health and safety concerns take on a rather bizarre twist. For example, psychiatrist Martin Greenberg found that "more than a few men purchase weapons during a pregnancy." Most of them get rid of those weapons after the baby is born.

I had seen the ultrasound and knew that the baby was fine. And I'd already read that at this point in the pregnancy, there was very little chance of a miscarriage. But still, I worried. I quizzed my wife about how much protein she was eating; I reminded her to go to the gym for her workouts; I even worried about the position she slept in. All in all, I was a real pain. (I was right about the sleeping

- Listen to her complain and commiserate with her, dropping in an occasional "You're amazing," or "That must be incredibly uncomfortable."
- Install smoke and carbon monoxide detectors in your house.
- If she's had a child before, don't tell her that she looks bigger this time than she did last time, even if she does.
- Make a new will that includes your baby.
- Don't complain about any physical pain you're having while she's still pregnant.
- Join a health club together.
- Tell her she's sexy.
- Clean out closets to make room for baby things.
- Stay away from comments like, "Didn't you just eat/cry a few minutes ago?"
- Call or text her during the day—just to tell her you love her.
- Offer to carry her bags.
- Do *not* tell her how great you think Angelina Jolie looks after having so many children.
- Load her iPod up with her favorite music to listen to in the labor room.
- Say "No" if she asks if she's acting crazy. Ditto if she asks whether whatever she's wearing makes her look fat.
- Don't ask what to make for dinner, just do it. Take a cooking class if you have to.
- As the pregnancy progresses, pick stuff up off the floor. It's going to get harder and harder for her to bend over.
- Do a little sexting.
- Buy her a pregnancy journal.

position stuff, though: sleeping on the back is a bad idea. The baby-filled uterus presses a major vein—the *inferior vena cava*—and could cause hemorrhoids or even cut off the flow of oxygen or blood to both your partner and the fetus. It's rare, and anyway, most women will feel uncomfortable enough that they'll move long before any damage is done. But if you're looking for something to worry about, you could do worse.)

A word of advice: if you're feeling overly concerned and protective of your partner and your baby, be gentle and try to relax a little. She's probably feeling some of the same things. Bull riding—even on a mechanical one—is definitely out. But your partner can use her computer as much as she wants without harming the baby (although all that typing might lead to carpal tunnel). Airport metal detectors are no problem during pregnancy, and neither are luggage scanners, unless your partner is intending to climb inside of one. The most important thing you can do is encourage her to eat right, exercise, and drink plenty of water. Most of the rest will take care of itself. If you're still worried, discuss your concerns with her practitioner at your next appointment. But leave your gun at home.

STAYING INVOLVED

Focus on Her

Although every pregnant woman will need and appreciate different things, there is a lot more common ground than you might imagine. Basically, she needs three things from you now—and for the rest of the pregnancy (and beyond)—more than ever before:

- Expressions of affection, admiration, and support (both verbal and physical).
- Sensitivity to her changing physical condition (hunger, fatigue, muscle pains, and so on).
- Expressions of affection and excitement about the baby and your impending parenthood. Your support is absolutely critical.

According to psychologist Edward Hagen, all this actually has a concrete effect on your partner's emotional and physical health, as well as on the kind of mother she'll be after the baby comes.

Finances

PLANNING A COLLEGE FUND

It may seem hard to imagine now, but in eighteen years or so the baby you haven't even met yet may be graduating from high school and heading off to college. And so, at the risk of reinforcing the old stereotype that a father's role in his children's lives is primarily financial, it's time to talk about money. Over the past twenty years or so, college tuition and expenses, such as room and board, have gone up an average of 6–8 percent a year—that's a lot faster than inflation—and most experts believe that they'll continue to rise at close to the same rate for the foreseeable future. This means that by the time your child walks off the stage with his high school diploma, a bachelor's degree at an in-state public college will probably cost around $240,000, including tuition, fees, room, and board; for a

Digging Out of the Hole

Before you even start worrying about how you're going to finance the future, it's critical to spend some time making sure the present is taken care of. If you have huge debts, the place to start is by paying them off. Adopting a child or conceiving one artificially, for example, can cost a ton of money—$25,000–50,000 is not at all uncommon. If you borrowed against your retirement accounts, took out a second mortgage, or put it on your credit cards, start working on those before, or at least at the same time as, you start saving for your child's education. You have a responsibility to your child, yourself, and your family to stay in the best financial shape possible. But big debts—particularly on high-interest-rate credit cards—can undermine your whole family's long-term financial health.

If you need to, consult a professional who can help you put together a budget that includes servicing your debt and savings (see pages 108–9 for more on this). Get in the habit of putting something aside every month, even if it's just a few dollars. The best way to do this is through *dollar cost averaging*. This means that on a regular basis—weekly, monthly, quarterly—you contribute a fixed amount to the same mutual fund or other investment. When prices are up you're buying fewer shares; when prices are down, you're buying more.

The problem with this or any other regular savings plan, though, is remembering to do it. If things get tight—as they have plenty of times at my house—the education checks can get "overlooked" or "rescheduled." Having it automatically taken out of your paycheck is a great—and somewhat less painful—way to go. If you can get control of your finances now, who knows: you might even be able to afford to have another kid.

private college, you could be looking at more than $540,000. (The College Savings Plans Network has a simple—but horrifying—calculator at www.collegesavings .org/collegeCostCalculator.aspx.) No wonder a growing number of Americans are saying they think that a college education isn't worth the expense. Now hang on a second before you panic. Things aren't as bad as they might seem. Here are some important factors to consider:

- The numbers above are based on average sticker prices. There are plenty of lower-cost institutions where your child can get a marvelous education.
- Two-thirds of college students receive some form of financial aid (including grants, loans, scholarships, and work-study programs), which can cut tuition

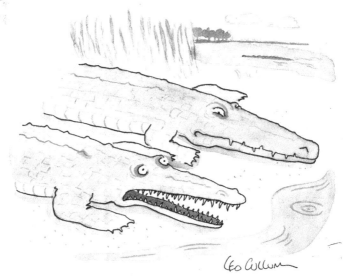

"I just found out what braces cost."

and fees by as much as 50 percent. (Of course, even at half off, those numbers are still pretty shocking.)

- You don't have to—and probably shouldn't—pay for your child's education in cash. You're unlikely to buy a house for cash, right? So why would you pay cash for an education that costs about the same?
- A college education is a good investment. According to a new report from the Federal Reserve Bank of San Francisco, a college graduate with a bachelor's degree will earn about 61 percent more per year than a high school grad. People with master's degrees earn twice as much as high school graduates, and having a professional degree triples earnings. MIT economist David Autor puts it a little differently, saying that the true cost of a college degree is actually about *negative* $500,000. In other words, even after all the expenses, someone with a college degree will earn half a million dollars more over his career than someone without one. There are also some hidden economic benefits. For example, people with college degrees are much more likely than high school grads to work at jobs where they get employer-paid health insurance and access to retirement plans.
- There are quite a few nonmonetary benefits to going to college. When compared to high school grads, those with degrees are healthier (they exercise more, smoke less, and are less obese) and more active in their communities (doing volunteer work, voting, giving blood).

But let's focus on the money. Unless your child gets a full-ride scholarship or attends a military college, you're still going to have to figure out how to finance her education. And your first step is to start socking away as much money as you can into your own retirement accounts. Wait, what? How does feathering your own retirement accounts help put your kid through college?

Here's how it works:

- Money you invest in your retirement accounts is often at least partially tax deductible and always grows tax-free until you start withdrawing it. It also reduces your AGI (adjusted gross income), which means less income for the financial aid departments to look at. In contrast, investments made in your child's name are after-tax dollars, and interest and dividends may be taxable as income or capital gains at your rate.
- The more assets your child has, the less eligible she'll be for financial aid. Schools will assume that 20 percent of your child's assets will be available for educational purposes but only about 6 percent of yours. Money in your retirement accounts doesn't count at all.
- Plenty of financial-aid options are available: student loans (usually at below-market rates), grants, fellowships, work-study programs, and so forth.
- You can borrow against the equity in your home or against the equity in your retirement accounts.
- If you'll be over 59½ by the time your child starts college, you'll be able to withdraw money from your IRA or other retirement account without incurring any penalties. If you're under 59½, you can make penalty-free withdrawals for qualified educational purposes. Keep in mind that you may still need to pay taxes on any withdrawals.

The bottom line, as certified financial planner Jackie Weitzberg so elegantly puts it, is, "You can always finance college, but you can't finance your retirement."

Of course, this approach may not work for everyone. You may have already maxed out all your retirement options or you may be wealthy enough that there's not much chance that your child will qualify for financial aid. Or maybe you just want to put some money away for your child to use later. In these cases, there are still a number of options. We can't possibly cover them all here, but we've focused on a few of the most common ones. Before you make any big decisions, I urge you to talk over your choices with a financial planner and/or an accountant to make sure that the plan you're considering fits in with your overall financial objectives.

529 PLANS

Creatively named after an IRS regulation, these plans will be the best option for most people. 529s come in two flavors: savings plans, which let you make contributions to an account that's to be used only for college-related expenses; and prepaid plans, which let you prepay some or all of the future costs of tuition and lock in a lower price. Let's look at each in a little more detail:

529 SAVINGS PLANS

The rules for 529s vary from state to state, but they're all pretty similar. As with Roth IRAs, you make contributions with after-tax dollars, but the earnings are completely federally tax-exempt, as long as they're used for qualified educational expenses (usually tuition, room and board, and fees). Each state has at least one 529 plan and you can sign up for almost any one you like. Contribution limits vary by state, and some states offer income-tax deductions and other benefits to residents (the College Savings Plans Network, www.collegesavings.org, has detailed info for each state's plans and lets you do head-to-head comparisons).

These plans are especially attractive because there are no income restrictions. Plus, the money can be used at any accredited, post–high school institution, anywhere in the country. This includes state and private colleges, community colleges, or even vocational schools. If your child doesn't go to college, you can transfer the account to another member of your family—including yourself.

With 529s, the money is in your name even though your child is the beneficiary. This means that you can withdraw it (with a penalty, of course) if you really need to. And since the 529 account is really a parental asset, it will have a smaller impact on your child's ability to get financial aid than if it were in his name. One way to ensure that the 529s don't affect aid eligibility at all is to have a grandparent or other trusted relative open the account. Anyone can contribute to it, but because it's in someone else's name, it won't be counted as your asset.

In each state, 529 programs are managed by a different financial services organization—e.g., Fidelity, Schwab, or Vanguard—and you'll usually have a number of investment options, ranging from the very aggressive to the completely conservative. There's usually also an option for an age-based plan. For example, a newborn's account might have 90 percent in a growth stock fund, 5 percent in an international stock fund, and 5 percent in bonds. By the time your child turns sixteen, the mix will have gradually shifted to something like 15 percent in growth stocks, 5 percent in international, 45 percent in bonds, and 35 percent in money markets. Look into your state's plan first, because it may offer benefits to residents. But if you don't like it, you may be able to invest through another state. And be sure to check into the fees charged by the managing company; they're all over the place and can make a huge difference.

529 PREPAID TUITION PLANS

Some states have plans that allow you to prepay all or part of your child's state college tuition costs. How much you pay depends on when you expect your child to start college and on current interest rates. Some private colleges offer similar programs.

These plans usually promise a pretty good return for the money, but there are lots of loopholes that can inflate prices and reduce the money you'd get back if your child ends up not going to school at all or decides to go somewhere else.

If you're thinking about a private college, you might consider the Private College 529 Plan (privatecollege529.com). With this plan, you buy a certificate today for a semester (or part of a semester) at any of nearly three hundred private colleges. The plan guarantees that you'll be able to cash that certificate in for a semester of college anytime within the next thirty years, regardless of what the current prices are. Buying certificates doesn't guarantee that your child will actually be admitted to any of the colleges, and your investments aren't FDIC insured.

OTHER COLLEGE SAVINGS OPTIONS

COVERDELL EDUCATION SAVINGS ACCOUNTS (OR COVERDELL ESAS)

If you and your partner together make $220,000 a year or less, you can put away a maximum of $2,000 each year into an account for each of your children. Your contributions aren't deductible from your income like an IRA, but they grow tax-free. Distributions are tax-free too, as long as the money is used to pay for education, room, board, books, and related expenses. If you end up not using the money at all, you can roll it over into a new account for another family member. Another interesting advantage to Coverdells is that you can use the money to pay for elementary and/or high school expenses if you need to. If you make more than $220,000, the amount you can contribute to your child's Coverdell goes down. However, someone else who meets the income threshold may be able to make the contribution in your child's name instead.

Watch out, though. If you're thinking you'll need financial aid, this account will be considered an asset and will reduce the amount of aid your child is eligible for (but since the asset is in your name, the impact will be smaller than if it were in the child's name, as it would be with a UTMA or UGMA; see below for more on this). More important, you cannot contribute to a Coverdell ESA and a prepaid tuition or state-sponsored savings plan in the same year without incurring some major penalties. Given that those other plans have much higher contribution limits, you might be better off putting your money there instead of here.

Beware of Good-Hearted Relatives

Because IRS rules for Coverdells, prepaid tuition programs, and life in general are often confusing and contradictory, there's way too much potential to get yourself into major tax trouble. So let your parents and any other potentially generous relatives and friends know that they should check with you *before* opening up any accounts in your child's name. And if you aren't absolutely sure what to do and how, have an accountant or financial planner take a look.

CUSTODIAL ACCOUNTS

There are two types of custodial accounts: UGMAs (Uniform Gift to Minors Act) and UTMAs (Uniform Transfer to Minors Act), which are basically the same thing. The big advantage of these accounts is that there are no lifetime contribution limits or annual income limits for the giver, although going over the IRS's annual gift tax limits could have tax consequences for the giver and the receiver. And like Coverdells, the money in UGMAs and UTMAs can be used for high school and even elementary school education expenses.

There are a few disadvantages to these accounts. First, unlike some of the other choices in this section, the gains are subject to federal taxes every year. The first $1,000 or so is tax-exempt and the next $1,000 is taxed at the child's rate. Everything after that is taxed at your rate—until the child turns eighteen (or older, if he or she is a full-time student and a dependent). Second, whatever gets put in there becomes an irrevocable gift to the child—and can never be transferred to any other child or beneficiary. As the custodian, you can invest it any way you want, but you can't take it out unless it's to be spent on something that directly benefits the child, such as education or summer camps. Spending it on yourself could land you in court. Third, when the child reaches the "age of majority" (usually eighteen or twenty-one, depending on the state), the money becomes his to spend any way he wants. You have absolutely no control anymore. And finally, because money in these accounts is considered the child's, it may reduce the amount of college financial aid you're eligible for later. If you already have an UGMA or UTMA, you may be able to roll it over into a 529.

LIFE INSURANCE

While you might think that this is a little early to be worrying about life insurance, you couldn't be more wrong. Because there are a lot of life insurance options, and because each of them is right only in certain circumstances, we're not going to go into much detail here. Suffice it to say that you and your partner should get life insurance if you don't have any, or meet with your agent to discuss if and how your new baby will change your insurance needs. The point is that if, God forbid, either of you dies unexpectedly, the survivor shouldn't have to worry about having to get a better job just to keep up the mortgage or private-school tuition payments.

Because insurance agents are salespeople, you may want to have a more neutral party (your financial planner, for example) evaluate how much and what kind of insurance you need first. That way you can walk into your meeting with the insurance agent with both eyes open.

There are two basic kinds of life insurance: *term* and *cash value*. Each is further divided into several subcategories.

TERM

Comes in a variety of flavors:

- Renewable (if you keep your death benefit the same, the premiums will rise, but if you develop a health problem, you may get canceled altogether)
- Level (you can lock in death benefit and premium levels, sometimes for as long as thirty years)
- Decreasing (death benefit decreases every year but the premium stays the same)

Term policies are, as their name indicates, in effect only for a specified period of time. They're also pretty cheap, especially in the early years. If you're young and don't have a lot in the way of assets, a level term policy is a good way to take care of your family if something should happen to you. As you get older and hopefully richer, you may find that you need less—or more—insurance. Of course, you'll check with your financial advisor before making any big decisions, right?

CASH VALUE

There are an increasing number of cash-value insurance products available, all of which essentially combine term insurance with some kind of investment. Part of your premium goes to buy term insurance; the rest goes into a fund. Depending on the plan, you'll have more or less control over how the fund is invested. Your investments accumulate tax-free; plus you can borrow against the fund—usually at pretty competitive rates—if you need to.

You can set your premium at virtually any level you want. But because the cost of the underlying term insurance is rising every year, you may reach a point when your payment isn't enough to cover the cost of the insurance. When that happens, the shortfall is taken out of your investment fund, which will reduce your cash value.

Getting Professional Advice

Over the course of the next twenty years or so, you're going to be spending a lot of your hard-earned money on health, life, and disability insurance; college investment plans; and retirement plans. The way you spend all that money will have a powerful—and long-lasting—effect on you and your family. So unless you're a financial planner, stockbroker, or insurance agent yourself, you've got no business making major financial decisions without advice.

Finding someone to give you that advice isn't always easy. Your goal is to find someone whom you like and believe will have your best interests at heart. Here are a few things you can do to help weed out the losers:

- Decide what you want your advisor to do. Will you be expecting your financial planner to advise you on taxes, wills, and trusts in addition to investments? Do you want daily updates or is once a week or once a quarter good enough? Do you want your advisor to execute trades for you, or just tell you what to do and leave it to you to perform the transactions through a discount broker? The more the advisor does, the more you'll be paying.
- Get references from friends, business associates, and other people whose opinions you trust. Alternatively, the Financial Planning Association (www.plannersearch.org) will give you references to some local certified financial planners. The National Association of Personal Financial Advisors, (www.napfa.org) makes referrals to fee-only (as opposed to commission-based) planners. Select at least three potential candidates and set up initial consultations (which shouldn't cost you anything). Then conduct tough interviews. Here's what you want to know:
  - Educational background. Not to be snobby here, but the more formal the education—especially in financial management—the better. In addition to a bachelor's degree (at least), certified financial planners (CFPs) go through a rigorous training program, and the CFP certification can help you differentiate between someone who's really a planner and someone who just sells stocks and insurance.
  - Licenses. Is he or she legally able to buy and sell financial products such as stocks, bonds, mutual funds, and insurance?
  - Level of experience. Unless you've got money to burn, let your niece break in her MBA on someone else. Stick to experienced professionals with at least three years in the business.

- Profile of the typical client. You want a planner who has experience working with people whose income level and family situation are similar to yours.
- Compensation. Financial planners may get paid on commission, charge an hourly rate or a flat percentage of however much they're managing, receive fees from companies they recommend, or some combination of the above. None of these options is necessarily better than any other (although many experts believe that you'll be happier, and possibly richer, with someone who charges a fee rather than a commission). The important thing is that you understand where the compensation is coming from, how much it's likely to be, and how it's calculated.
- Get a sample financial plan. You want to see what you're going to be getting for your money. Be careful, though: fancy graphics, incomprehensible boilerplate language, and expensive leather binders may be used to distract you from the report's lack of substance.
- A self-assessment. How well has the planner done for clients like you when the economy has been hot? How about when things aren't so hot? Most people will have returns of 2 percent one year, 14 another, and 0 yet another. Be very suspicious of anyone who promises a regular return (unless all your money is in a CD). Remember Bernie Madoff?
- References. How long have customers been with the planner? Are they happy? Better off? Any complaints or criticisms?
- Financial planners are overseen by two organizations, and your future planner should be regulated by either (or possibly both) the Financial Industry Regulatory Authority (FINRA, which regulates financial products such as insurance and stocks) and the Securities and Exchange Commission (SEC, which regulates financial advice), Also check with your state's securities regulator. The North American Securities Administrators Association (www.nasaa.org) has a list of state agencies; click on Contact Your Regulator.

The big drawback with cash-value policies is that the commissions and fees kill you. Commissions—which are built into your costs—routinely run as much as 100 percent of the first year's premium. And management fees are often much higher than the industry average. Oh, and let's not forget about the early cancellation fees, which can take a serious bite out of your cash value if you turn in the policy fewer than ten years after getting it.

So which is better? After long discussions with a number of insurance people and financial advisers, here's what I think: Get yourself a guaranteed-renewable, ten-year-or-more, level-premium term policy. That way your policy can't be canceled if you get sick, and you won't need a physical exam every year. Then set up a good savings, investment, and retirement plan for your family. If you've got enough knowledge and expertise to do it on your own, great. If not, get an expert to help you (see pages 108–9).

There is one exception to this rule: if you have an especially large estate (including real estate and retirement accounts), a cash-value policy is a good way to leave your heirs the wherewithal to pay off federal estate taxes. Unfortunately, it's hard to be more specific than "especially large" because Congress keeps changing the rules and the limits.

Whether you opt for term or cash value, be sure to go with a carrier you can count on being around when the time comes to pay up. The traditional way to do this was to go with a company that's top rated by one of the big ratings agencies: A.M. Best (ambest.com), Fitch (fitchratings.com), Moody's (moodys.com), and Standard & Poor's (standardandpoors.com) Unfortunately, in recent years those agencies have lost some of their credibility by receiving money from the insurance companies whose financial strength they rate. Nevertheless, companies that receive the ratings agencies' top marks are generally pretty safe bets.

DISABILITY INSURANCE

As long as you've got insurance on your mind, take a long, hard look at disability coverage. If your employer offers a long-term disability policy, sign up now. If not, or if you're self-employed, talk to your broker about getting one. A long-term disability could be more devastating to your family's finances than death.

LIFE INSURANCE FOR CHILDREN

This one is pretty simple. In most cases, taking out a life insurance policy on a child is a complete waste of money. The point of insurance is to provide for the survivors. A policy for a child can protect against future problems that might make getting insurance impossible later, but that's extremely unlikely. You're better off spending the money on insurance for you.

WHERE TO GET INSURANCE

If you work for a big company or belong to a union, you probably already have at least some life and/or disability insurance. And you may even be able to get additional coverage for great rates and without having to take a physical. You may also be able to get small policies for little or nothing if you're a member of certain organizations, open up a bank account at the right place, and so on. But before you spring for any "guaranteed issue" insurance (the kind you see advertised on late-night TV and don't have to take a physical for), do a little shopping around. You're usually paying a large premium for the guaranteed issue part, and there tend to be a lot of loopholes (such as, if you die within the first two years, all you get is your premiums back). You may be able to get the same amount of coverage for a lot less.

No matter how much coverage you get this way, though, these policies should never be all you have. If you suddenly leave your job, close your checking account, or whatever, you could find yourself without any coverage.

If you have an insurance broker, start there. But don't be shy about shopping around. Costs for the same policy can vary by as much as 200 to 300 percent. There are a number of online services that can help you compare policies and get the one that's best for you.

And while you're considering how much coverage you need, be sure to look into Social Security. Most people completely overlook the survivor benefits they'd be entitled to if their spouse died. If you factor in Social Security—assuming it isn't bankrupt by the time you need it—you may actually need a lot less insurance than you think.

OH, BUT WAIT. WE'RE NOT DONE YET . . .

Since we're already talking about depressing things, there are a few other documents you really shouldn't be without.

WILLS

A will is a document that spells out how you'd like to divide your assets if you die. In most cases, it'll all go to your partner. Or, if she gets hit by the same bus, everything will go to your child(ren). You can also appoint a guardian to look after the children's interests. For many young families without a lot of assets, a simple will is good enough for a while. But get on this right now. Not having a will leaves way too much to chance. Each state has its own rules about who inherits what when someone dies intestate (without a will). In addition, a probate judge—who has no idea what your wishes may have been—could appoint yet another stranger to be your child's guardian and manage the inheritance. Wouldn't you feel a little better if *you* were making these decisions? Another thing to keep in mind about wills is that they're contestable, which means that it could be held up in court for years. And, naturally, a lot of the costs will come out of your assets.

TRUSTS

A trust is similar to a will, but it gives you more control over how your assets are used. You can, for example, set up a trust so that your child can have access to the money only after age thirty-five, only if it's used for educational purposes, or only if she marries a left-handed calf roper. Another nice benefit of trusts is that they're incontestable, and as long as they're properly structured and funded, they'll stay out of probate.

HEALTH-CARE DIRECTIVE

You'll use this document to appoint someone to make health-care decisions for you if you're incapacitated.

DURABLE POWER OF ATTORNEY FOR FINANCES

This document designates someone to make financial decisions if you're not able to. It could be the same person you appointed for health-care decisions or someone else.

I know this sounds like a lot of paperwork (it is) and a lot of money (it doesn't have to be). The good news is that you may be able to create these documents yourself, guided by some of the excellent do-it-yourself resources at www.uslegalforms. com. They set up a basic package for readers of this book at www.uslegalforms. com/mrdad. If your situation is complicated, it might be worth hiring a good attorney—one who specializes in wills and trusts—to take you through the process or do it for you. One of the most common mistakes do-it-yourselfers make is that they forget to fund the trust. Setting one up is great, but it won't do you much good if your accounts and home aren't in it.

Finally, if you're in the military and are deploying, you'll need to complete these documents without fail, right away. Fortunately, you can get legal help for free on base.

The Lights Are On and Somebody Is Home

WHAT'S GOING ON WITH YOUR PARTNER

Physically

- May feel the baby's movements—and she knows what they are
- May have occasional, painless tightening of the uterus (called Braxton-Hicks contractions) or "false labor" (during real labor, the cervix begins to open; in false labor, it doesn't)
- Continuing darkening of nipples, appearance of dark line from belly button down the abdomen
- Breasts are getting larger and may "leak" a little when she's sexually excited— and even when she's not (hopefully you can tell the difference)
- Navel changing from innie to outie
- Vision changing; she's retaining so much fluid these days that it's changing the shape of her eyeballs, and contacts may irritate or no longer fit
- Hormones are causing all sorts of trouble: she's forgetful, her fingernails may be brittle, and her skin may be splotchy, but her hair probably never looked better (pregnant women tend to lose less hair than nonpregnant women)

Emotionally

- Very reassured by the baby's movements and less worried about miscarriage— although those worries may come rushing back if she stops feeling the baby move
- Developing feeling of bonding with the baby and may spend a lot of time day- dreaming about her
- Overwhelmed by the flood of advice coming in from all sides
- Sensitivity about her changing figure

- Increase in sexual desire
- Increasingly dependent on you
- Feelings of jealousy (after all, it was her private pregnancy until now)
- Enjoying some of the benefits of being pregnant—people giving up seats on public transportation, grocery clerks helping with her bags, and more

WHAT'S GOING ON WITH THE BABY

Your banana-sized baby's eyelids are still sealed, but her eyebrows and lashes are fully grown in and you might be able to see some hair on her head. Her skin is losing its transparency, and she may get occasional bouts of hiccups. By the end of this month she'll be about nine inches long and weigh in at close to a pound. She kicks, punches, grabs at the umbilical cord, sucks her thumb, and has developed something of a regular sleep pattern—waking and dozing at set intervals (although she'll be sleeping 90–95 percent of the time). She'll spend a lot of her awake time doing somersaults. Best of all, she can now hear what's going on outside the womb.

WHAT'S GOING ON WITH YOU

"Oh My God, I'm Going to Be a Father"

I have to admit that even after seeing the baby on the sonogram, I still found it hard to believe I was really going to be a father (how hard could it be to Photoshop a sonogram?). But when my wife grabbed my hand and placed it on her belly, and I felt that first gentle kick, I knew the whole thing was true. And as usual, after the initial excitement passed, I found something to worry about.

More Interested in Fatherhood

After that first kick, I suddenly became consumed with the idea that I just wasn't ready to be a father. I still wanted children—nothing had changed there—but I realized that in only four months I would face the biggest challenge of my life, and I didn't know a thing about what I was getting into. I felt as though I were about to attempt a triple backflip from a trapeze—without ever having had any lessons, and without a safety net.

I had already done a lot of reading, but I felt I still didn't know what fathers are really supposed to do. Doesn't it seem a little strange—scary, really—that you need a license to sell hot dogs on the street or to be a beautician, but there are absolutely no prerequisites for the far more important job of being a father?

Feeling the baby's first kicks may make you much more interested in reading about pregnancy, if you haven't been doing so already. You may also find yourself wanting to spend more time with friends or relatives who have small kids, or just watching how other men interact with their children. You'll probably notice that younger dads (those under about twenty-four) spend a little less time with their kids—playing, teaching, reading—than older dads (those over thirty-two). You may also start becoming aware of the negative, stereotyped images of fathers that are so common in the media. We'll talk a lot more about that in "Fathering Today," starting on page 281.

Turning Inward

You've had a lot to think about lately—your family's finances, your new role as a father, your partner's (and your baby's) safety. So don't be surprised if you find yourself preoccupied with your own thoughts—sometimes to the exclusion of just about everything else, even your partner.

Just as it was for her, this sort of "turning inward" is perfectly normal. The problem is that while you're focusing on everything that's going on inside your head, your partner (who has been pretty focused on *herself* until now) is now starting to focus on you too. She may be feeling insecure and may need to be reassured that you aren't going to leave her or be feeling emotionally needy and crave confirmation of your love for her. Notice her subtle (or not so subtle) hints and make sure she gets the attention she needs. If she doesn't, she may think you don't care. As Arthur and Libby Colman write, "A man who ignores his partner's anxieties may find they escalate rather than abate with a condescending 'Everything is going to be all right, dear.'"

At the same time, though, don't forget about your own needs. It can be extremely tempting to try to get away from the external pressures by distancing yourself from your partner (you can't, of course, get away from your internal pressures). If you can, tell her what's on your mind; it'll probably make you feel a lot better. (If you're having a tough time opening up, you might want to review the "Your Relationship" section on pages 86–90.) If she doesn't react well, reassure her that even though you might be a little preoccupied, you still love her and you'll still be there for her.

STAYING INVOLVED

Prenatal Communication: Can You Hear Me Now?

As we've discussed elsewhere, good communication with your partner is critical throughout the pregnancy. But what about communicating with your unborn child? While the very idea may sound a little wacky, research has shown that

What's Really Going On in There?

No matter where you stand on the pro-life vs. pro-choice debate, there's absolutely no question that your fetus is a living being who, like the rest of us, reacts to her environment. Your baby will be born with a full set of senses: touch, hearing, sight, smell, and taste. But those senses don't just show up at birth, completely out of the blue. They begin to form very early on in the pregnancy, and the fetus starts trying to use them immediately. The more practice she gets, the more developed the senses will be at birth. (Senses that aren't used tend to atrophy. In animal experiments, for example, when fetal chicks are prevented from moving inside their egg, cartilage turns to bone). Let me introduce you to the cast of senses, in order of appearance.

- Touch. About two months into the pregnancy, your baby's skin—which is considered the body's largest organ—is fully formed. Sensitivity starts with the cheeks and lips, and just a few months ago, if they were touched, the baby would turn away. Starting right about now (five months), the baby will turn *toward* the touch (after birth, that's called the *rooting reflex*, and it's designed to help the baby find the breast. When touched on the mouth, the baby turns toward the stimulus—usually a nipple, but it works with a finger too—and starts making sucking movements). The palms of the hands, soles of the feet, and genitals are next, followed by the rest of the body. To help develop their sense of touch, fetuses spend a lot of time exploring themselves—grasping the umbilical cord, stroking the face, sucking on fingers, and kicking and banging against the walls of the uterus. If the baby has a womb-mate or two, the fetuses often explore each other, sometimes poking, other times holding hands.

- Movement and balance. If your partner is up and about, the fetus will spend a lot of her day gently sloshing around in the uterus. Interestingly, the amount of movement the fetus experiences during pregnancy makes a big difference after the birth. Italian researcher Carlo Bellieni recently did a study of the children of ballerinas who didn't stop dancing while they were pregnant. "They needed to be rocked to sleep more energetically than the others," he says. Another researcher, Janet DiPietro, found that fetuses that are very active in the womb are more irritable as babies.

- Smell and taste (some lump the two under the heading "chemosensation"). Your baby's mouth and tongue developed a few months ago. And at this stage, her taste buds are just about as sensitive as yours. For the past month or two, your baby has been gulping down impressive amounts of amniotic fluid, peeing it right back out, and drinking it up again (it's best to get that image out of your mind). The amniotic fluid that flows through your baby's mouth and nasal passages changes flavor constantly, depending on what your partner eats. (The connection between diet and amniotic fluid is pretty strong. In one study, Julie Mannella and her colleagues found that adults were able to smell garlic in amniotic fluid collected from women undergoing amniocentesis who had eaten garlic just forty-five minutes before the test.) But mixed in there among the curry and chili peppers and peanut butter sandwiches are some odor molecules that are distinctly Mom. And after birth, the baby's sense of smell helps her adjust to life outside the womb. Mom's nipples smell (to the baby) like amniotic fluid, and that scent helps attract the baby to the breast. Babies definitely prefer the smell of their own fluid to anyone else's (hey, who wouldn't?). And when they start eating real food (at around six months after birth), they prefer foods that their mother ate while pregnant.

• Hearing. If your baby's ears are filled with amniotic fluid and any external sounds would have to pass through your partner's abdomen, how much could a baby hear in there anyway? Well, despite what you'd think, the uterus is a pretty noisy place—and has been since early in your partner's pregnancy.

Armed with ultrasound machines, researchers Peter Hepper and Sara Shahidullah found that fetuses first start reacting to outside sounds as early as fourteen weeks. Their hearing range is rather limited, though, with mid- and low-frequency sounds (like your voice) getting through better than high-frequency ones. By about thirty-five weeks, fetuses not only can hear both high and low frequencies but can actually tell the difference between the two. In one study, an obstetrician inserted a microphone into a woman's uterus while she was in labor and recorded the external sounds that could be heard from the inside. He got clear recordings—not only of voices and the mother's internal body sounds but also of Beethoven's Ninth Symphony, which was being played in the delivery room.

Hearing noises is one thing, but are fetuses affected in any way by what they hear from within the womb? Absolutely. Nearly a hundred years ago, a German pediatrician by the name of Albrecht Peiper observed that fetuses would kick when a car horn was blown. And if you ask your partner, she'll probably tell you that the baby moves around more when she's listening to music, and may kick sharply if a door slams nearby or a car backfires.

Several researchers have found that the fetus's heart rate changes in response to sounds. Rock music, for example, tends to produce an increase, while classical lowers it. And developmental psychologist William Fifer and

What's Really Going On in There? *continued*

his colleagues noticed that the fetus's heart rate increased when a stranger was speaking, but decreased when Mom was. His conclusion? "The fetus not only hears and recognizes the sound, but is calmed by it." Babies aren't just passive listeners, either; they're actually learning from what they hear.

Immediately after birth, for example, babies try to imitate some of the sounds they heard in the womb. Kathleen Wermke, a researcher at the University of Würzburg in Germany, compared recordings of three- to five-day-old French and German newborns. She found that the babies' cries mimicked the language intonation of their parents, with the French babies ending their cries on an upward note and the German babies ending on a downward note. For more on this subject, see "Prenatal Communication," pages 115, 118–22.

- Sight. Your baby's eyes will be fused shut for another month or two. Even after her eyes open, it'll still be pretty dark inside of Mom. (Reminds me of that great Groucho Marx line: "Outside of a dog, a book is man's best friend. Inside of a dog, it's too dark to read.") Nevertheless, she can do some visual processing. For example, if you were to shine a bright light on your partner's belly (which you shouldn't actually do), your baby's heart rate would accelerate and she would turn away from it. Because of the lack of practice, eyesight will be your baby's least developed sense when she emerges from the womb. At first, things will be a little blurry, although she'll be able to see objects—or people—ten to fifteen inches away fairly well. But in six to nine months, her eyesight will be pretty much up to snuff.

months before they're born, fetuses are extremely responsive to what they're hearing from the outside. Not only that, they're actually *learning* from it.

In one study, Peter Hepper, a psychology professor at Queen's University in Belfast, Ireland, found that newborns whose mothers had watched a particular soap opera while they were pregnant stopped crying when they heard the show's theme song. Babies who hadn't been exposed to the show had no reaction when they heard the music.

And in one of my favorite studies of all time, researcher Anthony DeCasper asked sixteen women to make a tape of themselves reading a poem called "The King, the Mice, and the Cheese," and two different tapes of Dr. Seuss's *The Cat in the Hat.* Then, during the last six and a half weeks of their pregnancies, the women were instructed to choose only one of the tapes and play it three times a day for their unborn child. When the babies were just three days old, DeCasper offered them a choice between the tape they'd heard over and over and one of the other tapes. Since three-day-old babies aren't particularly good about speaking up, DeCasper used a "suck-o-meter" (a specially rigged pacifier that enabled the babies to determine which tape they'd get to hear merely by changing their sucking speed) to allow the children to express their preferences. Fifteen out of the sixteen babies chose the tape they'd heard while in the womb. If nothing else, this research ought to convince you that even before they're born, babies' lights are on and there's somebody home.

Even more amazing, fetuses can tell the difference between two languages and exhibit a strong preference for their native one. Newborns will stare longer at people who are speaking the same language that Mom spoke while she was pregnant. Similarly, French researcher Jacques Mehler and his colleagues had a completely bilingual woman record several phrases in French and Russian, then played them to a few dozen brand-new French babies. Using a device similar to DeCasper's suck-o-meter, the babies adjusted their sucking so they could hear the French instead of the Russian.

So why should you try to communicate with your growing fetus? First of all, because it's a lot of fun. In the evenings, I used to place my hands on my wife's belly and tell the current resident all about what I'd done during the day. Sometimes I'd even do "counting" exercises: I'd poke once and say (loudly), "One." Most of the time, I'd get an immediate kick back. A few seconds later, I'd poke twice and say, "Two." Frequently, I'd get two kicks back. I've often wondered whether this little math game could be the reason my oldest got an A in AP calculus in high school.

The second reason to try some prenatal conversations is that they can help you establish a bond with your baby before the birth. It may even help make the pregnancy seem a little more "real." I have to admit that in the beginning, the idea of talking to a lump in my wife's belly seemed silly. But after a while I got used to it and began to feel a real closeness with the baby. Another father I spoke with felt that by communicating with his unborn daughter, he was able to establish a loving relationship with her while she was still inside. And when she was born, he described their first encounter as "like meeting someone face to face with whom you had only spoken on the telephone."

If you're in the military and you're going to miss large chunks of your wife's pregnancy, one of the best things you can do before you deploy is to record yourself reading a couple of nice, rhythmic stories or poems. Then ask your wife to play them for the baby every day—before and after the birth. If you're already gone and you have access to Skype or phone, you can do a live read—just ask your wife to put the headset or speaker close to her belly. I've heard from a number

Slice of Pie, Dad?

One topic that you'll probably spend a lot of time thinking about is what, exactly, being a father means, and how important fatherhood is to your sense of who you are. I'm not a big fan of self-help exercises, but here's one that's actually extremely effective.

First, take a minute to think of all the different roles you play and how they come together to form your identity. For example, you're a husband or spouse, friend, son, mentor, father-to-be, worker, coach, relative, athlete, and so on.

Next, take a sheet of blank paper and draw a large circle in the middle. Imagining that the circle (which researchers refer to as a pie) represents the whole you, slice it up into pieces that are proportional to the importance you place on each of your identities. There are no right or wrong ways to do this exercise, and every man's pie will be divided differently. What's especially interesting, though, is that the number and size of your slices will change over time. If you had done this exercise a year ago, you might not have had a "father" slice at all, or if you did, it would have been pretty small. But as the reality of fatherhood gradually sinks in, that slice will grow and grow. When that happens, other slices will have to get smaller—or disappear completely. At least for a while.

Once you've finished this pie, grab another sheet of paper, draw another circle, and divide it up according to the weight you place on each of the fatherhood roles you expect to play and the kind of dad you want to be. When Cherine Habib and Sandra Lancaster had a group of Australian expectant dads do this, they came up with seven possibilities.

I've added a few more to the mix: reliable presence, breadwinner, coach, co-parent, disciplinarian, mother's emotional supporter, mother's helper, playmate, primary caregiver, protector, provider, reluctant father, role model, teacher, and uncertain/confused father.

You're probably not going to use all of these attributes—and feel free to add any you think are missing. As with the first pie, don't get too used to the way your pie looks; the number and size of the slices will change with time.

of deployed service members who have done this, and many of them have been amazed that the first time they spoke to their baby, he or she turned to face them, having clearly recognized their voice. You'll find dozens of other tips on how to stay involved from a distance in my book *The Military Father: A Hands-on Guide for Deployed Dads.* Communicating with your unborn child will also help him or her start developing a bond with you. Many fathers are justifiably envious of the immediate bond newborn children have with their mothers. It seems, though, that this bond may have more to do with the mother's voice (which the baby has heard every day for nine months) than anything else.

In another of DeCasper's suck-o-meter studies, nine out of ten newborns selected a story recorded by their own mother over the same story recorded by another woman. And other research has shown that for their first few days newborns prefer their mother's voice to their father's; if she whispers in one ear and the father whispers in the other, the baby will most likely turn toward the mother.

But that's no reason to give up. When you speak to your baby before he's born, he "learns to recognize the tone, pitch, and speech patterns that are unique to you, and will instantly identify your voice after birth," says Dr. Sarah Brewer, author of *Superbabies.* This means that if you whisper in one of your baby's ears and some stranger whispers in the other, the baby, who "recognizes" you, will turn toward you 80 percent of the time.

Communication with the fetus isn't limited to words, of course. Boris Brott (yes, he's a relative, but I've never met him), a famous Canadian orchestra conductor, traces his interest in music to the womb:

As a young man, I was mystified by this ability I had to play certain pieces sight unseen. I'd be conducting a score for the first time and, suddenly, the cello line would jump out at me: I'd know the flow of the piece before I turned the page of the score. One day, I mentioned this to my mother, who is a professional cellist. I thought she'd be intrigued because it was always the cello line that was so distinct in my mind. She was; but when she heard what the pieces were, the mystery quickly solved itself. All the scores I knew sight unseen were ones she had played when she was pregnant with me.

In an effort to harness the power of prenatal communication, several physicians, obstetricians, and entrepreneurs have developed organized communication programs. Psychiatrist Thomas Verny claims that by singing and talking to the fetus, "parents create a positive intrauterine environment, reducing the level of anxiety-producing hormones that lead to frenetic activity and even ulcers in the unborn." And Dr. F. Rene Van de Carr maintains that his "Prenatal Classroom" provides systematic stimulation that may "actually help the growing fetus' brain become more efficient and increase learning capacity after birth."

Sarah Brewer goes even further. "Your baby's brain is literally shaped by the stimuli and nutrients received from his environment," she says. "By enriching his prenatal environment with additional stimuli, you can encourage the growth and development of his brain cells (neurons) so they develop more complex 'communication antennae' (dendron trees), more 'satellite dishes' (dendritic spines), and stronger synaptic connections." Translation: it may make your baby smarter.

Perhaps the most dramatic claims, though, are made by developmental psychologist Brent Logan, whose BabyPlus technology uses what he calls the "cardiac curriculum" to pump a set of increasingly complex heartbeatlike sounds into the mother's womb. Logan may really be on to something with the heartbeat thing. It's the one sound that fetuses hear even more than their mother's voices. And after birth, many newborns are soothed by recordings of their mothers' heartbeat (recordings of other people's hearts don't work nearly as well). Interestingly, although scientists have documented this, ordinary people seem to have known it all along. About 80 percent of mothers—whether they're right- or left-handed—naturally hold babies on the left side, where the baby's head can be nearer the heart. Even artists—a far less stodgy group than researchers and scientists—have noticed the left-side bias: studies of classical paintings and sculptures have shown that 80 percent of the people depicted carrying babies hold them on the left side. Those carrying inanimate objects, however, do so half the time on the right, half on the left.

Whether it's the heartbeats or something else, Logan says his "graduates" frequently learn to talk as early as five or six months and to read at eighteen months (most kids don't usually talk until they're at least a year old and don't usually read until they're five or six).

Besides all of this, Logan, Brewer, and other researchers have found that prenatally enriched babies tend to:

- cry less at birth
- be more alert at birth
- form attachments to Mom and Dad more quickly
- have longer attention spans and better concentration
- hold their heads up unassisted sooner
- have remarkable (for babies, anyway) physical strength
- sleep better
- mature more quickly
- be less likely to develop dyslexia
- demonstrate advanced musical and creative talents
- have an IQ in the 125–150 range (average is 100)

To be fair, you should know that there are plenty of people who claim that there is absolutely no benefit at all to any of this prenatal communication stuff. That said, if you're interested in finding out more, take a look at the Resources appendix.

Sex

Pregnancy can do funny things to your libido. Some expectant fathers are more interested in sex and more easily aroused than ever before. Others are repelled by the very idea. Whether you're feeling either of these ways or something in between, rest assured that it's completely normal.

In this section, we'll talk about the sexual issues that may come up in the first six months of your pregnancy. Late-pregnancy sexual issues are covered on page 179.

WHY YOU AND/OR YOUR PARTNER MIGHT BE FEELING *INCREASED* SEXUAL DESIRE

- After about the third month, her nausea and fatigue are probably gone, making sex more appealing—for both of you.
- You may find her pregnant body (with its larger breasts and fuller curves) erotic. If so, you certainly aren't alone. This is so common that there's actually a word for it: *maieusiophilia.*
- Your partner may be proud of her more ample figure and may be feeling sexier.
- You may be turned on by the feeling of power and masculinity at having created life.
- Your partner may be turned on by the confirmation of her femininity and by the awe at what her body is doing. She may also be aroused by how much she's arousing you.
- Throughout pregnancy, you both may experience a newfound feeling of closeness that frequently manifests itself sexually.
- One or both of you may be having more erotic dreams.
- The increased vaginal lubrication and blood flow to her pelvic area may make your partner's orgasms more powerful and easier to reach. (If that were happening to you, you'd want to have sex more often too.) It may also stimulate her to masturbate more than usual, or if she didn't (or says she didn't) before, she might start.
- If you experienced a miscarriage in an earlier pregnancy, you may have been abstaining from sex for the first trimester. Now that it's safely behind you, all that pent-up desire may have gotten you both to the point where you're about ready to explode.
- She's pregnant with a boy. According to neuroscientist Lise Eliot, women carrying boys have higher levels of testosterone (which is linked with increased sex drive) in their blood than those carrying girls.

A Few Things to Remember about Prenatal Communication

- Respect your partner. You've got a right to speak with your child, but she's got a right to privacy. If she's not completely into the idea, you might want to tell her that Logan and others have found that women who are carrying prenatally stimulated babies seem to have shorter labors and a lower C-section rate. In addition, certain kinds of stimulation may reduce the risk of breech births (where the baby comes out feet first instead of headfirst). Because they like sounds so much, some fetuses will "chase" after music playing through headphones placed against the mother's abdomen. The theory is that if you move the headphones to the bottom of the abdomen during the last month or so of the pregnancy, a stubborn yet music-loving breech fetus could be convinced to shift its head downward, right where it's supposed to be.
- Try to overcome the feeling that what you are doing is absolutely ridiculous. The idea that communicating with unborn babies could actually benefit them has been around for more than a thousand years.
- Don't whisper. Speak to the fetus loudly enough so that a person standing across the room could hear you clearly.
- Don't do it when you're feeling bored. The fetus will pick up on your tone of voice.
- Don't go overboard. Fifteen to twenty minutes, twice a day at most. Fetuses need plenty of time to rest, even more than newborns or kittens.
- Set up a routine. Try to do it at the same time every day so that the baby will get used to the idea that something's going to happen. Pat your partner's

WHY YOU AND/OR YOUR PARTNER MIGHT BE FEELING *DECREASED* SEXUAL DESIRE

- In the first trimester, your partner may be too nauseated or tired to be interested in sex. In the second trimester, she may feel too uncomfortable or too awkward to want to have sex (about 25 percent of pregnant women feel this way). But most say that the second trimester—months 4, 5, and 6—is the best time of the pregnancy, sexually speaking.
- She may think that you don't find her attractive and don't want to have sex with her.
- You may not, in fact, be attracted to a woman whose body has been transformed from fun to functional.
- You may think your partner isn't feeling attractive and wouldn't be interested in sex.

belly before you start to let the baby know you're out there. Use the baby's name (if you know it).

- Mix it up. Playing the same piece of music or reading the same poem or story every day is great, but be sure to keep the rest of the program different. When fetuses hear the same thing over and over, they just block it out.

- Have fun. No specialized training or advanced degrees required. Try some games, like gently patting your partner's belly and announcing to the baby, "I'm patting you now." Or play DJ with your iPod shuffle or your CD collection—give a gentle rub and say, "Get ready, baby, you're about to hear some jazz," or classical, hip-hop, salsa, country, rock, or whatever. It's a little much to expect your baby to remember a lot of individual artists, but hey, genres could work.

- Don't get your expectations too high. Most of the prenatal communication systems make claims that your baby will be taller, smarter, more beautiful, come out of the womb fully dressed and speaking three languages, or whatever. Not long ago, I got a call from a publicist who insisted that if a baby went through the entire curriculum described, the company would guarantee that the child's SAT scores would be 15 percent higher. Excuse me? Higher than what? The absurdity of the claim was completely lost on her. Seems to me that if you're expecting a superbaby and you get a healthy but perfectly average baby, you're going to feel disappointed. And I can't think of a worse way for a baby to start off her life outside the womb than by being a disappointment to Dad.

- You or your partner may be afraid that sex will hurt her—or the baby. In fact, there's nothing to be afraid of. The baby is safely cushioned by its amniotic fluid–filled sac, and unless your partner has cramps or bleeds during sex or her doctor feels there are extenuating circumstances, sex during pregnancy is no more dangerous for your partner than at any other time. The two of you may find this information reassuring. If you do, great. If not, now may be the time to talk about it and try some different sexual positions (your partner on top, both of you lying on your side, or your partner lying close to the edge of the bed and you standing) and different ways of bringing each other to orgasm (oral sex, vibrators, and so on). Often simply making a few such changes can go a long way toward alleviating your fears.

- Although in most cases sex is required to become a parent, you and your partner may feel, as it gradually sinks in that you are about to become parents, that parents aren't supposed to be sexual. (Even though we are all living proof that our parents had sex at least once, it's somehow hard to imagine the two of them, in bed, naked…)

- You or your partner may feel that sex serves only one purpose: creating children. And once you've done that, there's no more need for sex—until you want more kids.
- She may actually find it painful.

WHAT THE EXPERTS SAY

As you can see, the range of feelings about sex is broad. But if you still aren't convinced that you're not the only one feeling the way you do, here are a few interesting things researchers have found out about expectant couples' sexuality during pregnancy:

- According to psychologists Wendy Miller and Steven Friedman, expectant fathers generally underestimate how attractive their partners feel, and expectant mothers consistently underestimate how attractive their partners find them. (The bottom line is that most men find their pregnant partners' bodies erotic, and most pregnant women feel quite attractive. But many men and women fail to convey these feelings to their partners.)
- According to the Cowans, expectant fathers have more psychological inhibitions about physical intimacy during pregnancy than their partners do.
- The old myth that pregnancy somehow desexualizes women is just that—a myth. In fact, Miller and Friedman found that there are no significant differences in the level of sexual desire or sexual satisfaction between expectant men and women.

When to Be Particularly Careful

If your partner is at risk for, or has a history of, premature labor, *placenta previa* (when the placenta covers the cervix), or an incompetent cervix (when the cervix is not strong enough to hold the fetus inside until truly ready to be born), talk to her doctor before you hop in the sack. Nipple stimulation and orgasm have a direct impact on the uterus and could possibly trigger some contractions. If your partner has any of these conditions or is at risk for going into labor early, use a condom when you have sex. No, it's not a birth control thing. Strange as it sounds, there's a slim chance that one of the hormones in semen (prostaglandin) may cause contractions.

WHEN YOU AND YOUR PARTNER ARE OUT OF SYNC

Of course, you and your partner may not always be on the same wavelength. She may feel like having sex just when you're feeling put off by her Rubenesque figure. Conversely, you may want to have sex at a time when she's simply not interested. Here are a few suggestions that might help:

- Talk. At these and so many other times during your pregnancy, communicating with your partner is essential. As Arthur and Libby Colman so wisely write, "Unless the couple can talk about their sex life, their entire relationship may suffer, and that in turn will compound their sexual problems."

- Try some nonsexual affection, such as snuggling, touching, or just hugging each other. And say up front that that is what you're interested in doing, because it isn't as easy as it sounds. Professors Cowan and Cowan have found that many couples need practice finding sensual ways to please each other short of intercourse. And both men and women hesitate to make affectionate overtures if they aren't sure they're ready to progress to intercourse and are worried they'll be misinterpreted.

- Be nice to each other. Being critical of her figure will make her feel less attractive and less interested in sex. Instead, tell her how hot she looks and do a few more things from the list on pages 96–99—especially any of the cleaning, cooking, and other household tasks. They don't call it *choreplay* for nothing.

- Try something completely off the wall. Some fascinating new research has found that oral sex may actually make the pregnancy safer. Work with me here. Gustaaf Dekker, a professor at the University of Adelaide, did a study comparing forty-one women who had preeclampsia (a condition marked by dangerously high blood pressure) and forty-four who didn't. He found that 82 percent of the women without preeclampsia gave their partner regular blow jobs, but only about 40 percent of the women who had the condition did. According to Dekker, "The protective effect of oral sex was strongest if the woman actually swallowed the semen rather than coughing it onto the pillow." So now, when he's counseling couples who have had trouble in the past carrying a pregnancy to term, he tells them, "Semen exposure is good, and you could think of oral sex." Hey, I'm just saying: could be worth a shot. But don't hold your breath.

This doesn't have to be a one-way street, either. Sex researcher Amy Sayle found that women who are not "high risk" (check with her doctor to be sure) and who have regular orgasms during pregnancy have a lower risk of premature delivery than women who don't. And researcher Rachel Alicesteen found that couples who talk about sex—compared to those who don't—actually have sex more often. As you might expect, Alicesteen also found that the more sexual pleasure a couple experiences during the pregnancy, the more satisfied they are with their relationship.

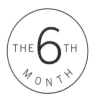

Work and Family

WHAT'S GOING ON WITH YOUR PARTNER

Physically

- Period of greatest weight gain begins
- Increased sweating
- Increased blood supply gives her that pregnant "glow"; it may also be giving her some sciatica, numbness and tingling in the hands, or even carpal tunnel syndrome as all the extra fluid compresses some of her nerves
- Swelling of the hands and feet
- Fatigue, dizziness, and a runny nose are not uncommon
- A constant, nagging backache—especially if she's carrying twins or more
- Some incredibly bizarre food cravings (see page 130 for more on this)
- She's getting a full-body aerobic workout; her heart and lungs are working 50 percent harder than before she was pregnant and not surprisingly, she's a little short of breath
- A little bit of urine leakage when laughing, coughing, or sneezing

Emotionally

- Moodiness is decreasing
- Continued forgetfulness and even some short-term memory loss (see pages 130–31 for more on this)
- Feeling that the pregnancy will never end
- Increased bonding with the baby
- Still very dependent on you

- Wondering what kind of mom she'll be, and how the way she was mothered will affect her own parenting

WHAT'S GOING ON WITH THE BABY

The baby looks pretty trim—he hasn't started putting on much fat yet—and is starting to get covered with *vernix*, a thick, waxy, protective coating. His eyes are beginning to open, he coughs and hiccups, and if you were inside the uterus, you could see his unique footprints and fingerprints. The movements of your now foot-long two-pounder are getting stronger—no more of those butterfly kicks—and he can hear, and respond to, sounds from the outside world. Baby girls develop eggs in their ovaries this month, and according to some researchers, this is when your baby's emotions begin to form. He learns about love through the comfort that your voice (and your partner's) gives him. And when your partner is feeling stressed or angry or sad, the baby gets a tiny jolt of the same hormones that are affecting Mom.

WHAT'S GOING ON WITH YOU

Reexamining Your Relationship with Your Father

As the reality of your prospective fatherhood unfolds, you'll probably find yourself contemplating how you'll juggle the various roles—parent, provider, husband, employee, friend—that will make up your paternal identity. As mentioned in earlier chapters, you may be spending more time reading about parenting and watching how your male friends, family members, or even strangers do it.

But eventually you'll realize that your own father—whether you know it or not—has already had a profound influence on the kind of father you'll be. You may also find yourself nearly overcome with forgotten images of childhood—especially ones involving your father. Just walking down the street, I'd suddenly remember the times we went camping or to the ballet (he's a very well-rounded guy, culturally speaking), how he taught me to throw a baseball in the park, and the hot summer afternoon he, my sisters, and I stripped down to our underwear in the backyard and painted each other with watercolors. There's nothing like impending paternity to bring back all the memories and emotions of what it was like to be fathered as a child.

Not all childhood memories of fathers are positive, of course. Some men's images of their fathers are dominated by fear, pain, loneliness, or longing. Either way, don't be surprised if you find yourself seriously reexamining your relationship

A Few Positively Odd Things Your Partner Might Be Experiencing

PICA

You've probably heard all about pregnant women's strange and oddly timed food cravings—such as pickles and ice cream at two in the morning, or strawberries and garlic for breakfast. As repulsive as some of them may be, cravings like these are completely normal. Some pregnant women, though, crave laundry starch, wax, gravel, dirt, coffee grounds, paint, ashes, clay, cigarette butts, and even the smell of gasoline. Needless to say, such cravings are anything but normal. They are part of a fairly rare condition called *pica*, which generally affects only kids one to six years old and pregnant women (yet another reason I'm glad I'm not a woman). Women who grew up or live in the South or in rural communities seem to be at greater risk, as are women who suffered from pica as children. Some people believe that these wacky cravings are the body's way of satisfying its nutritional needs; there is, for example, plenty of iron in clay. The problem is that there's also a lot of really dangerous stuff in it.

Other experts discount the nutrition angle completely; if she's missing some nutrients, she needs to eat better or take some vitamins. So if you catch your partner licking ashtrays, or if she wakes you up in the middle of the night asking for a handful of gravel or a candle to chew on, offer her a healthy snack, get her to sleep, and call her doctor first thing in the morning.

MOMNESIA

As if that wasn't weird enough . . . if your partner has been forgetful lately, or seems to be losing a lot of things—including her memory—it may be because her brain is shrinking. Yep. Anita Holdcroft, an English anesthesiologist, found that during pregnancy, women's brains actually get 3–5 percent smaller.

with your dad. Was he the kind of man you want as your role model? Was he the perfect example of the kind of father you *don't* want to be? Or was he somewhere in between? Many men, particularly those who had rocky, or nonexistent, relationships with their fathers find that the prospect of becoming a dad themselves enables them to let go of some of the anger they've felt for so long.

Don't be surprised if you start having a lot of dreams about your father. Researcher Luis Zayas found that an expectant father's uncertainty about his identity as father, his actual role, and the changed relationship with his wife and

Now that you know this, it's probably best that you keep it to yourself. After all, there's really no nice way to tell someone that her brain is shrinking. You could mention it in the hope that your partner will forget it right away, but if she doesn't, you're in big trouble. And anyway, the shrinkage seems to be attributed to the brain cells being compressed—not to an actual loss of cells. And, oh yes, it generally clears up within a few months after the birth. (Several researchers have recently disputed the pregnancy brain-shrink theory—also called "mommy brain" or "momnesia"—but most mothers will tell you that they've had issues with memory, concentration, and the ability to think straight.)

THE SWEET SMELL OF . . .

If you've had a suspicion that your partner seems, well, a little more odiferous lately, you're probably right. A pregnant women's digestive system operates a lot more slowly than yours, which means that everything she eats has more time to ferment. For beer, wine, cheese, and bread, fermenting is a good thing. But in humans, it causes gas. And the longer the fermenting goes on, the smellier the farts. Your partner may try to cover it up by blaming it on the dog or the sewage treatment plant just down the road. But you can disarm the situation by simply saying, "Thank you." According to some new research about farting (yes, amazingly, there is such a thing), hydrogen sulfide, the stuff that gives rotten eggs—and farts—their delightful aroma, may offer some significant health benefits, including reducing blood pressure, improving survival rates for victims of stroke or heart attacks, and treating diabetes, arthritis, and dementia. Beans, anyone?

family are some of the "psychic threads of fatherhood" that are fundamentally related to the man's relationship with his own father and are frequently present in his dreams.

So, whether you're awake or asleep, as you're thinking about your dad, remember that what's really going on is that you're worried about what kind of a father *you* will be when your baby arrives.

There's no question that the way your dad parented you will influence the kind of father you become. But despite all those silly aphorisms like "The acorn never

Turning the Tables on Mom

We've talked a lot about how just about everything your partner does affects your baby. But can the fetus affect the mother in return? This could very well be. Claire Vanston, a Canadian researcher, did a fascinating study on the brain function of women throughout pregnancy and beyond. She tested the women five times: during pregnancy at twelve weeks, twenty-four weeks, and thirty-seven weeks, then six weeks after the baby was born, and several months after that. She found that "women pregnant with sons consistently outperformed women pregnant with daughters" on several tests of working memory. And the boy/girl difference was there from the first test all the way through the last. As to why this happens, no one knows yet. But it's still pretty interesting, isn't it?

falls far from the tree," whether that influence is positive or negative is completely up to you.

According to researchers Kory Floyd and Mark Morman, father involvement is based on a combination of modeling and what they call "compensation effects." On the one hand, if you feel that your dad did a good job parenting you, you'll use him as a model for your relationship with your own kids. On the other hand, if you were dissatisfied with the fathering you received, or you feel that your relationship was unaffectionate or distant, you'll "feel compelled to remake the fathering experience into something more positive" for your own children.

What's especially interesting is that your dad's relationship with your mother (when you were a boy) may also influence your fathering behavior, but not in the way you might expect. According to researchers John Beaton, William Doherty, and Martha Rueter, you'll be more committed to being an involved father if your parents "disagreed about how you should be raised." Apparently, in disagreeing with your mother, your dad was demonstrating that he wanted to be involved on his own terms. And you'll want to do the same thing.

Bottom line: if you work at it, you can be the father you want to be, rather than the one you think fate (and possibly genetics) might have planned for you to be.

A Sense of Mortality

I've always been more than just a little fascinated by death—I love the movie *Harold and Maude*, and I wanted to paint my room black and hang an "R.I.P." sign over my bed when I was a kid (my parents wouldn't let me). But it wasn't until my wife got pregnant for the first time that death became something more than a mere abstraction. Suddenly it occurred to me that my death could have a serious impact on other people.

This realization had some interesting and fairly immediate results. The first thing that happened was that I became a much better driver—or at least a safer one. Overnight, yellow lights changed their meaning from "floor it" to "proceed with caution." I began to leave for appointments a few minutes earlier so I wouldn't have to hurry, wove in and out of traffic less, and found myself not quite so annoyed with people who cut me off in traffic. But besides becoming a better driver, I began to look back with horror at some of the risky things—parachuting, scuba diving, joining the Marine Corps—I'd done before I'd gotten married, and I began to reconsider some of the things I'd tentatively planned for the near future—bungee jumping, hang gliding. After all, now there were people counting on me to stay alive.

My preoccupation with my own mortality had other interesting consequences as well. I found myself strangely drawn to my family's history; I wanted to learn more about our traditions, our family rituals, the wacky relatives no one ever talked about. I even put together a family tree and began bugging my relatives

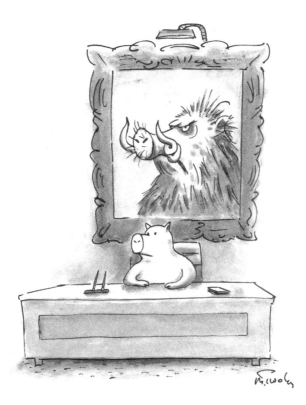

about their birth dates. I didn't realize it at the time, but it's quite common for expectant fathers to experience a heightened sense of attachment to their relatives—both immediate and distant—even if they weren't particularly close before.

This really isn't so unusual, especially when you consider that one of the main reasons we have kids in the first place is so that a little piece of us will live on long after we're gone. I guess the hope is that one day seventy-five years from now, when my great-grandson is expecting a child, he'll start to explore his roots and want to get to know more about me.

Feeling Trapped

As we've already discussed, you and your partner probably aren't feeling the same things at the same time. Earlier on in the pregnancy, your partner may have turned inward, preoccupied with how the pregnancy was affecting her.

You may have felt a little (or a lot) left out. By now, though, your partner may be "turning outward"—concentrating less on herself and the baby, and more on you. Meanwhile, you may have just begun the process of turning inward that we began discussing last month (page 115). You're going to be a father in less than four months, and you've got a lot of things to think about, many of which you need to work through on your own. The potential problem here is that just as you begin to focus on yourself, your partner is becoming increasingly dependent on you. She may be afraid that you don't love her anymore and that you're going to leave her. Or she may be worried—just as you are—about your physical safety. Although being doted upon is nice, it can sometimes get out of hand. And your partner's increased dependence on you may cause you to feel trapped. As Arthur and Libby Colman found, a pregnant woman's "sudden concern may make a man feel over-protected, as though his independence is being threatened." If you are feeling trapped, it's important to let your partner know in a gentle, nonconfrontational way. And don't even joke about wanting to pack your bags and leave. At the same time, encourage her to talk about what she's feeling and what she wants from you.

STAYING INVOLVED

Having Fun

Besides being a time of great change—physical as well as emotional—pregnancy can be a fun time, too. Here are a few ways to amuse yourselves:
- Take lots of pictures. I took regular shots of my wife—from the front and the side, with emphasis on the belly—holding a mug-shot-style card labeled "Pregnant Woman Number 1 (2, 3, and so on)." For another series of photos, she stood

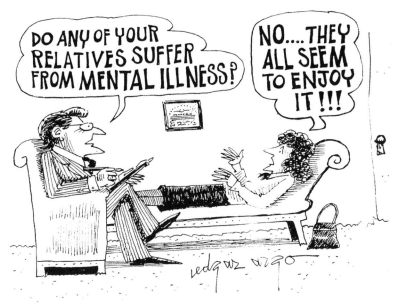

up while I lay on my back between her legs and took pictures of her soft under-belly. Be sure to take note of the critical day the belly completely blocks your view of your partner's face. Take as many pictures as your partner will pose for, but at the very least, try for once a month until the eighth month, then once a week after that.

- Get some special clothes. His-and-hers "Yes sir, that's my baby" T-shirts and "Father-to-bee" hats (featuring a picture of a bumblebee) are favorites in some circles.
- Get some exercise—together. Taking a water aerobics or swimming class together can be a lot of fun. You'll be amazed at how agile pregnant women can be when they're floating in water. Unless you're quite confident about your partner's sense of humor, it's best to stifle your comments about whales—beached or otherwise.
- Start a clipping file or scrapbook for the baby. Digital scrapbooks, blogs, and Instagram are great, but when your child grows up, he may be curious about what paper and DVDs (which will probably have disappeared completely by then) looked like. So while you still can, put together a file with newspapers and magazines, DVDs of a few of your current faves, books, and maybe even a list of popular songs, political issues, and prices for a variety of items (cell phones, computers, food, movie and theater tickets, and so on).
- Start planning birth announcements. See pages 158–59 for more details.
- Make a plaster belly cast. Believe it or not, this is my all-time favorite. It's a little complicated, but well worth the trouble. Long after the baby is born, you, your

partner, and your friends will be absolutely amazed that your partner was ever that big (and the baby that small). If you're interested in trying it, you can pick up kits at places like Toys Я Us, check out www.proudbody.com, or just Google "plaster belly cast." An important warning: don't even *think* about making a cast of your partner's belly using any kind of plastic, rubber, or resin. No matter what anybody tells you, these products can be harmful to both your partner and the baby.

Work and Family

FAMILY LEAVE

Let's face it: while your partner is pregnant, it's going to be kind of tough for you to put in a lot of quality time with your unborn child—a little before work, a bit more after work, a few hours on weekends. But what about after the pregnancy? Is a few hours a day going to be enough time to spend with your child? If it were, you probably wouldn't be reading this book. Contrary to the common stereotypes, work/family balance is *not* just a women's issue. It's something that most working dads strive for too. But it's not easy.

Today, according to a new study by the Boston College Center for Work and Family, 70 percent of working dads say their role in the family is to be both the involved dad and the provider. It's no big surprise, then, that 60 percent of working dads in dual-income households say they experience work/family conflict, according to the Families and Work Institute. That's up from 35 percent in 1977 (over the same time period, the percentage of women who say they have work/family conflict has stayed pretty much the same, at around 45 percent).

Despite all this, today's dads really want to make some changes. Consider the results of a few recent studies:

- Eighty-six percent of working dads say that their children are their "number one priority." Sixty-four percent say that being a father makes them a better employee, and, according to the Boston College Center for Work and Family, more dads say that having a flexible schedule that would allow them to spend more time with their family is of greater importance than career advancement or high income. In fact, according to monster.com, 82 percent of working dads searching for a job view companies more positively if they offer a flextime benefit.
- A Harvard University study found that among men between the ages of twenty-one and thirty-nine, seven in ten say they'd give up some pay to be able to spend more time with their families (men were actually more likely than women to

give up pay), and 68 percent would consider being a stay-at-home parent if money were no object.

Sounds pretty good, doesn't it? Well, unfortunately, despite their good intentions, only about 5 percent of new dads take any more than two weeks off after the birth of their child. And remember all those guys who say family is their top priority and rate family time as more important than career? Those same studies found that 76 percent of working dads would like to "advance to a position with greater responsibility with their employers" and 58 percent have "a strong desire" to be in upper management. Perhaps most ironic of all, while 58 percent of working dads (vs. 49 percent of men without children) say they'd like to work fewer hours, the dads put in an average of forty-seven hours per week on the job, whereas the nondads log only forty-four hours per week, according to the Families and Work Institute.

So what accounts for the contradiction between what men say and what they actually do? First of all, the vast majority of family-leave plans (including the Family and Medical Leave Act, which we'll talk about in a minute) are unpaid, which makes them unworkable for many families.

Over the past decade or so, there's been a definite increase in the number of companies that offer family-friendly benefits. But when it comes to *male* employees, the messages about whether it's okay to actually use those benefits are mixed at best. For example, about 14 percent of U.S. employers offer paid paternity leave. But even at those companies, less than half of eligible men take it. Put a little differently, fathers are only one-tenth as likely as mothers to use parenting leave, and one-sixth as likely to have ever used part-time work hours, according to researchers Julie Holliday Wayne and Bryanne Cordeiro.

Why? People generally see taking maternity leave (beyond the disability component) as a normal thing for women to do. But when a man requests family leave, he's no longer behaving the way men are "supposed" to. As a result, the people around him start to see him as more feminine (weak and uncertain) and less masculine (competitive and ambitious), according to Rutgers University researchers Laurie Rudman and Kris Mescher. Rudman, Mescher, and another team of researchers led by Joseph Vandello at the University of South Florida found that the penalties men pay for asking for family leave are quite heavy. They're seen as not serious about their jobs, they get lower evaluations from coworkers and managers, and they may get passed over for promotions and get smaller raises than male coworkers who act more like "real men" and don't request time off for family reasons. And, sadly, men are more judgmental of other men than women are.

137

The Family and Medical Leave Act

The Family and Medical Leave Act (usually referred to as the Family Leave Act or FMLA) is a relatively straightforward document, and I suggest you familiarize yourself with it before you start making too many plans. You can find thousands of references to it online, but for the latest, take a look at the Department of Labor's website, www.dol.gov/dol/topic/benefits-leave/fmla.htm.

Here's a quick summary of what it means for fathers:

- Who can take the leave? Any person who works for a public agency (federal, state, or local) or a private-sector company that employs fifty or more people within a seventy-five-mile radius. You must have been employed by that company for at least twelve months and have worked at least 1,250 hours during that time. This covers about two-thirds of the total U.S. labor force. If you're in the military, the FMLA may apply to you as well. Check with your CO and keep in mind that the needs of the service may trump your eligibility.
- How much leave can you take? Eligible employees can take up to twelve workweeks of leave at any time during the twelve-month period that starts the day your child is born or adopted. If you and your wife are employed by the same company, though, you may get only twelve weeks total.
- When do you have to take it? You can start anytime, as long as you finish within a year. Beyond that, whatever you can work out with your employer is fine. You can take twelve weeks in one chunk, work part-time for twenty-four weeks, take every Friday off for a year, or make some other arrangement.
- Is it paid? Employers are not required to pay you your salary while you're on

Yes, women have been dealing with a flexibility stigma for decades, and they pay a steep financial price when they move from the fast track to the mommy track. Corporate America should be ashamed. But according to Scott Coltrane and his colleagues at the University of Oregon, "Men who leave the workforce for family reasons can expect to earn 26.4 percent less later in their careers than they would have had they never left the workforce. Women face a 23.3 percent financial penalty."

But dads are certainly not giving up. Even those who don't take paternity or family leave manage to cobble together sick days, comp time, vacation days, and so on in order to be with their newborns. On average, that adds up to a little over a week. What it comes down to is what attorney Kari Palazzari calls the "daddy double-bind." Men are still expected to be the primary breadwinner, so "success" leave. But suppose your employer pays for six weeks of family leave: you're still entitled to take another six without pay. And even if your employer doesn't have paid leave, they may require you to burn through your sick time, vacation, and comp days before you can start using the leave.

- What about benefits? Your employer must maintain your coverage under the company's health plan for the duration of your leave.
- Is your job protected? In most cases, yes. Your employer cannot fire or replace you while you're on leave unless he or she can prove that your absence has caused "substantial and grievous economic injury to the operations of the employer."
- Do you have to give notice? According to the FMLA, you're required to give your employer at least thirty days' notice before taking your family leave. But the more notice you give, the more time everyone will have to get used to the idea.

Individual states may offer family-leave benefits that are more liberal than those of the federal program. In some states, for example, companies that employ as few as twenty-five people are required to offer their employees family leave. And a small number of states are now offering family leave that's paid (although you probably won't get anywhere near your current salary). And remember: these benefits are completely separate from the (potentially more liberal) ones your company may offer. Be sure to check with your employer's Human Resources department.

at work means spending less time at home. But today's dads are now expected to be actively involved in every part of their family life, and "success" at home requires spending less time at work. You can see that there's no way out.

The good news is that it looks as though some cracks are developing in what I like to call "the other glass ceiling"—the obstacles that make it hard for men to be with their children as much as they'd like.

Though a growing number of companies are discovering that offering flexible work arrangements (FWA) is the right thing to do, there are a number of concrete, bottom-line-affecting benefits that your employer probably doesn't know about. Go ahead and enlighten 'em.

- Businesses lose more than $150 billion a year due to absenteeism, employee turnover, health care, and workers' compensation benefits directly resulting from overworked, overstressed dads. Absenteeism alone costs an average of nearly $800 per employee every year—$80,000 per year for a company with a hundred employees.

- FWAs boost productivity. Stanford University economist Nicholas Bloom found that employees who telecommute are 13.5 percent more productive than employees who go into the office. Bloom says that one-third of the increase is attributable to the quieter environment at home. "Offices are incredibly distracting places," he says. The other two-thirds has to do with the longer hours people at home put in. They have no commute, they start earlier, take shorter breaks, and don't run errands at lunchtime.
- FWAs increase retention/reduce turnover. The telecommuters in Bloom's study quit their jobs at about half the rate of their peers in the office. Turnover is a huge expense. "The costs of hiring and training a new employee, and the slower productivity until the new employee gets up to speed in their new job," average about 20 percent of the worker's salary, according to economists Heather Boushey and Sarah Jane Glynn. For executives, the costs can exceed 200 percent of salary.
- FWAs improve recruitment. Companies find that offering FWAs helps attract top talent.
- FWAs improve employee morale and loyalty. When employees feel that their employer respects their need for flexibility, they're happier, don't take sick days when they're not sick, and are more committed to their employer's success.
- Loyal, happy employees are engaged employees—and engaged employees are profitable employees. Gallup recently analyzed data from 192 organizations in 49 industries, looking at the relationship between employee engagement and company performance. They found that companies in the top 25 percent in terms of employee engagement outperformed those in the bottom 25 percent in customer ratings, profitability, and productivity. The top 25 percent also reported fewer safety incidents, less shrinkage, and fewer quality defects. If that doesn't convince your employer, I can't imagine what would.

MAKING LONG-TERM WORK SCHEDULE CHANGES

So far we've talked about taking a few weeks off just after the birth of your child. But what about after that?

Not long after our first daughter was born, my wife left her big, downtown law firm and found a less stressful, three-day-a-week job closer to home. Almost everyone we knew applauded. But when I made the announcement that I, too, would be cutting back to three days a week, the reaction was quite a bit different. At work, I was hassled repeatedly by my boss and coworkers, and a lot of my

Family Leave If You're an Employee

- Take it. Every man I've ever interviewed who took paternity or family leave told me he'd do it again.
- Know your rights. Find out whether you're eligible under the Family and Medical Leave Act (see pages 138–39), your company's voluntary plan, or any other federal- or state-mandated program. There's often a disconnect between what you're legally entitled to and what your employer will let you know about, so ask around.
- Start talking to your employer now. If you're covered by a leave plan, start working out the details in a nonconfrontational way. If you're not covered by a leave plan, you may be able to arrange for some time off anyway.
- Come up with a plan. I have an MBA, and before I switched to writing full-time, I worked in business for many years. That's why, as big a pro-father/pro-family advocate as I am, I believe that when an employer hires you to do a job, they have every right to expect that job to get done—and it's up to you to figure out how that's going to happen while you're out on leave. Start by talking with your partner and figuring out an ideal-case scenario that works for both of you. Then come up with a plan and present it to your employer, along with a way to evaluate whether everyone's needs are being met. If everything's on track after a couple of weeks, keep it going. If not, revise the plan and try again. Acknowledging your employer's needs will make it a lot easier for them to acknowledge and support yours.
- Sell the benefits. If you're having trouble convincing your employer, take a quick look back at pages 139–40. Employers need to know that dad-friendly benefits aren't just something that's nice to offer (although they certainly are that); they're good business.

friends and relatives began to whisper that if I didn't go back to work full-time, my career might never recover.

I'm not suggesting that everyone should cut back their work schedules to three days a week. Clearly, that just isn't practical for most people (although it sure would be nice if you could, wouldn't it?). Frankly, you may never be able to resolve your work/family conflicts completely. Fortunately, there are a few ways you can maximize your time with your family, minimize your stress, and avoid trashing your career.

For example, depending on your job, there's a good chance that you don't really need to be cooped up in a cubicle Monday to Friday, 9 A.M. to 5 P.M., with a manager peeking over your shoulder making sure you're doing your job. According to the Society for Human Resource Management (SHRM), nearly 60 percent of employers offer some kind of flexible work arrangements—and nearly half of those companies make those arrangements available to a majority of their employees. (Great news, but still a long way from satisfying the 80–90 percent of working parents who say they want access to more flexible options).

There are a variety of FWAs, which human resources experts Barbara Wleklinski and Elizabeth Jennings divide into several categories:
- Time: When and how long you'll work.
- Place: Where you'll be doing that work.
- Task: What, exactly, you'll be doing.

Here are a few examples:

TIME-ORIENTED ARRANGEMENTS
- Flex time. You'll still work the same number of hours, but you might, for example, start at 5 A.M. and go home at 1 P.M. instead of the usual 9 to 5.
- Compressed workweek. The basic idea is that you put in extra hours on certain days in exchange for a day off. Typical arrangements include working four ten-hour days per week or working an extra hour every day for nine days and taking a day off every two weeks.
- Alternate workweek. You still put in your forty hours, but you might work Wednesday through Sunday and take Mondays and Tuesdays off.
- Part-time work. Less than a typical forty-hour week but usually more than twenty hours per week. You'll need to find out how many hours you're required to work so you don't lose your benefits.
- Family leave. You take off a chunk of paid or unpaid time.

PLACE-ORIENTED ARRANGEMENTS
- Work at home. You do your entire job from your home/home office.
- Telecommuting. If you're not a construction worker or a retail salesman, you might be a prime candidate for this option. Now don't get too excited: it's not as if you and your boss will never see each other again. Most telecommuters are out of the office only a day or two a week. But be careful: if you think you'll be able to save money on child care or have your baby sit on your lap while you crunch numbers, you're sorely mistaken.

  Besides the convenience aspect, one of the major advantages of telecommuting is that you don't have to shave and you can work in your underwear (unless you're working somewhere other than your house). There are, however,

Creating a More Family-Friendly Workplace for Dads
If You're an Employer (or Supervisor)

- If you don't have father-friendly policies, get some. See pages 139–40 for some of the benefits. If you need help putting a program together, email me at armin@mrdad.com.
- Spread the word. At the very least, let all of your employees—especially the men—know that you support their desire to find a better balance between their work and family lives, and that family-friendly policies aren't just for women. Then put your money where your mouth is. Start by taking family leave yourself. The ultimate responsibility for helping men get more involved with their families rests at the top—with male managers. If you demonstrate that it's okay for men to put their families first, everyone else will follow your lead.
- Encourage other men to take leave (whether it's official or not). Most of your male employees will be reluctant to approach you with their family-leave plan. If you know they're expecting, raise the issue with them first. Chances are, they'll be grateful. If you can afford to make the leave paid, so much the better.
- Encourage flexible schedules. This doesn't mean that your employees will work less, just that they'll have more control over when and where they do their jobs. Whatever you spend on technology to allow your people to work remotely will more than pay for itself in increased productivity, loyalty, and so on.
- Educate your workers. Have an occasional brown-bag lunch at which dads get together to discuss their work/family issues. You—and they—will probably be amazed that a lot of other people are facing the same issues.
- Don't forget about employees who don't have kids. It's easy to think of work/life balance as something that affects only parents. But single, childless, and older workers have plenty of personal and family issues to deal with. And supporting them with flexible schedules and everything else we've talked about in this section will pay off in many of the same ways, such as being able to attract more top-quality workers and increasing productivity, morale, and loyalty.

a few disadvantages. Primary among them is lack of human contact; you may hate that train ride into the city or the annoying guy in your carpool, but after a few months alone in your house, you might actually miss them. You might also miss going out to lunch with your coworkers or even just bumping into them in the halls. And if you have a tendency to obsess about your work (as I do), you'll have to train yourself to take frequent breaks. I can't tell you how many times I've realized—at ten o'clock at night—that I haven't eaten all day, and that the only time I went outside was to take the newspaper in from the porch.

Though working at home will allow you to spend more time with your baby and partner, there can be some interesting conflicts. Several dads I spoke with told me that they felt a lot of pressure to hang out with the family, but also a lot of guilt at not getting as much work done as they (or their employer) thought they would.

TASK-ORIENTED ARRANGEMENTS

• Job sharing. You and another person divide up the responsibilities of the job, usually at a prorated salary. You'd probably use the same office and desk. A typical job-share schedule might have you working two days one week and three days the next, while your workplace partner does the opposite. Or one of you might work the mornings and the other afternoons. Either way, be very careful to negotiate a continuation of your health benefits. Many employers drop them for less-than-full-time employees.

• Job splitting. You keep some, but not all, of the tasks in your job description and offload the rest to someone else.

A FEW OTHER OPTIONS

There are two other FWAs to consider. One is gutsy but still pretty conservative, the other is just plain gutsy.

• Become a consultant to your current employer. There are lots of tax advantages, particularly if you set up a home office. At the very least, you'll be able to deduct auto mileage and a hefty percentage of your phone and utility bills. But be sure to check with an accountant first; the IRS uses certain tests to determine whether someone is an employee or a consultant. If, for example, you go into the office every day, have a secretary, and get company benefits, you're an employee. Also, remember that if you become a consultant, you'll lose your benefit package. So be sure to build the cost of that package (or the amount you'll have to pay to replace it) into the daily or hourly rate you negotiate with your soon-to-be-former employer.

- ROWE (Results-Only Work Environment). Basically you work whenever, wherever, and however you want—as long as you get the job done. This option can only work if your employer is not only incredibly flexible but also incredibly clear on what you're supposed to accomplish. At the same time, you have to be extremely well organized and self-directed.

A WORK/FAMILY SOLUTION YOU MIGHT NOT HAVE THOUGHT OF

There are a number of the child-care options you and your partner will have to sift through sometime soon. But what if you'd both really prefer to have your child raised in the arms of a loving parent? Most families that make the decision to have a parent stay home automatically assume that it has to be Mom. Sometimes, though, that just won't work. She might have a more stable career than you, make more money, or simply have no interest in staying home. Well, all is not lost. If you and your partner truly want to have your children raised by a parent, the solution may be only as far away as the nearest mirror: you.

Now before you throw this book down and run out of the room screaming, take a minute to consider the idea. Actually, take longer than that—take at least as much time considering this option as you would any other. You may discover that it's not as crazy as it sounds. Brad Harrington and his colleagues at Boston College Center for Work and Family found that more than half of new fathers would "seriously consider" being a full-time, at-home dad. Let's start with some of the benefits:

- You won't have to agonize over picking the right babysitter or nanny or daycare center.
- It could be cheaper. Full-time daycare for an infant in major metro areas can exceed $18,000 per year. Add in the dry cleaning you won't need to do as often, the three-times-a-week take-out meals you won't be needing, car expenses, train tickets, bridge tolls, and so on, and staying home could end up being a wash.
- You'll have a wonderful opportunity to get to know and build a strong relationship with your child.
- You'll be giving your child what you think is the best possible upbringing.
- You'll be able to help give your partner some peace of mind, while advancing her career at the same time.

Still with us? Deciding to be a stay-at-home dad is a big decision, one that will affect everyone in your family. If you're even remotely considering it, start by asking yourself the following very important questions:

- Can we afford it? Although you'll undoubtedly save on some things by working at home, if you're really committed to the idea, there are all sorts of ways

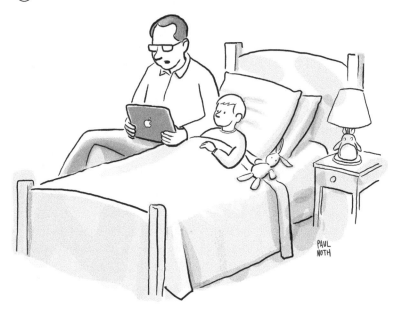

"And then Winnie the Pooh decided that it was time to check Daddy's e-mail again."

to cut your expenses. For example, buy food in bulk, eat out less often, raise your insurance deductibles, take staycations (vacations closer to home), make presents instead of buying them, get rid of the housekeeper, move to a smaller house or a place where the cost of living is lower.

- Can I take the career hit? This is a big one, since earning power and masculinity are inextricably linked in so many people's minds. (If I'm not making money, I'm not a good man/father, the thinking goes.) If you can get over this hurdle, you may still be able to keep a finger or a foot in the work world by teaching, consulting, writing, or starting a home-based business. But don't be hasty. If you decide to reenter the workforce later, you may find that the employment gap on your résumé could cause you some problems with potential employers, many of whom are going to be a lot less enlightened and a lot more closed minded than you.

- Can I handle the pressure? Some people will come right out and tell you that you really should be out there bringing in some money. After all, that's what guys are supposed to do, right? But even if you don't hear the actual words, you may feel the need to demonstrate that you're still a man, that even though you've chosen *not* to earn money (or at least not as much as you did before), you *could* if you really wanted to. Although some of that pressure may be external, some of it may be internal. Traditional sex roles do a real number on us, don't they?

- Do I have a job description? What are your responsibilities? Will you be doing all the laundry, shopping, and cooking? Some of it?

- Can I handle the workload? Staying home with a child is a lot more work than you think. It can also be a little mind numbing. (Having done the stay-at-home-dad thing for many years, I say this from experience. Sometimes, no matter how much fun you've had with the kids, you'll crave some adult conversation at the end of the day.)

- Am I selfless enough? You're not going to get a lot of personal time, and you'll have to put your children's needs above yours. Always.

- How do I deal with isolation? Being a stay-at-home dad can be a bit lonely. According to researcher Robert Frank, about two-thirds of stay-at-home dads feel isolated, compared to only about one-third of stay-at-home moms. There's also not a lot of social support for men who decide to stay home, and you won't see many other guys around who are doing it.

- Is my skin thick enough? Women—whether they're moms, nannies, babysitters—tend not to welcome men into their groups at parks or playgrounds or malls and the other places people take their kids during the day. You'll have to deal with people's stereotypes about dads (very few of which are positive). You'll have to get used to the funny looks and stupid comments you'll hear from people who see you with your kids in the middle of the day. ("Hey, are you babysitting today?" is one that always bugs me. "No, bozo, I'm not babysitting, I'm taking care of my children.") And you'll have to deal with people's criticisms and critiques of your parenting—the kinds of "advice" and comments no one would ever make to a woman.

- How thick is my partner's skin? When you're the primary parent, your child will run to you when he wants a hug or has a skinned knee. And if Mom tries to provide that hug or apply a Band-Aid', he may push her away. I've been on both sides of this, and I can tell you that it hurts. A lot.

- Do I have a reentry plan? It's a good idea to have a rough plan for how long your at-home stint will last, and what you'll do afterward.

In reality, you won't be quite as alone in making this choice as it might seem. At least two million stay-at-home dads are doing it every day, and the number is rising all the time. If you need some support, you'll find some great resources for at-home dads in the Resources appendix.

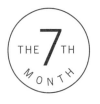

Entering the Home Stretch

WHAT'S GOING ON WITH YOUR PARTNER

Physically

- Increasing general physical discomfort (cramps, dizziness, abdominal achiness, heartburn, gas, constipation, and so forth)
- Itchy belly, puffy face
- Increasing clumsiness and decreasing stamina
- Her hip joints are expanding and she's having to learn to walk in a new, awkward way, which may explain why she's a little more susceptible to muscle pulls and general klutziness
- Some thick, white, vaginal discharge (it's called *leukorrhea,* and is completely normal)
- Increased Braxton-Hicks (false labor) contractions

Emotionally

- May be getting kind of used to the emotional ups and downs of pregnancy
- Decreased moodiness
- Forgetful
- Dreaming/fantasizing about the baby
- Concerned about work—not sure she'll have the energy to go back, and anxious about how to balance roles of mother, wife, employee . . .
- Feeling energized and eager to get things ready for the baby—or completely overwhelmed by everything there is left to do
- Fearful about the labor and delivery

WHAT'S GOING ON WITH THE BABY

The baby's lungs are maturing, and if she were born today, she'd have an excellent chance of survival. She's getting a little cramped inside now—especially if she's got a womb-mate. Her eyes are fully open, and her irises react to light and dark. She can now move in rhythm to music played outside the womb. The fat she's putting on has made her skin a little less red and wrinkly, and she's bulked up to two or three pounds and measures thirteen to fifteen inches long. Her brain is developing incredibly quickly, but the surface of it is still fairly smooth and she's not really capable of much rational thought (given her living situation, that's probably a good thing).

WHAT'S GOING ON WITH YOU

Increasing Acceptance of the Pregnancy

As we've discussed earlier, for most expectant fathers the process of completely accepting the pregnancy is a long one—with the baby becoming progressively more real over the course of the nine months. "It's like getting the measles," said one man interviewed by researcher Katharyn May. "You get exposed, but it takes a while before you realize that you've got it." Another researcher, Pamela Jordan, found that despite seeing the fetus on a sonogram, many men don't really experience their children as real until they meet them face-to-face.

Visualizing the Baby

The growing reality of the pregnancy is reflected in men's dreams as well. Researcher Luis Zayas has found that in expectant fathers' dreams in the early and middle stages of the pregnancy, "the child is not represented as a person. Instead, symbols of the child are present." But as the pregnancy advances to the final stage, expectant fathers—consciously and unconsciously—produce clearer images of their children.

If you want to get a little bit of insight into one of the differences between mothers and fathers, ask your partner to describe herself with the baby. Chances are, she'll talk about a brand-new, fresh-from-the-oven baby. Now do the same thing yourself. More than 90 percent of the expectant fathers in my research (myself included) describe a scene in which they're engaged with a three- to five-year-old child, holding hands, leaving footprints on the beach, playing catch, reading together, or doing something else interactive.

It's a fascinating difference, one that I think is the result of hardwiring. Women, perhaps because of the physical link between themselves and the fetus, have no problem seeing themselves as mothers. And mothers can simply *be*. But for us, fatherhood is about *doing*—teaching, mentoring, preparing our children to meet the world. If you're ever out at a park or some other place where new parents are hanging out, carrying their babies in front packs, you'll see a perfect example of this being-vs.-doing approach. Moms almost always carry their babies facing in. Dads almost always carry them facing out, as if to say, "Hey, baby, this is your world."

Speculating about Gender

In case you hadn't noticed, our society is fixated on gender. These days, 50–60 percent of expectant couples find out their unborn baby's sex. And those who don't, eventually—or constantly—speculate about it. Is your partner carrying the baby high? Wide? Low? Are the baby's kicks hard enough to move your hand, or are they more gentle? Is your partner's complexion clear, or does she have a little acne? Does she crave salty foods or sweets? Is the hair on her legs growing more quickly than usual? And are *you* putting on weight or staying steady? There are literally hundreds of absolutely, positively surefire ways of determining what flavor your baby will be. Each has a fifty-fifty chance of being right, and before your baby is born, you'll hear every one.

A lot of the speculating people do about their unborn children is based on common stereotypes and prejudices that almost all of us have about gender long before our kids are born. Take the baby's kicks, for example. Expectant mothers who know they're carrying a boy often describe the baby's movements as

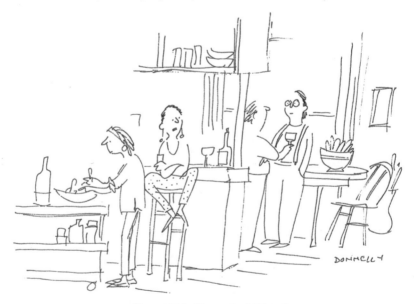

"I want kids. He wants children."

"vigorous," "earthquake-like," or even just "very strong." They describe girls' kicks as "very gentle," "not terribly active," or "lively but not excessively energetic." Truth is, there aren't any differences between boys' and girls' fetal activity levels (however, boys do tend to be more active as two- and three-year-olds).

Preconceived notions (so to speak) such as these may also have an influence on expectant parents' preferences. "Parents usually say they don't care what gender their child is as long as it's healthy," says Carole Beal, author of *Boys and Girls: The Development of Gender Roles*. "But the truth is that couples have a definite preference for the sex of their child." That preference is usually for a boy, and it's expressed by both men and women. Generally speaking, dads prefer boys because they feel more comfortable with them or because they feel that a boy would carry on the family name. Mothers may prefer boys because they know—instinctively or otherwise—how much it means to their husbands.

Interestingly, more women than men call their unborn baby "it." However, both men and women prefer to call the baby by some kind of nickname. In my case, the nicknames I gave our in-utero daughters stuck with them long after they were born. I called our oldest "The Roo"—as in kanga—because she kicked so hard she could knock an open book off my wife's belly. The next one was "Pokey" because, unlike her sister, she preferred to jab and poke. And the youngest is "Lumpty," because her first ultrasound picture looked like Humpty Dumpty.

Some expectant fathers (and mothers) are actually afraid of getting a child of the "wrong" gender, feeling that if they do, they won't be able to have the parenting experience they'd imagined. For many men, their images of themselves as parents are closely linked to the gender of their children. As boys, most of us spent a great deal of our childhood doing things, such as running, jumping, wrestling, and playing football. So it's natural to imagine ourselves doing the same with our own children. Yet some men feel uncomfortable with the idea of wrestling with their daughters, believing that playing physically with girls would somehow be inappropriate. The truth of the matter is that not only is it safe and appropriate to play physically with girls, it's quite beneficial for them in some unexpected ways (see pages 278–80 for more on this).

Your preferences may have a major impact on a lot of other people. According to Beal, boys tend to bring fathers into the family more: fathers of newborn boys actually visit the nursery more often and stay there longer than fathers of girls. In addition, couples who have girls first often have more children, trying to have a boy. But those who have boys first often end up with smaller families. Some experts speculate that this is at least in part due to the perception that boys are more "difficult." And two researchers in Stockholm, Sweden, recently found that

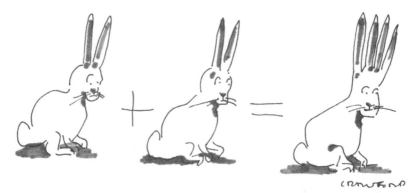

men are generally more satisfied with their role as fathers when their babies—boys or girls—are the gender they'd hoped for.

At the same time, there's evidence that children who did not turn out to be the gender their parents preferred have worse relationships with their parents in childhood than preferred-gender kids. That is especially true for kids whose parents had wanted a boy but got a girl.

The sex of the baby can have some interesting and surprising effects on the parents. For example, having daughters increases a parent's likelihood of cutting back on smoking, drinking, and abusing drugs. And the more daughters the better. "Every additional daughter rather than son makes a person approximately 6% more likely to quit smoking and 7% less likely to have an alcohol or drug problem," writes University of York (England) researcher Nattavudh Powdthavee. On the other hand, researchers Gordon Dahl and Enrico Moretti found that unmarried expectant couples are more likely to get married before the birth if they know they're having a boy than if it's a girl. Among married couples, divorce rates are lowest for those who have only boys and highest for those who have only girls. Divorced women with all-girl offspring are less likely to remarry, and if they do, they're more likely to get divorced again. And in countries where polygamous marriages are relatively common, women who have given birth to girls are more likely to be in polygamous relationships than mothers of boys.

It's going to be tough, but if you find yourself preferring one gender over the other—particularly if you're hoping for a boy—try to stop. If you can't, do yourself and everyone else a favor and keep it to yourself. If your child turns out to be the "wrong" gender, chances are he or she will eventually find out about it (probably from an unthinking friend or relative whom you once told in complete confidence). Besides the problems I just raised in the previous paragraphs, the feeling of being inadequate, of "letting you down," and even of being secretly rejected or loved less, may haunt your child for many years, especially in adolescence, when self-confidence is often at a low.

Fear of Falling Apart During Her Labor

Men are supposed to be strong, right? Especially while their wives are pregnant. And any sign of weakness could be taken as an indication of, well, weakness. Perhaps it's those old societal pressures that make most men dread labor—not only because they aren't looking forward to seeing their partners in pain and they know they'll be helpless to do anything to stop it, but because they're afraid that they'll simply fall apart. And everybody knows that real men don't crack under pressure.

If you're worried about how you'll perform during your partner's labor, do yourself these favors:

- Read the "Classes" section on pages 160–69—especially the "What If You Feel Like You Don't Want to Be in the Delivery Room at All?" section at the end. The more you know about what to expect during the labor and delivery, the less likely you are to worry that you won't be able to handle things.
- Lighten up. It's perfectly natural to be afraid for your partner's and baby's life. Actually, it would be rather surprising if you weren't.
- Remember that it rarely happens. In Jerrold Shapiro's study of more than two hundred expectant fathers, none of them fell apart during their partner's labor.
- Keep talking to your partner and let her know how you feel. The more supported and understood you are, the less likely you'll be to feel the need to do everything absolutely perfectly.
- Focus on the team. Your partner wants you—more than anyone else—to be there with her, to help get her through her labor. Knowing that you're a critical part of the process may help you pull it all together.
- Talk to some other dads who've experienced it. Most fathers who have will say it was some combination of tiring, exhilarating, amazing, boring, scary, exciting, bloody, annoying, and just about any other positive or negative feeling you can come up with. And just about all of them will also tell you they wouldn't have missed it for the world.

STAYING INVOLVED

Choosing a Name

Naming a child may sound like an easy task, but it's harder than you think. And you'd better start thinking about it soon because the second question you're going to hear after the baby comes (the first being "Boy or girl?") is "What's the baby's name?" Here are a few things you might want to keep in mind as you begin your search:

- Think about the future. That name that strikes you as unbearably cute right now might be unbearably ridiculous when your child gets nominated to the Supreme Court. Take the real-life case of the Jackson 5 (not the one Michael Jackson was in as a child): Appendicitis, Laryngitis, Meningitis, Peritonitis, and Tonsillitis. I'm sure those names seemed to their parents like a great idea at the time. As did Anne Aass, Jo King, Ray Gunn, Stan Still, Barb Dwyer, Paige Turner, Carrie Oakey, Ben Dover, and Justin Case—all of which are real names, found by researchers digging through birth certificates in the United States and Britain.
- Watch out for rhyming names (Jane Payne, Bill Hill).
- Watch out for initials. Before you make your final decision, think about what your baby's initials could spell. Terms like BFF, FBI, BLT, and SAT might or might not cause problems. But do you really want to saddle your child with HIV, STD, DNR (do not resuscitate), LOL, TMI, or WTF? Think about it.
- Do you need—or want—to honor a relative?
- Do you want a name that indicates your ethnic or religious background?
- Do you want something unique yet manageable?
- Do you want something easy to spell and/or pronounce?
- How do you feel about the nicknames that go with it?
- How does it sound with the last name? How would the nicknames sound with the last name?
- No, you can't use numbers. (There was a real-life court case a while back about a guy in Minnesota who tried to change his name to a number. He lost.)
- Make sure you have at least one middle initial. People with a middle initial are perceived by others as smarter and more intellectual—whether they actually are or not—and having two makes them seem even smarter, according to Wijnand A. P. van Tilburg of the University of Southampton (who has two) and Eric R. Igou of the University of Limerick, who, poor guy, has but one.

HOW TO PICK 'EM

Start by making a list of the ten boys' and ten girls' names you like best. Exchange lists with your partner and cross off all the ones on her list you couldn't possibly live with. She'll do the same to your list. If there are any left, you're in business. If not, keep repeating the process until you come up with names acceptable to you both. Some couples who cannot agree on two names decide instead to let one partner choose the name if it's a boy and the other choose the name if it's a girl (and let the loser choose the next child's name).

Not only is this little exercise fun, but it will also give you and your partner some interesting insights into each other's minds. My wife, for example, had never really taken my interest in mythology seriously until the names Odin (the chief god in Norse legends) and Loki (the Norse god of mischief and evil) showed up on my top-ten list. I don't know what I'm more grateful for, that both those choices were vetoed or that all three of my children are girls.

Another approach—albeit an odd one—to picking names is offered by Albert Mehrabian in his book *The Name Game.* Mehrabian surveyed two thousand people, asking them to judge several thousand first names and rate them according to success, morality, health, warmth, cheerfulness, masculinity/femininity. Not surprisingly, Mehrabian found that certain names evoke certain stereotypes. Bunny, for example, scored high on femininity, but low on morality and success. Ann and Holly were highly rated in all categories. For boys, Grover and Aldo were big losers in all categories, while Hans (go figure) was rated highly across the board.

That ought to give you plenty to start with. But if you still need a little help, there are literally hundreds of resources out there that can give you access to tens of thousands of names, their history, meanings, popularity, and more. A lot of websites have search engines designed to help you wade through the endless possibilities. The ones at www.greatdad.com and nameberry.com are among my favorites. We've listed some more in the Resources appendix.

FAMILY PRESSURES/TRADITIONAL CUSTOMS

In many cultures (or families), your choice of names may be severely limited by tradition:

- Among the Kikuyu people of Africa, the family's first son is named after the father's father; the second son, after the father's grandfather; the first daughter, after the father's mother; and so on.
- In Burma, each day of the week is assigned a different letter of the alphabet and children's names must begin with the letter of the day on which they were born.
- In Thailand, the parents may ask a nearby priest—or even a fortune-teller—to give their child just the right name.
- Jews of Eastern European extraction generally don't name babies after living people because of the traditional fear that the Angel of Death might take the baby instead of the older namesake. Jews of Spanish or Moroccan descent don't have the same worries.
- If there is someone on either side of a family who absolutely has to be honored with a name for the sake of family peace, you may be able to find a reasonable compromise. Harry Truman's parents, for example, gave him the middle initial S—no name, no period, just the initial—to satisfy both grandfathers (whose names were Solomon and Shippe).

What's in a Name? Waaaay More Than You Ever Thought

Some *onomasticians* (people who study names) claim that a child's name has a direct and profound effect on the kind of life, and success, he or she will have. Of course, there's a big difference between causation and correlation (meaning that just because two things seem related doesn't necessarily mean that one caused the other). Nevertheless, here are a few examples of some positively bizarre name-life connections.

- In one study, fifth- and sixth-grade teachers were asked to grade identical essays called "What I Did Last Sunday." The essays "written" by Michael and David were given one full grade higher than those "written" by Elmer and Hubert. Similarly, Karen and Lisa outperformed Bertha by one and a half grades.

- Nicholas Christenfeld and his colleagues identified a connection between life expectancy and people's three-letter initials. People with positive initials (like HUG, VIP, or WOW) live almost five years longer than those with negative initials (like BAD, ZIT, or RAT). Ernest Abel and Michael Kruger analyzed nearly 2,000 major league baseball players whose initials were acronyms or words, and who died before 1950. They found that players who had positive initials (like ACE and WIN) lived thirteen years longer than players with negative or neutral ones (like BUM or SOB). In fairness, I should mention that other researchers have disputed the life expectancy effect.

- Boys who have peculiar names (Armin, for instance) have a higher incidence of mental problems than boys with common ones or girls with peculiar ones. Leif Nelson and Joseph Simmons looked at ninety years' worth of pro baseball stats and found that players whose names begin with K (scoring shorthand for "strikeout") actually do strike out more (in 18.8 percent of their plate appearances) than other players (17.2 percent of appearances).

- Students whose names begin with A or B have higher grade point averages than students whose names begin with C or D. Oh, and it goes further than that. According to Nelson and Simmons, students whose names begin with A or B and go on to law school are much more likely to get into top schools (as ranked by U.S. News & World Report) than those with C or D initials.

- In a study by British researcher Philip Erwin, photographs of women labeled with names that score high on attractiveness scales (such as Jennifer, Katie,

Julia, and Christine) were rated as far more physically attractive than the identical photos labeled with "unattractive" names (like Ethel and Harriet).

- People generally like their names a lot. So much, in fact, that names may influence where your children live, what they do for a living, and the causes they support. For example, Brett Pelham, Matthew Mirenberg, and their colleagues discovered a disproportionate number of Mildreds in Milwaukee, Jacks in Jacksonville, Philips in Philadelphia, and Virginias in Virginia Beach. There's a similar connection between name and career: a disproportionate number of dentists are named Dennis or Denise, and a surprising number of geoscientists are named George. Just looking at hardware stores and roofing companies, hardware store owners were about 80 percent more likely to have names starting with H than R, and roofing companies were 70 percent more likely to be owned by people with first names starting with R than H.

The name effect applies in a number of other unexpected areas as well. For example, René Bekkers, a researcher at VU University Amsterdam, found that female alumni are more likely to make a donation to their alma mater when they're solicited by a student with a phonetically similar first name initial (Jane would be more likely to donate when called by Jenny or George than by Roberta); male alumni are more likely to donate when solicited by a student with a field of study similar to their own first name (George would be more likely to donate when called by a geology student than a computer nerd); and both males and females are more likely to give when their first name is similar to the name of the university (Jennifer would rather donate to Penn, and Harry would rather donate to Harvard—even though neither school really needs the money).

Others have found that people who share an initial with a disaster (hurricanes Katrina and Rita, for example) are more likely to donate to disaster relief; that teams made up of people with the same name or same first initial outperform those with random names; that investors are more likely to buy stock in a company that has a name similar to their own (Alphonse is more likely to buy Apple stock than Coke); and that people are more likely to engage with others on social media (in particular following on Twitter or adding to Google+ circles) when their names are the same or similar.

THE LAST-NAME GAME

If you and your partner already have the same last name, you haven't got anything to worry about; if you don't, there could be a few complications. Perhaps I spent too much time in Berkeley, but I've known people who have done at least one of the following when they had kids:

- Given the kids the man's last name (probably the most common)
- Given the kids the woman's last name (less common)
- Used the woman's last name as the child's first or middle name
- Given the kids a hyphenated last name (but when Mary Jane O'Flaherty-Ignetowski marries Roberto Goldberg-Yamahito, what will their children's last name be?)
- Made up a completely new last name
- Given the boys the man's last name, and the girls the woman's

Birth Announcements

WHEN TO ORDER

Since you don't know the weight, height, or (less commonly) sex of the baby before he or she is born, there's not much sense in having birth announcements printed until then. And in the era of mobile everything and social media, there may not be any sense in printing them at all. But running around trying to decide how you're going to get the word out to everyone you know is about the last thing you're going to want to do when you're sleep deprived out of your mind. So now's the perfect time to start shopping.

There are two basic types of birth announcements: hard copy and electronic.

The hard copy variety can be as low-tech as a preprinted card with blanks to fill in, which you can get at stationery or office-supply stores. You can also go to an online store or photo-printing site and use one of their standard designs or upload your own custom artwork. Select your design now, then log on and drop in the baby's vital statistics as soon as you know them. If you're going the hard-copy route, try to get the envelopes now and address them—or at least print up some labels—while your lives are still relatively calm.

The electronic route will probably be a little less labor intensive. All you need is your digital camera and web access and you can tweet, send e-vites, and update your blog, Facebook, or Google+ page from almost anywhere.

WHAT TO INCLUDE

As medical science becomes more exact, birth announcements will probably contain your baby's IQ, SAT scores, future profession, spouse's name, and number of

Baby Showers

Not too long ago, baby showers—like so many other baby-related activities—were considered "for women only." But today, if your partner's relatives or friends organize a shower for her, there's a good chance you'll be invited too. (But don't hold your breath waiting for your friends or relatives to plan one especially for you.)

The vast majority of baby showers take place several weeks or months before the baby is born, and the idea behind them is obvious: give the new parents a selection of baby clothing, furniture, toys, and the latest gadgets so the soon-to-be newborn can come home to a well-stocked nursery. If your relatives and friends are so inclined, enjoy—a shower can be a wonderful way to share your excitement about the coming event with others. Just don't forget to keep track of who gave what—after the birth, when you get around to those thank-you notes, all those yellow sleepers and *Where the Wild Things Are* dolls can look disconcertingly similar.

I've always thought, though, that having a baby shower before you've got a real baby in hand is kind of creepy—too much like tempting fate. After all, what if, God forbid, something were to happen to the baby? A friend of mine, when his wife was seven months pregnant, put a new patio in his backyard and carved the name of his yet-to-be-born son (they'd done an amnio) in the wet concrete. I could hardly bring myself to go back there until after the baby was safely home. Anyway, if you join me in the anti-shower camp, you may find that some people will be offended by your not wanting one. In such cases, try to steer them toward a post-birth shower instead (call it a "Welcome Baby" or "Baby Birthday" party if you want to stay away from the word "shower"). Be firm. Stressing how much more fun it will be for the guests to get presents for a baby whose name and gender are known may also make the no-shower news easier to swallow.

children. But for now, all you really need to include is the baby's name, date and time of birth, weight, length (since they can't stand up, babies don't usually have "height"), and the names of the parents. Oh, and in all the rush, don't forget to include a photo of the baby.

WHERE TO SEND 'EM

Family and friends are the obvious recipients. When it comes to more casual acquaintances and business associates, however, take it easy. Many people will feel obligated to send a gift if they receive a birth announcement, so don't send one to anyone from whom you wouldn't feel comfortable getting a gift. Exceptions include people who request an announcement as a memento, employers or employees who have already given you and/or your partner a baby gift and/or shower, and people to whom your parents and in-laws ask you to send announcements.

Classes

Until the late 1960s, there really was no such thing as childbirth education. Basically, all you had to know to have a baby was where the hospital was located. And all that expectant parents did to prepare for the arrival of their baby was set up a nursery. Women checked into the hospital, labored alone in stark, sterile rooms, received general anesthesia, and woke up groggy and tender, not knowing the sex of the child they'd delivered, and sometimes even the number of children. Meanwhile, men were left to pace anxiously in hospital waiting rooms until a nurse came to give them the happy news. Fathers who tried to buck their nonrole in the birth of their children were in for a real surprise.

In 1522, a German guy named Dr. Wertt (no one knows what kind of doctor he was) wanted to learn about childbirth and see midwives in action. So he dressed up as a woman and slipped in to watch a delivery. Unfortunately, someone saw through the disguise and raised quite a stink. Poor Wertt was burned at the stake. Seems a touch harsh, doesn't it?

More than four hundred years later, not much had changed. Dr. Robert Bradley, who originated the Bradley method, cites the 1965 case of a man who was arrested and fined for having "gained unauthorized admission to a hospital's delivery room in an attempt to witness the birth of his second child." Hey, at least he wasn't burned to death.

In her book *The Experience of Childbirth,* Sheila Kitzinger, a pioneering birth educator, quotes from a publication put out by the British Medical Association in 1959: "The last requirement of all for a successful delivery at home is the husband— the poor father. If he is of the right mentality, and very few are, he may sustain his wife's morale during the first part of her labour. Otherwise, he is best employed making tea, keeping the kettles boiling, and answering the front doorbell."

And in 1975, Evelyn and Bruce Fitzgerald, Debra and Michael Greener, and at least eight other couples who had gone through a Lamaze course were told by Porter Memorial Hospital in Indiana that hospital policy prohibited "the presence of any person or persons in the Delivery Rooms located in the Obstetrics Ward other than members of the Medical Staff and Nursing Staff." In other words, no dads allowed. The Fitzgeralds and the other couples sued, and asked the court to decide a fairly simple question: does a father have a constitutional right to be present—per the wishes of himself, the mother, or their physician—in the delivery room of a public hospital during the birth of a child? The answer was no.

Over the years, the situation gradually changed, and today, as I'm sure you're well aware, it's hard to find a man who hasn't already, or isn't planning to, attend the birth of his children (according to recent statistics, over 90 percent of fathers-to-be are present at the birth) and just about everyone involved in the process—from parents to doctors—has given the word *preparation* a whole new meaning. Mothers and fathers frequently attend prenatal OB/GYN visits together, and many embark on a reading program reminiscent of cramming for college exams. In addition, most expectant couples sign up for childbirth preparation classes.

When my wife got pregnant for the first time, one of the first things we did was read everything we could get our hands on. By the time the baby was born, we'd probably read enough magazine and newspaper articles, books, and pamphlets to qualify for a degree in prenatal education. But unlike my various "real" degrees, which were fairly useless once I got out into the real world, my education in childbirth and parenting served me quite well.

SELECTING A BIRTHING CLASS

When the first childbirth preparation classes appeared in the late 1960s, the emphasis was on how to have a "natural," unmedicated childbirth. Recently, however, the focus has changed somewhat. While natural childbirth is still the goal of most classes today, the overriding principle is that the more you learn about pregnancy and the birth process—from good nutrition and exercise to the types of pain medications most frequently given to laboring women—the less you have to fear and the more in control you'll feel.

Although a lot of people use the terms *Lamaze* and *childbirth preparation class* interchangeably, there are in fact quite a few very different childbirth methods. What distinguishes one from another is the approach each takes to dealing with pain. Here's a little information about the most common methods.

LAMAZE

In the early 1950s, French obstetrician Ferdinand Lamaze took a trip to the Soviet Union to check out the latest medical advances. He was especially interested in *psychoprophylaxis*, which the Russians were billing as a revolutionary way of relieving childbirth pain. Psychoprophylaxis was too big a mouthful, so people started calling it the Pavlov method, since it was based on Ivan Pavlov's (yes, the guy with the dogs) theory that learned reflexes can be overcome by repetition and training. In this case, the learned reflex is pain and the way to overcome it is by focusing on something else—the woman's own breathing. According to historian

John Bell, instructors were supposed to "emphasize that Pavlovian science and a benevolent Soviet government had freed women from the curse of labor pain."

Unfortunately, benevolent or not, the Soviets weren't terribly popular in the Russophobic West in the 1950s. So the method was renamed Lamaze. Oddly, though, the method's supporters have backed off the painless part. According to an article on www.pregnancy-info.net, "Contrary to what many people may believe, Lamaze does not actually aim to make the labor process less painful." And an article on www.durhamlamaze.com adds that Lamaze classes help women understand the value of pain and learn how to respond to pain in ways that both facilitate labor and increase comfort. Hmmm.

Today, Lamaze doesn't focus solely on drug-free, if not entirely painless, labor and delivery. The object is to give expectant parents the knowledge they need to be able to make well-founded decisions. You can take classes privately or at just about any hospital. Visit www.lamaze.org.

BRADLEY

Like Lamaze, the Bradley method believes in educating and preparing the expectant parents for the labor and delivery experience. But instead of trying to distract the woman's attention from her pain, Bradley believes that she should just "go with it." If she feels like groaning, she's encouraged to groan; if she feels like screaming, she's encouraged to scream. The Bradley method also devotes a lot of attention to exercise and nutrition. Over 90 percent of Bradley graduates have "natural" births. Bradley was the original "husband-coached" childbirth method and does more to include the father than any of the other methods. Visit www.bradleybirth.com.

HYPNOBIRTHING/MONGAN METHOD/DICK-READ

Grantly Dick-Read, an English obstetrician who, like most of his colleagues in the early part of the twentieth century, used chloroform to ease his patients' labor pains, developed a theory that fear is the source of pain during labor and delivery. Here's how it works: when someone's afraid, the "fight or flight" instinct kicks in, drains blood away from organs that don't need it—such as the face—and pumps it to the organs that need it most, such as the legs. (Hence the expression "white as a sheet.") Fear also diverts blood away from the uterus (if you have one), leaving it unable to function correctly, which results in pain. "Severe pain does not have to be an accompaniment of labor," they say. Get rid of the fear, then—by relaxation techniques, affirmations, or even hypnosis—and the pain will be reduced as well. Dick-Read's theory—which is still very much in vogue today—was so radical at the time that it got him bounced out of the British Medical Society. Visit www. hypnobirthing.com.

"Coach"—Don't Use That Word

Almost all of the most common childbirth methods now refer to the man as the childbirth "coach"—a term that seems to have been coined by Dr. Bradley. Today most expectant fathers (at least those who take childbirth classes) and their partners view themselves in those terms, but I agree with Professor Katharyn May that there are some very compelling reasons to erase the word from your non-sports vocabulary.

- We all know what happens to coaches when things don't go according to plan…
- The coach concept focuses attention on your role during the brief period of labor and delivery but minimizes how important you've been throughout the pregnancy and how important you'll be to your child after the birth.
- The coach concept reinforces the sexist stereotype that you're some kind of prop, rather than a unique individual who's in the process of sharing a challenging life experience with your partner. It also places way too much pressure on you by implying that you should be providing direction if things don't go quite the way they're supposed to during labor and birth. Does anyone seriously expect that, after maybe twenty hours of classes and absolutely no medical training, you're going to know how to handle a true emergency? So if anyone calls you "coach," tell them you're not—you're the child's father.

McMOYLER METHOD

Started by an experienced labor and delivery nurse named Sarah McMoyler, this method is aimed at the needs of today's busy parents and picks up where the others leave off. McMoyler's main emphasis is on education: since labor and delivery are completely unpredictable, it's best to learn about everything and anything that could possibly happen on that big day. Students are encouraged to work *with* the medical team and trust them, instead of being suspicious. With McMoyler, there's no such thing as failure. Natural childbirth is the goal, but if things don't go according to plan (and they rarely do), there's no guilt and no regret. If you walk out of the hospital with a healthy baby and a healthy mom, you win. Visit www.thebestbirth.com

LESS COMMON METHODS

- Leboyer is based on the philosophy of Frédérick Leboyer, a French obstetrician, who contends that the bright lights and noise of today's delivery rooms

163

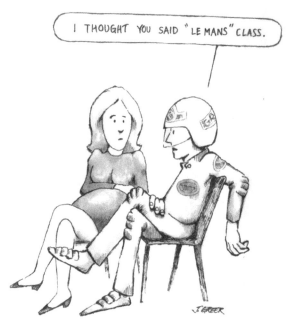

are quite stressful and upsetting for a newborn. Leboyer babies are generally born in dimmed rooms, often with the mother fully or partially submerged in warm water.

- Birthing From Within is a spiritually focused approach based on the philosophy that childbirth is a profound rite of passage, not a medical event. Visit www. birthingfromwithin.com.
- BirthWorks is based on the idea that women's bodies were designed to give birth and that the knowledge about how to give birth already exists inside every woman. Visit birthworks.org.
- Alexander Technique focuses on freedom of movement, balance, support, and coordination. Visit www.amsatonline.org.

Childbirth classes usually run five to nine weeks (although McMoyler classes are conducted over two half days or one very full one). Your practitioner is probably the best source of recommendations and information on where childbirth classes meet and how to sign up. If you can't find one you like, check their websites for web-based classes.

Whatever you do, take one as soon as you possibly can. The knowledge you'll get will help ease some of your anxieties for the rest of the pregnancy. Before you sign up, though, it's important to reach an agreement with your partner about the childbirth philosophy that best fits your family. Does your partner want drugs if they're offered? How 'bout you? (No one will be offering you any drugs, no matter how badly you may want them—the question is whether you'd prefer that she get medical pain relief or do without.) I've heard of cases in which the woman wants an epidural and the dad gets angry because he had his heart set on a natural birth. There are also instances when the dad can't stand to see his partner in pain anymore and suggests drugs, and she gets angry with him. If you can't reach an agreement, suck it up and give her 51 percent of the vote. It's best to talk these things out in advance, though. A woman in the throes of a difficult labor should really not be making major decisions.

PREPARING YOUR OLDER KIDS

While millions of second- and third-time parents sign up for some kind of childbirth classes, very few of them ever consider that their older children might need some preparation as well. Here are a few things you can do to help get those big sisters- and brothers-to-be ready:

- Sign them up for a class too. A lot of hospitals offer classes for soon-to-be older siblings.
- Try to have them spend some time with new babies.
- Give them some practice. Use a life-size doll to show them how to hold an infant and support its head. Demonstrate the proper way to touch a baby and explain the need to be gentle, but do not poke, or prod, or hit the doll to illustrate behavior to avoid. You'll just be showing the big kid exactly how to do what she's not supposed to do.
- Get them excited. Show them pictures of new babies, have them make a drawing for the new baby, even let them pick out some furniture or clothes or the color of the new baby's room.
- Prepare yourself for some disappointment. Most brand-new older siblings are thrilled—for a while. When the novelty wears off, they're going to want to go back to being the center of the universe. See the "Helping Older Kids Adjust to

Infant CPR

Another class you should try to fit in this month is baby CPR (if you wait until after the baby comes, you'll never get around to it). Hopefully, you'll never have to use the skills you'll learn, but learn them anyway—for your own peace of mind and for your baby's safety. You can find out where to sign up from your birth class instructor, your baby's pediatrician (if you've picked one already), the hospital you've chosen, or your local American Red Cross.

What Childbirth Classes Don't Teach You

Most childbirth prep classes are taught in groups and give you an opportunity to ask questions about the pregnancy in a less hurried environment than your practitioner's office. They also allow you to socialize a little with other expectant couples and compare notes. But there are a couple of things you probably won't learn there.

- Socialization isn't worth much for the father. In the first birthing class I took, the teacher lectured most of the time, and the socializing consisted of the women discussing how much weight they'd gained, how painful their backs were, the color and consistency of their vaginal discharges, and how many times a night they had to get up to pee. From my perspective, that was a complete waste of time. What was helpful for me was the educational part of the class itself. By the time we'd finished, I felt that whatever happened, whether we had an unmedicated birth or a medicated one, whether my wife had a C-section or an episiotomy (an incision to enlarge the vaginal opening), I'd at least have some idea what was happening and what to do.

- Dude, it's not just about Mom. Over the years, I've interviewed many men whose experiences were very similar to mine. Generally speaking, they felt all but left out by the instructors, who focused almost exclusively on the mothers. Of course, that's important. But she's not the only one becoming a parent. As British researchers John Lee and Virginia Schmied put it, "Men are not present at the birth solely to support women—they are there in their own right, as father of the child." Sure, guys learn some important things, but with their concerns all but ignored, they usually walk out feeling more like mommy's little helper than dads.

Their New Sibling" section on pages 264–66 for tips on how to help the kids—and yourself—through this transition.

GETTING SOME EXTRA HELP

Reading this book will help you prepare yourself for the emotional and physical experiences you and your partner will be going through during pregnancy and birth. But while the two of you are actually in the midst of labor, you're both in a state of trauma. You're both under pressure, and you both need support—physical as well as psychological.

Your partner has you to help her through. And she has her practitioner and the rest of the medical team. But what about you?

What's the solution? Set up a time to hang out with the other guys in the class. I've taught classes for expectant dads for years, and I can guarantee you that men simply will not talk about the issues that really concern them if there's a woman—especially a spouse—in the room. A two-hour get-together with a group of men who are going through the same thing will be far more meaningful than the rest of the coed class.

If you get any resistance on this from your partner, tell her what Australian researcher Andrea Robertson says: "It is unfair to expect men to provide practical help and emotional support if their own needs are not being met during what is an anxious time for both parents." And as John Lee and Virginia Schmied have found, when men have a chance to explore their feelings about pregnancy, childbirth, and parenting (which isn't going to happen in a regular class), they're "more involved with their spouse and participate more with housework after the baby is born."

Finally, it's okay to question authority. No matter how much you've read or how thorough your class is, something you don't understand is bound to happen during the labor or delivery. When it does, don't become a wallflower and let the practitioners take control of the whole process (unless it's a true medical emergency). Your child—not the doctor's or the nurse's—is about to be born, and you have the right to get your questions answered. So ask someone to explain what's happening and what they're doing, every step of the way. If you miss something the first time, ask again. Keep in mind, though, that there's a big difference between being assertive and being annoying or confrontational, so be nice.

Each time my wife was in labor, I tried to do everything they'd taught me in the classes we'd taken: I reassured her, held her, told her stories, massaged her back and legs, mopped her brow, encouraged her, "helped" her breathe, and fed her ice chips. It was absolutely exhausting and sometimes scary, and I sure could have used a break (and an occasional back rub), but there wasn't anyone around to do it.

Fortunately, however, there is a way to help ease the burden—both yours and your partner's—of the trauma of labor and delivery: get yourselves a doula.

WHAT IS A *DOULA*?

As we discussed on page 19, a doula is someone who's supposed to be there throughout labor, to give your partner *and* you emotional and physical support.

According to Dr. Marshall Klaus, the doula concept is hardly a new one. For hundreds of years, pregnant women in more than 125 cultures have gone through labor with another woman at their side the whole time. This used to be the case in the U.S. as well. But in the 1930s women began to have their children in hospitals instead of at home, and everyone but the laboring woman and her doctors was barred from the delivery room. In 1980 Dr. Klaus and his colleagues reintroduced the doula concept in the United States and gave it its name.

I've got to confess that when I met with Dr. Klaus, my first reaction was: no way. I've got too much invested in this pregnancy, and nobody is going to come between me and my wife during this critical stage. But as I continued talking to Dr. Klaus and reading the research on doulas, I began to change my mind.

It turns out that the presence of a doula can have some rather dramatic effects, potentially shortening the length of a woman's labor and reducing the odds she'll need pain medication, forceps delivery, or a Cesarean section. Considering my wife's history of long, painful labor, I began to feel that having a doula around the next time might be the way to go.

But I still had questions: Would a doula do anything for me? Wouldn't she just push me out of the way? Not according to Dr. Klaus. "We make the mistake of thinking that a father can take a birthing class and be prepared to be the main source of support and knowledge for the entire labor. That's just unreasonable. A doula can reach out to the man, decreasing his anxiety, giving him support and encouragement, and allowing him to interact with his partner in a more caring and nurturing fashion." In one interesting study a researcher compared couples who had a doula present with others who didn't. The study found that men in both groups spent about the same amount of time with their partners.

Back on page 19, I talked about some of the problems associated with doulas. But there are plenty of people—including medical professionals—who swear by them. One of the main advantages is that your partner will have more consistent support. The doctors and nurses are usually juggling five or six patients at the same time, meaning that they won't be able to focus very much on your partner and you. Shift changes just make the care even more disjointed. So if you're feeling that you really want someone (besides you) to be there throughout the whole ordeal, a doula may be the way to go. (Keep in mind that doulas do not deliver babies—that's something your practitioner and the medical team will handle. When it comes time to push, it's nice if your partner can be guided through by a nurse who's had a chance to get to know her. That's harder to accomplish when a doula is present.)

Doulas—Some Basic Q's and A's, Dos and Don'ts

- What do they charge? Most doulas charge a flat fee. The national average is around $700, although the range can be anywhere from $300 to $1,500, depending on where you live, how long she'll be with you, and what you want her to do. This usually includes one or two prenatal visits, labor and delivery—from whenever you first feel you need the doula until one to three hours after the birth—and a few postpartum visits to answer any questions you or your partner might have and to help your partner get started breastfeeding.
- Will my insurance company pick up the tab? There's no hard and fast rule about this. But more and more insurers are finding that paying for a doula can significantly reduce their other birth-related costs. You may also be able to pay your doula through your company's flexible spending program or a Health Savings Account. But check with your company's HR department or your insurer to confirm.
- Where can I find one? Ask your partner's practitioner to recommend a doula he or she has worked with. You can get referrals from Yelp, DONA International (www.dona.org), DoulaMatch.net, or Doula World (www.doulaworld.com).
- Interview any prospective doula. You want someone who shares your vision for how you'd like the birth to go. Flexibility is key. You don't want someone who's going to storm out of the room in a huff if your partner decides she wants an epidural.
- Have her meet the rest of the team. If the doula and your partner's OB or midwife don't already know each other, giving them a chance to meet before labor starts can go a long way toward avoiding problems later.
- Confirm that she's on board for you too, and that she acknowledges you as your partner's primary support person.

WHAT IF YOU FEEL LIKE YOU DON'T WANT TO BE IN THE DELIVERY ROOM AT ALL?

Years ago, no one expected men to be involved in their partners' pregnancies or to be there for the births of their children. But today, men who aren't jumping up and down about the idea of being in the delivery room are generally considered insensitive Neanderthals. The problem with such a black-and-white approach is that, as Katharyn May says, "there's a fine line between finding options for father participation, and pressuring men to adopt levels of involvement which may be unwanted or inappropriate for them."

The truth is that not all of us feel the same need to be involved, and the last place some men should be is in the delivery room. You may be squeamish during medical procedures, prone to fainting at the sight of blood or needles, or worried about losing control during labor. You may not want to see your partner in pain, or you may simply be feeling ambivalent about the pregnancy. You may be worried that you'll feel useless and get shoved off into a corner somewhere. Or you might even be feeling resentful about the pressure other people are putting on you to get involved.

You may be frightened by what you saw in some of the movies you viewed during your childbirth prep class, or you may worry (as a number of new dads have told me) that you won't be able to get those images of a baby coming out of a vagina out of your mind. It's important to remember that these feelings—as well as any other reasons you might have for just not wanting to be there—are not only completely normal, they're shared by more men than you might think.

If you're feeling less than overjoyed about being involved in the labor and delivery, don't beat yourself up too badly or allow yourself to feel like a failure. You're not. In fact, as many as half of all expectant fathers have at least some ambivalence about participating in childbirth. Clearly, being forced into a role that isn't comfortable for you will do you and your partner more harm than good. But there are a few things you might want to try that could help you get over some of your concerns.

- Talk to other fathers. Other dads you know may have been through something similar and may have some suggestions. Even if they don't, it's often very reassuring to get some living proof that you're not alone.
- Talk to your partner. Let her know what you're feeling and why. At the same time, reassure her about your commitment to her and to the baby.
- Understand what your partner is thinking. Instead of being sympathetic, she may interpret your apprehensiveness as a sign that you don't care about her or the baby.
- Do it for her. No matter how well you explain it to your partner, your desire to miss the birth or to miss the classes is probably going to hurt her. If you can stomach it at all, at least try to take the class—it will help her feel more understood, and you might just learn what it is that's been bothering you.
- Consider a doula. See pages 167–69 for information about doulas.
- Don't worry about how your child will turn out. While there's plenty of evidence about the positive impact on children of early paternal bonding, your not being

there for the actual birth—whether it's because you didn't want to or because you simply couldn't—will not cripple your children; you'll still be able to establish a strong relationship with them. Just make sure you're there right after the birth.

- Don't give in to the pressure. If, after everything is said and done, you still don't feel comfortable participating, don't. But be prepared: your family, friends, and medical practitioner will probably suggest that you just quit pouting and do what you're "supposed to." If you're among the 10–15 percent of adults who pass out at the sight of blood, or the 10 percent who have a phobia of needles, and that's why you'd rather not be in the delivery room, you might want to tell your critics about the tragic case of Steven Passalaqua. Passalaqua, whose wife was in labor, was asked by hospital staff "to hold and steady his wife" while an anesthesiologist "inserted an epidural needle into her back." Seeing the needle caused Steven to faint, and he hit his head on a piece of molding at the base of the wall. He died two days later. Of course, that's an extreme case, but it ought to get people off your back for a while.

A Note for Deployed Dads

What can I say? You want to be there, your wife wants you to be there, but Uncle Sam needs you somewhere else right now. Despite the distance, though, there are a number of things you can do to stay connected with your wife (and, later, your baby).

- Make sure your wife knows every possible way to contact you, just in case she needs to reach you quickly.
- Talk to your CO about whether you can get a few days off. The military does offer some paternity leave, but exactly how much you'll be able to take is impossible to pin down. The good news is that it won't count against your regular thirty days' leave. The bad news is that it's trumped by the needs of the military, so there's no guarantee that you'll actually make it. However, just having made the effort shows your wife that you're committed to her and the baby and will boost your stock in her eyes.
- Check into whether you can set up a real-time phone or video conference for the delivery. It's not the same as being there, but in this case, close counts for a lot. If you have access to high-speed Internet and a webcam, get signed up with one of the many free, real-time video services, such as Skype or Google+ Hangouts. I've heard wonderful stories from service members who used video conferencing to watch the birth of their baby, see the kids in their Halloween costumes, or even participate in parent-teacher conferences. You could, I suppose, use this technology to keep an eye on what the painter's doing during your remodeling project too.

Banking on the Future: Cord Blood and Tissue

Unless you're a paramedic or an emergency room doctor, you probably don't have a lot of opportunities to save lives. But for a few minutes after your baby is born you'll have a chance to do just that. Best of all, you'll be able to do it with something you otherwise might have thrown out: your baby's umbilical cord.

The blood inside the umbilical cord is an incredibly rich source of *stem cells*, which can be used to treat dozens of conditions, including leukemia and a number of blood- and immune-system-related disorders such as sickle-cell disease. Tissue inside the cord contains different types of stem cells, which have the ability to transform into all different types of cells and could be used to treat a far broader range of conditions. As technology advances, researchers are looking at cord blood and cord tissue as potential cures for everything from torn ligaments and diabetes to heart disease, Alzheimer's, and spinal cord injuries.

So what can you do? Well, you have two basic choices: donate the cord blood and tissue so some other person can benefit, or store them for your own family's use. Let me give you some of the pros and cons of each of these options:

- Public donation. This is a free option. Your partner will need to register between weeks twenty-eight and thirty-four of the pregnancy. Assuming enough blood can be collected (usually three to five ounces) and the mother meets certain requirements (for example, she must be free of HIV, most cancers, diabetes, and a number of other conditions), your baby's cord blood and tissue (not all public donation sites accept tissue yet) will be analyzed and frozen for storage. It will then be listed in a national registry where surgeons from all over the world can search for matches for patients who need stem-cell transplants. Unfortunately, because of the high costs of collecting and storing cord blood, there are only about two dozen facilities in the United States that can take donations. If your baby won't be born in one of them, there are a number of mail-in options.
- Private banking. If you can afford it, private cord blood banking can be an

---

- Read as much as you can about what's left of the pregnancy—how the baby is developing, and what your wife is going through. When you get close to the due date, start in on a book that covers childbirth and infancy. Again, you want to understand as much as you can about what's happening with your wife and baby. And don't forget to think about yourself too. You may not be able to see excellent insurance policy—especially if you have a family history of leukemia or any of the other diseases that can be treated with cord blood, and/or your child belongs to an ethnic minority or is multiracial. People of a mixed-race heritage historically have a much harder time finding bone marrow matches than Caucasians. Privately banking your newborn's cord blood and tissue is the only way to provide a 100 percent guarantee that you will have access to stem cells that are a perfect match for future medical treatments. Initial costs for cord blood typically range from about $1,500 to over $2,000. For tissue banking, add another $1,000 or so. Annual storage fees range from about $130 to over $300.

The public-vs.-private decision is one that only you and your partner can make. Both methods are medically safe and painless for the mother and baby, because the cord blood and tissue are collected after the baby is born. If you're having trouble deciding or need more information on your options, the Parents' Guide to Cord Blood Foundation (www.parentsguidecordblood.org) has great resources, including a searchable map of public and private donation sites for an unbiased review of the options.

If you're interested in donating your baby's cord blood, start by talking with your partner's OB now. Most public banks like to get the testing and screening processes started before the thirty-fourth week of pregnancy. You should also make contact with the National Marrow Donor Program (www.marrow.org), which maintains the largest listing of cord blood units in the world. They have a huge amount of excellent information about stem cells and cord blood donation on their website.

If you're interested in exploring private banking, start with your partner's OB. You should also do some research right now to find the best possible bank. Important factors to consider include the company's financial stability (less chance it will go out of business), its age, the number of samples it currently stores, and whether it provides a complete listing of fees.

or hold your baby, but fatherhood is changing you too, and it's nice to know how. The more up-to-date you are on where everyone is, the easier it will be for you to plug into the routines when you get home. This book and the sequel, *The New Father: A Dad's Guide to the First Year*, will walk you through everything you need to know.

- Send presents, love notes, and jewelry. Flowers may seem like a complete waste of money, but send some anyway.
- If you haven't deployed yet, do as many of the following as you can before you go:
  - Burn a CD or DVD, or record an audio or video on your phone of you reading some simple children's books. Before the birth, ask your wife to play them near her belly. Once the baby is born, she can play that same CD/DVD; plus you can record new stories, songs, poems, or whatever, until you're able to take over the story-reading duties yourself. This will help the baby recognize you—well, your voice anyway—when you come home. If you need help getting any of this set up—or you didn't get a chance to do it before you shipped out—it's not too late. Check out United Through Reading (www.unitedthroughreading.org).
  - Don't take a shower just yet…Right before you leave, wear a few shirts to bed and have your wife keep them around (unwashed) until after the birth. Like kittens and puppies, young humans acquire a lot of information about their world through their sense of smell, and the hope is that if your baby is exposed to your smell, it'll be easier for him to bond with you when you get home.
  - Strike a pose. Have your wife or someone else take pictures of you doing your favorite things, eating your favorite foods, hanging out with your favorite people, and so on. Print out the best shots, laminate them, and get them bound together. This will give your child a chance to get to know a little bit about you—and gnaw on you—while you're away.
  - Ask your wife to send things to keep you in the loop. Before the birth, this could be an ultrasound picture or a recording of your baby's heartbeat. After the baby comes, photos, worn outfits, and a full-length cutout of the baby are nice. If someone filmed the birth, she may want to send that video along too. But think about whether you really want to see your wife in incredible pain that you can't do anything to stop.
  - Send more presents, flowers, and a gift certificate for a spa day. Poetry, even bad poetry, is appreciated.
  - Ask a friend to take the childbirth class with your wife if she hasn't already lined up someone else.
  - Ask friends to help. And make sure they understand what you mean. Most people define help as holding the baby for a few minutes, cooing, and then giving him back. Your definition of help should include laundry, shopping, meal preparation, or reroofing the garage.

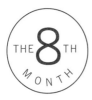

Making a List and Checking It Twice

WHAT'S GOING ON WITH YOUR PARTNER

Physically

- Even stronger fetal activity
- Heavier vaginal discharge
- Overall discomfort getting more severe
- Frequent urination
- Sleeplessness—can that really be a surprise?
- Increased fatigue
- Shortness of breath as the baby takes up more room and presses against her internal organs
- Water retention, and swelling of the hands, feet, and ankles
- More frequent Braxton-Hicks contractions

Emotionally

- Feeling special—people are giving her their seats on buses or in crowded rooms, store clerks go out of their way to help her
- Feeling a bond with others, like a member of a secret club (strangers keep coming up to tell her about their own pregnancy experiences or to touch her belly); she might also be scared by all those horror stories or angry at the unsolicited touches
- Feeling exceptionally attractive—or ugly
- Relieved that the baby would survive if born now

- Worried about whether the baby will be normal, what he'll look like, whether she'll be able to cope with the responsibilities of motherhood, and whether her body will ever get back to normal
- Afraid her water will break in public

WHAT'S GOING ON WITH THE BABY

At this point, most babies will have assumed the head-down position that they'll maintain for the rest of the pregnancy. He's getting big and fat: eighteen inches long, five pounds (a little less if he's sharing his quarters with a sibling), and his body now looks a little more like it belongs with that huge—and probably pretty hairy—head. With practically no room to maneuver around, the baby's movements are becoming a little less frequent but often so powerful that you can often tell which part of his body is doing the poking. His little heart is pumping something like 300 gallons of blood every day (yours pumps around 2,000), and his sense of hearing is getting so good that he now responds differently to your partner's and your voices. Chances of survival outside the womb are excellent.

WHAT'S GOING ON WITH YOU

Dealing with the Public Nature of Pregnancy

As intensely private as pregnancy is, it's also inescapably public. Your partner's growing belly can bring out the best—and the worst—in people. Perfect strangers will open doors for her, offer to help her carry things, give up their seats in crowded subway cars and buses. In some ways, people's interest in pregnant women and in the process of creating life is heartwarming. But there may come a point when this outpouring of interest in her status and concern for her comfort begins to feel like an invasion of privacy.

People would often come up to my wife when she was standing in the checkout line at the grocery store and start chatting. The "conversations" would usually begin fairly innocuously, with questions like "So, when are you due?" or pronouncements about the baby's gender. But after a while the horror stories would inevitably come out—tales of debilitating morning sickness, ten-month pregnancies, thirty-hour labors, emergency C-sections, anesthesia that didn't work, and on and on. And as if that weren't enough, people would, without even asking, start touching, rubbing, or patting her belly as if she were a Buddha statue or a magic lantern.

Perhaps the strangest thing about the public nature of pregnancy is that a surprising (to me, anyway) number of women seem to take it all in stride. I kept waiting for my wife to bite some belly-rubber's hand off, but she never did. Not everyone stays so calm, though. I've heard stories of women reacting to being groped by strangers by screaming, wearing "keep your paws off my belly" T-shirts, slapping their hand, telling them of a highly contagious disease that's transmitted by touch, or even reaching out and fondling their belly in return. Why anyone tolerates this is a mystery to me. Can you imagine how you'd react if someone did the same thing when your partner *wasn't* pregnant? Or if you decided to touch some woman's breasts because they looked so inviting?

For men, this touching business can bring out feelings of anger and protectiveness: "Nobody touches my woman!" If this happens to you, it's best to take your cues from your partner. If she doesn't mind, try to relax. But prepare yourself. You're going to have to deal with a very similar situation after she gives birth, when complete strangers come up and start fondling your baby—without even washing their hands.

Panic

Just about six weeks before our first daughter was born, I suddenly had a great epiphany: our childless days were about to be over. It wasn't that I was worried about becoming a father—I already felt confident and prepared for my new role: I'd read a lot of material about becoming a parent, my wife and I had been taking childbirth classes, and we'd thoroughly discussed our concerns and fears. What struck me was much more superficial: once the baby came, it would be a long time before we'd be able to go to movies, plays, or concerts (or just about anyplace where you might have to be quiet), or even stay out late with our friends.

As it turned out, my wife was feeling the same thing at about the same time, so during the last two months of the first pregnancy, we ate out more often, went to more movies, saw more plays, and spent more late evenings with friends than in the next three years combined. A lot of expectant dads who are worried about the impending loss of their social lives find themselves looking up and visiting old friends they haven't seen for years.

In addition to trying to pack a lot of fun activities into the final few months of the pregnancy, you might want to consider cramming in a few practical things as well. For instance, when you (or your partner) are cooking a meal, try to double or even triple the recipes and freeze what's left over in two-person servings. Believe me, during that first postpartum week, defrosting a container of frozen spaghetti sauce is a lot easier than making a new batch from scratch.

Nesting

After morning sickness and 2 A.M. cravings for pickles, perhaps the most famous stereotype about pregnancy is a woman's "nesting instinct." Most women, at some point in their pregnancies, become obsessed (often unconsciously) with preparing the house for the new arrival: closets and cupboards are cleaned, and furniture that hasn't been budged for years suddenly has to be swept under.

Although much has been made of the woman's instinct, a number of studies have shown that almost all expectant fathers experience some sort of nesting instinct themselves. It often plays out in stereotypical provider-protector behavior: worrying about finances and the family's physical safety. Most expectant dads start thinking a lot about—or become obsessed with—saving money, and many finally get around to important things they've been avoiding dealing with, like getting life insurance and writing a will.

A lot of nesting dads start eyeing minivans in a way they never have before. And some end up buying a vehicle with every conceivable safety feature, from sensors that help you avoid collisions, monitor your blind spot, and keep you in your lane to the most advanced airbag and seatbelt systems and the latest in military technology, including drive-flat tires and bulletproof glass (okay, we can skip the military stuff, but you get the point).

Many men spend a lot of time assembling—or even building—cribs, changing tables, and other baby furniture; shopping for baby supplies; painting and preparing the baby's room; rearranging furniture; and even trying to find a larger living space for their growing families. Other guys take care of all those things that have been on their to-do lists for months: cleaning the gutters, getting the car tuned up and its tires changed, installing fire and smoke alarms, finally learning to square dance. For some men, these activities are a way to keep busy and to avoid feeling

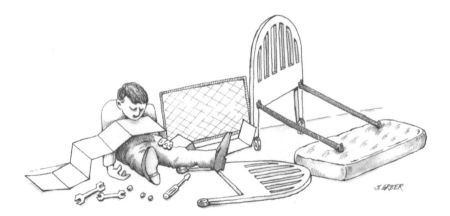

left out. But for others, they represent something much more fundamental. As Pamela Jordan writes, "These nesting tasks may be the first opportunity the father has to do something for the baby rather than his pregnant mate."

Sex—Again

While the second trimester is frequently a time of increased sexual desire and activity, during the third trimester your sex life is bound to suffer. The most common reasons for this are:

- A mutual fear of hurting the baby or your partner.
- Fear that your partner's orgasm might trigger premature labor.
- Your partner's physical discomfort.
- Your partner's changing body makes the "usual" sexual positions uncomfortable.
- Your sense of changing roles. Soon your partner will no longer simply be your partner; she's going to be a mother—someone just like your own mother. Remember that as she begins to see you as a father, she may have similar (often subconscious) thoughts.

Unless your partner's doctor has told you otherwise, sex still poses no physical risk to the baby or to your partner. As we discussed on pages 123–26, if you're both still interested in sex (and I've heard from a lot of dads whose sex drive actually increased toward the end of the pregnancy), now would be a good time to try out some new and different positions. Again, if you and your partner aren't in sync, sexually speaking, it's critical to talk things through.

Several researchers have noted that a small number of expectant fathers have affairs during the late stages of their partners' pregnancies. But these "late-pregnancy affairs" rarely happen for the reasons you might think. Jerrold Shapiro found that most men who have had a late-pregnancy extramarital affair share the following characteristics:

- They felt extremely attracted to their partners and were very interested in "affectionate sexual contact" with them.
- They felt particularly excluded from the pregnancy and birth process.
- The affair was with a close friend or relative of the woman. (This would indicate that the person with whom the man had the affair was also feeling excluded from the mom-to-be's life during the pregnancy.)

Expectant mothers also have affairs during their pregnancies. In fact, Shapiro suggests that women are just as likely to have affairs as men. Couples who suddenly find themselves with no sexual outlet—and are feeling misunderstood by their partners—may be tempted to satisfy their needs elsewhere.

Birth Plans

Just about every expectant couple—together or individually—has a vision of how they'd like their baby to come into the world. Sometimes these dreams come true, but babies aren't particularly good about going along with the program. And in most cases—especially with first pregnancies—what actually happens during labor and delivery won't look very much like what you hoped it would. Which is why the words *birth* and *plan* really don't belong in the same document, let alone the same sentence.

Nevertheless, a lot of childbirth instructors and other folks still recommend that expectant couples write up a comprehensive birth plan that outlines every aspect of labor and delivery, lays out their demands for the way they want things to go, and makes it very clear that the expectant parents—not the medical staff—will be making all the decisions.

While birth plans may sound logical, they almost always cause more trouble than they prevent. You and your partner may feel bound by whatever you've planned, and if something unexpected (or contrary to the plan) happens, you'll be confused and tense, you may squabble with the medical team or each other, and you'll almost surely look back on the birth with some feelings of regret.

From the medical team's perspective, getting handed a rule-filled, demand-filled document immediately makes the rather intimate relationship they're going to have with you for the next few days adversarial rather than cooperative. Not a good idea.

Babies, meanwhile, have their own thoughts on the matter. The notion that an expectant couple might have some choice in the labor, delivery, and immediate postpartum-period procedures is a fairly recent one. But it's important not to get too attached to that sense of control.

Saul Weinreb, an OB and one of my medical advisors, puts it this way: "If you are comfortable with your care providers, and you share all of your thoughts and wishes and ideas about labor and what you expect, and you trust that they will be open and discuss your options, risks, benefits, etc. before they do any interventions, I have no idea why birth plans are necessary. If you haven't done the above, then a birth plan won't save you, it will only create tension. If you aren't comfortable with your providers, you haven't made a good choice, and you'll have problems whether you have a birth plan or not. Bottom line, they don't help anyone."

Some doctors and nurses I've spoken with half-jokingly say that the longer and more complicated the plan, the greater the chance of a Cesarean—after every possible intervention and drug has been used. And I mean *half*-jokingly.

Okay, so after all that, should you have a birth plan? Well, yes and no. Here's what I mean. Yes, you and your partner should absolutely go through the exercise of putting together a plan. Talk about your ideal scenario, your philosophy, and anything you can think of. Would you like to burn incense and have your baby ushered into the world by a troupe of Tibetan monks? Great. Have your partner give birth standing on one foot while riding horseback? Have the delivery filmed live for a new reality show? Have the entire medical team speak only Mandarin Chinese so that your baby will begin life bilingual? Have the baby licked clean by your pet schnauzer rather than cleaned up by the nurses? Wonderful.

Then, once you've got it all worked out and the wording is just perfect, fold it up and put it in your pocket. And keep it there. Feel free to use it as a cheat sheet in case you forget something, but do *not* show it to anyone else. Ever.

The idea here is to get you and your partner to set some goals and think about what you want for the labor and delivery while you still have clear heads. Remember, though, that things rarely, if ever, go the way they're supposed to. So, be flexible. Here are some topics the two of you may want to discuss. If you have questions about any of them, be sure to bring them up with your partner's practitioner now. There may be certain policies that can't be breached.

- Emergencies. Do you want the doctors or midwives to handle things on their own or would you prefer to have them explain what's going on? If your partner is unconscious or unable to make a decision, should the practitioners get your permission before doing anything out of the ordinary?

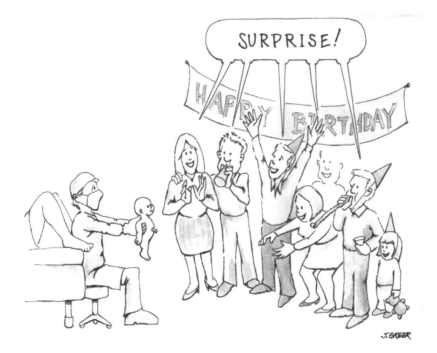

Should Your Older Children Attend the Birth?

Having older children attend the birth of the new baby can be a tricky thing. In general, it's probably okay to have children present both during labor and immediately after the birth (although depending on hospital policy, that may not even be an option). But there are several reasons why children—especially those under five—probably shouldn't be there for the birth itself.

- They may be frightened that their mother is being hurt, and that all of the blood and moaning might mean she's dying. The last thing you want is for your scared preschooler to be running to Mommy for comfort (or to comfort her). She's going to have a few other things on her mind.
- Even well-prepared children can have unpredictable reactions, and you and your partner won't want to have to be distracted by anyone else's needs but hers, yours, and the new baby's.
- The older child might be jealous of all the attention paid to the new baby.
- Aside from the fear factor, kids under four aren't able to understand what's really going on, and they certainly won't appreciate the specialness of the occasion.

If you're still thinking about having an older sibling there for the birth of his or her new sibling, be sure to discuss the idea with your doctor first. Then, get yourselves some visual aids—books, movies, or pictures of births, for

- Pain medication. Do you want the hospital staff to offer it if they feel your partner could use some? Or do you want them to wait for her to ask for it?
- Staying together. Do you and your partner want to remain together for the entire labor and delivery?
- Freedom of movement. Will your partner be able to labor in the hallways (or in the shower), and in whatever position she'd like? There's no reason to spend the whole time in bed. In fact, walking around as much as possible yields better results.
- Labor. If labor slows down, does she want to be offered oxytocin or other drugs to speed it up?
- Pictures and videos. Do you want to take them? Do you want someone else to? Do you want to be able to take them even if there's a C-section?
- Fetal monitoring. Does your partner want the baby's heart rate monitored by machines throughout her labor, or would she prefer that monitoring be done only when necessary?

example—and plan on having some long discussions with the child. It's important to keep in mind that watching Mom give birth will not be like anything they've seen on one of those PBS specials or on Animal Planet. Birth scenes (human or animal, but especially human) are usually carefully edited to avoid showing private parts, blood, and extreme pain. Encourage the child to ask questions; answer them; tell him what's going to happen; talk about acceptable and unacceptable behavior; and plan on spending some private time with him—older children can get really jealous.

Also, make sure there's an adult around to help each child who will be at the birth. This person should be prepared to talk to the child about what's happening and to take the child out of the room if necessary. Your place—and your focus—is with your partner.

If you've got a tween or a teen, your decision to have him or her in the delivery room will depend on a couple of factors.

- Maturity. Is the child able to handle seeing mom in pain? How do you think big bro or sis will respond if something completely unexpected happens and your partner needs an emergency procedure?
- Sex of the child. Your partner may not feel comfortable with a son being at the south end of the bed. For a girl, however, watching Mom give birth could be the best birth control you'll ever come across.

- Water breaking. Your baby has been swimming around in a sac filled with amniotic fluid. Before the baby can be born, that sac has to rupture. Ideally, that will happen on its own and, depending on the position of the baby, the fluid will gush or dribble out. Sometimes, though, the rupture may need to be induced manually.
- The birth. Do you want the doctors to try forceps or suction to speed up the delivery, or do you want to hold out for a while longer? Do you want any other people (friends, relatives, midwife, other children) to attend the birth? Will a mirror be available (so your partner can get a better view of the delivery)?
- Episiotomy. If your partner's vagina won't stretch enough to allow the baby's head through, the doctor may suggest making a small cut in the perineum—the space between the vagina and the anus. Some doctors do episiotomies as a preventative measure; others don't do them unless absolutely necessary. Some people believe that a small but natural tear in the vagina is better than a surgical cut. Others say that the cut helps control the tearing. Either way,

your partner should learn as much as she can about episiotomies and think about whether—barring emergencies, of course—she would want one, and if so, whether she would want it done with or without anesthesia.

- Cesarean section. In case of a C-section, can you stay with your partner, or will you have to be separated? Will you be separated only for the spinal or epidural anesthesia, or for the entire procedure? Where will you be allowed to stand?
- The baby. Who will cut the cord, and when? Do you want the hospital staff to take the baby away for cleaning and testing right after birth, or would you like him or her handed to you and/or your partner first?
- After the birth. Do you want the baby to breastfeed right away, or will you be bottle feeding? Do you want the baby with one of you all the time, or would you rather have him or her kept in the hospital's nursery? What about circumcision?
- Going home. Do you want to stay for as long as the hospital will let you, or do you want to go home as soon as possible?

I'm not saying that you should blindly follow every single thing a doctor, nurse, midwife, or hospital janitor tells you. Nurses love it if you tell them—in a nice way—about your ideal scenario. They love it when you ask questions—it shows you're interested and engaged and that you respect them. And they especially love it when you tell them that you're prepared to defer to their judgment in case of emergency. All you want is to be part of the process.

I know that despite everything I've said in the preceding paragraphs, some readers will want a written birth plan anyway. If you're in that category, that's okay, I'll get over it. But please keep the following guidelines in mind:

- In the first paragraph, indicate your flexibility should an emergency arise.
- Try not to make it sound like a legal document. That's a great way to make a doctor or other health-care provider very nervous and defensive. Your practitioner will not be comfortable if she feels her hands will be tied in the case of an emergency.
- Try to word your desires in a positive way. Avoid beginning every statement with "No" or "Do not."
- Refrain from including things in your plan that are not part of your birth site's normal procedures.
- Be sure to thank everyone for their respect and support.
- After you and your partner have hammered out a draft of your birth plan, show it to your doctor. Let him or her go over it and make suggestions.
- Remember that a birth plan is not a contract. It's a way for you to communicate your preferences to your partner's practitioners.

If you Google "birth plan," you'll find dozens of sample plans including some templates for which all you have to do is fill in the blanks.

Making Final Plans

REGISTERING AT THE HOSPITAL

Despite what you've seen on TV and in the movies, getting to the hospital doesn't have to be a frantic exercise at breakneck speed. Fortunately for men (but not nearly as fortunately for our partners), the onset of labor and the delivery itself are usually hours (if not days) apart, so if you plan carefully, there should be plenty of time to get everything done. And once you've got your bags packed and ready to go (see pages 188–91 for details), the next most pressing concern is registering at the hospital.

Most hospitals will allow—or may even require—you to register up to sixty days before the anticipated birth of the child (I've heard of some that ask you to register as early as the fourth month of the pregnancy). This doesn't mean that you're making a reservation for a particular day. All it means is that when you do show up at the hospital, you won't have to waste time signing papers while your partner is having contractions and screaming. So as soon as you can, check with your hospital's or clinic's administrative offices and/or website to find out their policy. Doing so is particularly important because besides making you fill out 785 forms, the hospital will have to get a verification of coverage and eligibility from your insurance company. And that can take some time.

FINDING A PEDIATRICIAN

I know, you don't actually have a baby yet, but you will soon, so you'd better start putting some real thought into picking a doctor for her. Most people take their kids to pediatricians, but plenty of family practitioners see babies too. During their first year, all three of my kids saw their pediatrician nine times—and they were all as healthy as horses. A typical first-year schedule includes visits a few days after you bring the baby home, two weeks after that, then once a month until six months, once in the ninth month, and again in the twelfth month. Clearly, since you're going to be spending a lot of time with your child's doctor, you should select someone you think you can get along with at least until your child turns sixteen or so. Given the state of health coverage in this country, your options may be limited. But if your plan gives you some flexibility, try to interview several prospective pediatricians. Here are some questions you should ask (you might want to write some of them down and bring them along to the interview):

- Are you affiliated with the hospital where the baby will be born? If not, that could be a deal breaker, or you might be able to change hospitals.
- Will you visit the baby at the hospital?
- What insurance do you take? Another potential deal breaker.
- What's your philosophy about vaccinations? Although the vast majority of pediatricians advocate routine vaccination, there is a vocal minority that doesn't. The debate is interesting but beyond the scope of this book. It's similar, in a way, to debates about the death penalty, abortion, cloth vs. disposable diapers, circumcision, and a few others. It's almost impossible for anyone on either side to change anyone else's mind.
- Where do you stand on breastfeeding? Current thinking is that babies should have nothing but breast milk for at least six months (longer is okay too). You'd be hard pressed to find a pediatrician who won't support breastfeeding. But you also want someone who's flexible enough not to make your partner feel bad if she can't breastfeed for some reason or decides not to.
- How many waiting rooms do you have? This may sound silly, but hospitals and medical offices are full of sick people—exactly the kind of people you'll want to keep your baby away from. Ideally they should have a waiting room for sick kids and another one for kids who are there for well-child visits.
- Do the waiting room toys get cleaned often? Another seemingly silly question, but do you really trust all those sick kids to cover their mouth and nose when they sneeze? And to keep their fingers out of their nose—and their ears and their butts? And to wash their hands before they touch any of the toys? Yeah, right.
- How long are routine office visits? For at least the first few visits you're going to have a ton of questions. Some doctors, though—particularly those in HMOs—see six or more patients per hour, meaning that appointments can be as short as ten minutes. Other doctors are more relaxed and can spend twenty minutes or more with you and your baby.
- How many doctors are in your practice? You may think that male and female doctors are the same, but your child may not agree. When she was about two, my oldest daughter absolutely refused to see her regular (male) pediatrician, and insisted on seeing a "girl doctor." Don't worry about offending your pediatrician—about 75 percent of kids prefer to see a doctor of their own sex.
- What about emergencies? Is there an on-call doc?
- What about nighttime and weekend hours? Does the practice have an advice line, staffed by a nurse, who can talk you off the ledge when you inevitably panic about something?

- What about non-life-threatening emergencies? Who's covering the phones and what happens if your child needs to be seen? During business hours, most practices will have a special line staffed by pediatric nurses who will be able to diagnose just about anything and who, if necessary, will make a same-day appointment.

GETTING TO THE HOSPITAL

Sooner or later—unless you're planning to have a home birth—you and your partner are going to have to get to the hospital. There are several ways of getting there, each with its own advantages and disadvantages:

- Walking. If you live close enough to the hospital, walking may be the best option. You won't have to worry about any of the disadvantages of driving yourself or getting a ride (see below). You will, however, have to deal with the possible embarrassment of having people stare at you as your partner leans up against the side of a building every three minutes and bellows. But she may actually like this option, since walking can help make the contractions of early labor easier to cope with.

  If you're walking, be sure to bring enough cash to take a cab—just in case things don't go the way they should.

- Driving yourself. No matter how much you've prepared, when labor really starts, you're going to be a little nervous, and that could potentially be dangerous when you're behind the wheel of a car. You could get lost, get caught speeding, or even cause an accident. Worst of all, while your eyes and mind are on the road, they can't be where they really ought to be—on your partner. And when you finally get to the hospital, you'll have to deal with parking—and later retrieving—the car.

  If you're driving, make sure you have a full tank of gas and that you've got the hospital programmed into your GPS (along with several alternative routes). Don't worry: if you get there a little early, they probably won't throw you out. Also, check with the hospital parking lot (if they have one) to find out their rates and hours of operation. You may be able to park, get your partner settled into her room, and then run down and move the car.

- Getting a ride—taxi, friend, or relative. If you're in the backseat of someone else's car, you'll at least be able to tend to your partner. Problems might arise, however, if your partner goes into labor at 2 A.M. and your friends or in-laws take more than a minute or two to roll out of bed. In addition, since most people have never driven a pregnant woman to the hospital, they'll be at least as nervous (probably more) than you would have been. And watch out for potholes; my wife assures me they're hell for a laboring woman.

If you're taking a taxi, have the phone numbers of at least three companies that can get a cab to your door within minutes, at any hour of the day or night. Also, be sure to have enough money (or your credit card) for the fare. If you're planning on having someone else do the driving, make sure you have a few backups. And if you're using a ride-sharing service such as Uber or Lyft, check to see whether they have any issues with transporting pregnant women.

WHAT IF YOU HAVE OTHER KIDS?

If you have other kids—especially young ones—getting to the hospital can be doubly stressful and requires extra planning.

Toward the end of my wife's second pregnancy, we decided that we'd take a cab to the hospital. We also decided that if she went into serious labor in the middle of the night, we'd signal our friends who had agreed to take care of our older daughter by calling them, letting the phone ring once, hanging up, calling again, and letting it ring three times.

So, at one in the morning, we made the phone calls, got into the cab, and arrived at our friends' house, where, holding thirty-five pounds of sleeping deadweight, I pounded on the door for five minutes before giving up (our friends had apparently slept through the secret signals). Fortunately, we'd made a backup plan, and when we got to the hospital, we called my parents and had them take their grandchild to their house.

AND FINALLY, SOME LAST-MINUTE DETAILS

- Keep your doctor's number by the phone.
- Keep your gas tank full. Have an extra set of keys stashed someplace, or cash for a cab ready.
- Make sure you've checked to see whether there are any road closures or construction projects along your route to the hospital. You can't always rely on GPS.
- Get ready at work. Labor usually starts without warning and can last a long time—sometimes more than a day. Be sure you've delegated urgent matters to a coworker or supervisor, and that your time-off plans are in order. (See pages 136–44 for more on work/family concerns.)

Packing Your Bags

FOR HER

- A favorite picture and/or anything else she might need or want to help her through labor and the birth.
- A battery-operated CD or MP3 player and some favorite music to help you both

relax during labor. I know this sounds so twentieth century, but some hospitals may not allow you to plug anything, including chargers, into their outlets.

- A bathrobe, a nightgown, or even one of your old T-shirts that she won't mind getting a little blood on. Or a lot.
- A large sports bottle (you know, the kind with the built-in straw) for sipping clear liquids.
- Warm, nonskid socks and/or old slippers (hospital floors can be slippery). Again, ones she won't mind getting bloody.
- A change of clothes to go home in—not what she was wearing before she got pregnant. Sweats or maternity pants are particularly good.
- A nursing bra.
- Her toiletries bag. Don't forget things like mouthwash, toothbrush and toothpaste, glasses, contact lens paraphernalia, hairbrush or comb, and a headband or ponytail holder or two.
- Leave the jewelry at home.

FOR YOU

- Comfortable clothes.
- Your e-reader or some magazines and a collection of your partner's favorite short stories to read to her.
- A swimsuit (you might want to get into the shower with your partner, and the nursing staff might be surprised at the sight of a naked man).

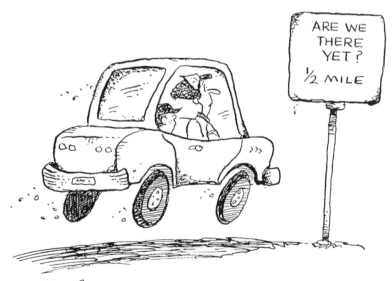

DAVE CARPENTER...

While You're Waiting

If your partner is at risk for giving birth prematurely, try to carve out a few minutes to do some research or make a few calls on the following topics. You're going to be plenty busy with other things, but the time you spend now will be well worth it.

- Contact Social Security and the Motor Vehicle Department. Since premature babies sometimes need extra (and expensive) medical care, Social Security may help you out. You may also be able to get a temporary handicapped parking pass, which should cut down on the time you have to spend looking for parking. You may be able to do some of this on the Web, but you may need to speak with or, gasp, see a real person.
- Find a doctor who has a lot of experience with premature babies. Check with the pediatrician you've already selected, your insurance carrier, or the hospital where the baby will be born.
- Find out about infant massage. Researcher Tiffany Field found that preemies who got three fifteen-minute periods of gentle massage a day grew 50 percent faster than preemies who didn't. Hospital stays for the massaged babies were also a week shorter (and a week cheaper).

- A camera, plenty of batteries, and memory cards or film.
- This book.
- A cooler filled with snacks. This is not for your partner. (She shouldn't be eating while she's in labor, but you'll need to keep your energy up.) You're not going to want to leave your partner, mid-contraction, to run down to the hospital cafeteria. If you have some extra room, bring along a small birthday cake and maybe even some Champagne for afterward.
- Cash. For vending machines, parking meters, cab rides, and so on.
- Chargers for your phone, tablet, MP3 player, and any other electronic gadgets you're planning to bring with you.
- Tennis balls for back rubs.
- A toothbrush, extra underwear, shaving kit, and the like. You'll probably end up staying at least one night.

FOR THE BABY

- An infant car seat (if you don't have one, the hospital won't let you leave). And make sure it's been properly installed.

- A little outfit to go home in—a sleeper or sleep sac is fine, just as long as it has legs so the car seat's harness can go between them. (It's a good idea to wash all new clothes before putting them on the baby.)
- Diapers.
- Several receiving blankets, weather-appropriate.
- Warm blankets for the ride home.

Preterm Labor/Premature Birth

In the vast majority of pregnancies, labor doesn't start until about the fortieth week. However, a small but significant number of babies (8–10 percent) are born prematurely—meaning sometime before the thirty-seventh week. More than half of twins and about 90 percent of triplets, however, are born prematurely. Interestingly, identical twin boys are more likely to be born prematurely than identical twin girls. This gender distinction doesn't seem to hold for fraternal twins.

The symptoms of premature labor are exactly the same as those of real labor (see page 214 for more)—they just happen before they're supposed to. If your partner has any of the following symptoms, she may be considered at high risk for giving birth early.

- An "incompetent cervix"—meaning that the cervix is too weak and may open, allowing the baby to be born too soon. Diagnosed early enough, an incompetent cervix can be "corrected" (and premature births prevented) by sewing the opening of the cervix shut.
- "Placenta previa" (when the placenta is covering up the cervix) or "placental abruption" (when the placenta has prematurely separated from the wall of the uterus).
- Any kind of surgery during pregnancy.
- She's carrying twins (or more). See "When Premature Labor Really Isn't" on page 193.
- There's too much or too little amniotic fluid.
- She didn't eat well during the pregnancy or is (or has recently been) smoking, drinking, or using drugs.
- She's been spending a lot of time on her feet. Several recent studies have found that pregnant women who spend five hours or more standing or walking every day are as much as three times more likely to deliver prematurely than women who are on their feet less than two hours a day. So if your partner is a waitress or nurse or runway model, she might want to switch to a desk job until after the baby's born. Moderate, recreational physical activity, on the other hand, has been shown to protect against preterm birth.

- Exposure to Diethylstilbestrol (DES). Many of the daughters of women who took DES to prevent miscarriage were born with abnormalities of the reproductive tract). DES was banned in 1971, so this won't affect your partner directly. However, there's some evidence that the granddaughters of women who took DES could be affected. Have your partner ask her mother.
- She's had a previous premature labor.
- She's carrying an unusually small fetus.

The bad news about premature babies is that if they're born too soon, they really aren't ripe yet. The fetus's lungs aren't fully developed until it's at least twenty-eight weeks old. Babies born before that time have a far higher risk of developing serious respiratory problems, including chronic lung disease, as well as neurological and cognitive problems. Babies born at twenty-eight to thirty-two weeks are far better off, but still at risk for vision and gastrointestinal difficulties.

Overall, premature and low-birth-weight babies are at risk for a number of short- and long-term problems. As infants, they may be less responsive to visual and auditory stimulation, and their reflexes aren't as sharp as normal-birth-weight babies. They may have trouble breathing, sucking, or swallowing, and are more likely to develop a chronic illness or to die of SIDS (Sudden Infant Death Syndrome). As they get older, they may have smaller vocabularies than other kids the same age, have shorter attention spans and lower self-esteem, and are more likely to fail in school or have to repeat a grade. As adolescents they often have more behavioral and psychological problems, and as adults they're more likely to suffer from depression.

Premature babies are also less likely to be breastfed. Breastfeeding boosts babies' immune system and protects them from developing ear infections, pneumonia, and stomach problems, and from becoming obese later in life. There's some evidence that breastfed babies have higher IQs and a lower risk of developing leukemia or diabetes.

The good news is that medical technology has advanced so much in recent years that the chances of survival are excellent. Ninety percent of thirty-week babies do quite well. And by thirty-five weeks, it's up to 99 percent.

Obviously, it's to the fetus's benefit to spend as many days as possible right where it's supposed to be: in Mom's uterus. Therefore, if your partner shows signs of being in real labor (see page 214), call her doctor immediately. Caught early, premature labor can sometimes be arrested (usually with the help of intravenous drugs), and the fetus will be able to stay where it belongs for a few more weeks.

After an arrested premature labor, your doctor will most likely order your partner to stay in bed for the rest of the pregnancy. She may even be put on a home fetal monitor to keep an eye on the baby. If this happens, be prepared to step in and take over all of the household responsibilities, as well as responsibility for other children if you have them. If you aren't in a position to do this, you may have to hire someone or ask friends or relatives to help out.

Your involvement is actually a lot more important than you might think. Researcher Michael Yogman tracked a group of preemies and found that at three years old, for example, the IQ scores of the kids with highly involved dads were six points higher than the ones with less involved dads.

When Premature Labor Really Isn't

If you're expecting twins (or more) and your partner goes into labor, chances are it's not premature at all. Although single babies spend an average of forty weeks under construction, most twins are born at about thirty-seven weeks. Triplets usually arrive at thirty-five weeks, and quads make their entrance a week earlier. Even if it turns out that you're going to be skipping the traditional ninth month, read the next chapter anyway—especially the "What's Going On with You" section—to make sure you aren't missing out on anything important.

The Nursery: Everything You Need and Why

There are literally thousands of things you *could* buy for your newborn's nursery, but you'll max out all your credit cards, clean out your IRAs, and have to take a second mortgage on your house to get them all. Most are simply unnecessary. You could, for example, buy a special machine that warms up the wipes you use to clean your baby's bottom. But believe me, your baby's bottom will get just as clean with room-temperature wipes. Here are some of the items you'll truly need or at least have a pretty good chance of using. You can probably save quite a bit by buying these things online, at garage sales, from friends, or at used-furniture stores.

Please remember that when acquiring *anything* for your baby, safety should be your primary concern. Before you spend a fortune on Queen Victoria's original bassinet or drag out the crib that you (or your parents or grandparents) slept in as a kid, consider this: your baby will do just about everything possible to jeopardize his or her own life (and scare the hell out of you), from sticking his head between the bars of the crib and throwing himself off tall changing tables to burying herself under a pile of blankets left in the corner.

So before you buy anything for your baby—whether it's new or used—make sure it complies with the most recent safety standards. Some of them are listed in the sections that follow. For additional guidance on the safest—and best-quality—deals, as well as product recalls, consult the latest *Consumer Reports Guide to Baby Products* (www.consumerreports.org) or Safe Kids Worldwide

Essentials to Have Waiting at Home

FOR THE BABY

Note: You'll have to increase the quantities somewhat if you have twins or more.

- Enough diapers to last for at least a week (you're not going to want to go shopping). Just so you know, your newborn will go through about a dozen every day. Do the math. If you're buying disposables, don't go out and buy a truckload of the infant size. Babies tend to bulk up pretty quickly, and you might be on to the next size before you go through all the smaller ones. If you know your baby will be big, you can skip the newborn size completely. If you're going with a cloth diaper service, a week's supply is typically eighty (for one baby).
- Baby soap and shampoo.
- Thermometer. You may want to invest in one that takes the temperature via the forehead or ear, or one that's part of a pacifier. Preventing your baby from squirming for three minutes while trying to keep a thermometer in her mouth or bottom is going to be an unpleasant experience for everyone concerned. Those old glass-and-mercury thermometers can be dangerous, so if someone gave you one, dispose of it properly or donate it to a museum.
- An ear bulb. These are usually used for rinsing adults' ears, but for babies, they're used for suctioning mucus from their noses. Well, what do you expect? They can't do it themselves.
- Nail scissors. Essential: a baby's nails are like tiny razors and grow like Jack's beanstalk.
- A first aid kit. You can get one from your local drugstore or online for about $20. But just to be sure, ask your pediatrician what should be in it.
- A diaper bag. It used to be that most diaper bags looked like oversized purses. They were pink or flowery and no self-respecting man would be caught dead with one. Fortunately, there are now quite a few more masculine options. Check out www.diaperdude.com and www.dadgear.com for some possibilities.
- Cotton swabs and alcohol for umbilical cord dressing.
- Some formula, just in case. But keep in mind that some breastfeeding experts think this is a bad idea, because it might be too big a temptation to give up breastfeeding.
- Pacifiers.
- Stroller.
- Fitted crib sheets.
- Bottles and a breast pump.

- 5 or 6 Onesies (those cute little one-piece suits).
- 5 or 6 pairs of booties (those stretchy socks).
- 3 or 4 undershirts.
- 3 or 4 outfits with separate top and bottom (that way you can wash only the part that gets dirty). Try to get the kind that have snaps.
- 3 or 4 nightgowns or sleep sacs.
- 1 or 2 coveralls with snaps.
- 4 or 5 baby blankets.
- 1 or 2 hooded bath towels.
- 1 or 2 sun or snow hats.
- 1 or 2 sweaters.
- Snowsuit (as needed).
- 0 shoes (people who don't walk shouldn't wear shoes—it can hurt their feet).

A word of advice: your baby will poop or vomit on his clothes every single day. More than once. So skip the silk T-shirts and the lamb's wool sweaters and stick with good-quality *washable* materials. And, as with diapers, don't invest a huge amount on newborn-sized clothes. Your baby will grow out of them in no time.

FOR YOUR PARTNER

- Nursing pads.
- Maxi-pads (she may need these for weeks).
- Any medication or dressing materials needed in the event of a C-section or episiotomy.
- Milk and vitamins, especially if she is nursing.
- Flowers, and favorite chocolates or other foods she might have avoided during pregnancy.
- A good book about your baby's first year of life. Modesty aside, my books *The New Father: A Dad's Guide to the First Year* and *Fathering Your Toddler: A Dad's Guide to the Second and Third Years* are the best resources out there for dads.
- A comfortable rocking chair or glider, for nursing.
- A breastfeeding pillow.
- For both of you, a general pediatrics reference book, such as *Caring for Your Baby and Young Child, Birth to Age 5*, from the American Academy of Pediatrics.

Green Babies

People generally select the products they buy based on price, quality, availability, and brand. In recent years, though, consumers are paying more attention to how products impact the environment, whether it's their home environment or the one we all live in. A number of recent national polls have found that around 70 percent of American consumers say that they would prefer to buy environmentally friendly products than non-environmentally friendly ones. However, only about 35 percent of consumers say that they would pay a premium for it, and only 25 percent actually do buy eco-friendly products (as you might expect, those numbers are higher for consumers aged eighteen to thirty-four and lower for older generations). So what does this have to do with you and your baby? Plenty.

You might be concerned that the paint you used in the nursery could emit toxic fumes. Or maybe you're worried about the bleaches in your laundry and you'd prefer that your baby wear nothing but organic fabrics. Or perhaps you're concerned about how disposable diapers are impacting the environment. Whatever your concern, there are environmentally friendly alternatives to just about any product you're currently using (although the most common reason given by those who don't buy green is that the products cost too much).

You can find some of these products at places like Walgreens, Sears, Whole Foods, Babies Я Us, and even Walmart, or at your local natural grocer. But the widest selection and the most resources are going to be online, at places like Green Home (www.greenhome.com) and EcoMall (www.ecomall.com/).

(www.safekids.org/product-recalls). And you can find out the latest standards and requirements for car seats and other travel-related equipment from the National Highway Traffic Safety Administration (www.nhtsa.dot.gov).

BABY FURNISHINGS

CRIB

Nothing says baby quite like a crib. And so it's no surprise that this is one of the first pieces of baby furniture an expectant couple thinks about. Some cribs are just cribs; others can be converted to a toddler bed or other furniture as your baby grows up. Here are some safety tips:

- No corner posts. Babies can accidentally strangle themselves if their clothes become caught on a post. New cribs are constructed without them, but if you have your heart set on using a vintage model, unscrew or saw off the posts. Anything more than 1/16 inch is too high.
- Slats or bars should be spaced no more than 2⅜ inches apart, and none should be broken or missing.
- Never place your crib near draperies, blinds, or anything else that has long, hanging, or wall-mounted cords. Babies can tear these down or become entangled in them.
- Keep the crib away from radiators, heaters, and area rugs. The last thing you want to do while holding your baby is burn yourself or slip.
- Do not get a crib that has sides that can be lowered. "Drop side" cribs seemed like a good idea because they made it easier for parents to get babies in and out. But they were responsible for thousands of injuries and dozens of deaths and are now banned. Some cribs have a feature that allows you to lower the mattress as your baby gets bigger and stronger.
- Any teething rails (the hard plastic caps over the top rails of the crib sides) should be firmly attached. They're going to get chewed on a lot, and you don't want them to come off.
- Before you buy, check the U.S. Consumer Product Safety Commission website (www.cpsc.gov) for recall info.

CRIB MATTRESS

Couples are often surprised that mattresses are usually sold separately from the crib. The theory is that some babies prefer firm mattresses while others prefer softer ones. Since your baby is going to be spending around fifteen hours a day on that mattress for a while, don't skimp—there's no reason why the one you buy now shouldn't last you through several kids. Just make sure it comes with a moisture-proof protector. A few safety tips:

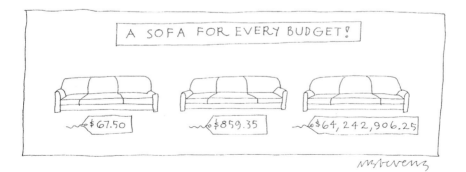

- The firmer the better. Studies have shown that there is an increased risk of SIDS (Sudden Infant Death Syndrome) if the mattress is too soft. For the same reason, never put pillows in the crib.
- The mattress must fit tightly into the crib (no more than one finger's width between the edge of the mattress and the side of the crib).
- You'll have a choice between innerspring and foam. Neither is necessarily better than the other. The main thing is to go for quality over price. There are a lot of cheapies out there that either won't last or are made using questionable materials.
- Consider flame-retardant coverings and organic or eco-friendly materials, if those things are important to your family.

CRIB ACCESSORIES
- Sheets: Get at least three of the fitted kind. They usually come in regular and organic.
- No bumpers: Even though they can't move very well, babies somehow manage to ram their heads against the sides of the crib—hard enough to leave an impression of the slats or bars on the top or back of their head. It supposedly reminds them of the feeling of having their heads smashed up against your partner's pubic bone for the last month or two of pregnancy. Until recently, crib bumpers (soft pads that ran along the inside of the crib) were pretty much de rigueur because they supposedly kept the baby's head from being bruised. But new research shows that they pose a severe suffocation hazard (babies may run into them with their face and not be able to back away) and entrapment risk (babies can get caught between the bumper and the mattress). Don't use bumpers of any kind—not even the mesh "breathable" ones, which eliminated the suffocation risk but left the entrapment issue. No bumpers may mean a few bumps and bruises to your baby's head, but she'll be a lot safer.
- Dust ruffle: Extremely optional, unless you're Martha Stewart.
- Mobile: Optional but nice. Some of the most beautiful (and most expensive) ones are made to be looked at from the side—where the person who bought it is standing. But remember whom the mobile is really for, and think about whether your baby is really going to be interested in looking at the bottom of a bunch of cars or the undersides of a group of jungle animals. Babies prefer high-contrast patterns to simply bright colors. You can get mobiles that merely hang, some that play incredibly annoying music when you wind them up, some that run on batteries, and some that ring bells or make other noises when the baby swats at them.

BASSINET (SOMETIMES CALLED MOSES BASKET)

For the first few months of your baby's life, you may want him or her to sleep in the bedroom with you. If nothing else, this arrangement will make breastfeeding a lot more convenient. Bassinets come in a variety of styles (wheels, no wheels, handles, no handles, rocking, non-rocking). But because they generally accommodate a baby for only three months or so, you'll be better off borrowing a safe one from someone and passing it on to the next new parents. To choose a safe one, use the same guidelines as for cribs: no posts, slats you can't get a soda can between. And as with the crib mattress, the one in a bassinet should be firm and fit snugly against the sides. And follow the manufacturer's weight and age recommendations.

SIDECAR OR COSLEEPER

These are essentially three-sided cribs that attach to the side of your bed (most likely on your partner's side). The idea is that breastfeeding may be easier with the baby close by.

CAR SEAT

A car seat may be the most indispensable baby item. (Again, you won't be able to take your baby home from the hospital without one.) This is a critical purchase, so don't skimp. Stay away from hand-me-downs unless they're practically new, have never been in an accident, and conform to the very latest standards. Some are designed to face backward; others only face front; some convert from one to the other. You may want to consider getting two—a small one (perhaps with handles so you can carry the baby around with you) that can be used until the baby reaches twenty pounds, and a larger one for later. There are also some car seat/stroller combinations out there. Check Parents Central (www.safercar.gov/parents) before you buy any car seat.

CHANGING TABLE

Changing tables come in an unbelievable variety of sizes and configurations. Some have drawers so that they can be used as a dresser when a changing table is no longer needed. The problem with drawers, however, is that you have to remember to take out what you need before you get started; when you're in the middle of changing the baby, the last thing you want to be doing is fumbling around blindly for a clean outfit. Be sure to get a foam pad for the top of the table and a couple of washable pad covers. You should also stock your changing table with a good supply of the following:
• Diapers

- Baby wipes
- Diaper rash ointment, such as A&D or Desitin
- Cotton swabs and water for cleaning the umbilical cord stump
- Baby shampoo and soap (a mild one like Neutrogena or Dove is best)

Note: Stay away from talc-based baby powders. They can cause breathing problems and lung damage if inhaled. Cornstarch-based powders seem to be okay, but there's no solid evidence that either one does anything to help with diaper rash. The most important things you can do are change diapers regularly and pat or air-dry your baby's bottom before closing the diaper.

PORTABLE PLAYPEN

Perfect for children less than thirty-four inches tall and lighter than about thirty pounds. Not only does it fold up compactly enough to check as luggage when you're traveling, but it can also be used at home—to keep your baby from crawling under your feet while you're cooking, for example. Some of our friends' children essentially lived in their playpens for the first eighteen months of their lives.

STROLLER

A good stroller can make life worth living, so don't waste your time or money on one that won't last. We took our oldest daughter and her stroller all over the world, and it was still in good enough condition three years later for her younger sister to use. Getting a quality stroller doesn't mean you have to buy the one with every available option. Stick to the basics, such as weight (you'll spend a surprising amount of time carrying the stroller—loading and unloading the car, getting on and off buses and trains, going up stairs, and so on), ease of folding, brakes, and balance (you don't want the thing tipping over backward with your baby in it). Finally, make sure the handles are long enough for you to push the stroller when you're standing up straight. Most strollers are made to be used by women, which means that if you're over 5'6" or so, you'll have to stoop a little to push. You might not notice it at first, but after a while, your back may give you trouble. Some smarter manufacturers have adjustable handles.

City dwellers who do a lot of traveling on subways or buses will want a sturdy but collapsible stroller—preferably one that you can fold with one hand while holding the baby with the other. Otherwise, it's next to impossible to get onto public transportation (at least without annoying everyone behind you). The stroller/car seat combos are especially bulky and hard to fold.

There are dozens of stroller manufacturers, and they come in a nearly infinite range of designs and functions. Some are designed for running. Some accommodate twins or more. Some look like Harley-Davidson motorcycles and convert to a child's bike after the stroller years are past. Some look generic, some have military camouflage, and some seem to serve no purpose but to show off how much money you have (or used to have, before you mortgaged your house to buy the stroller).

BATHTUB

A small plastic washbasin is better than a sink for newborns for several reasons. First, you probably won't want to have your new baby's little body in a place where you might have had raw meat or other food-borne sources of bacteria. And you certainly wouldn't want to have your baby pooping in a place where you might be putting food (of course you'd wash the sink before and after the bath, but still . . .). Second, you'll actually be giving your baby sponge baths, with the baby lying down in the tub, not soak-in-the-water baths. In the sink, you'd have to hold your baby with one hand and do the washing with the other. Squirmy, soapy babies are hard enough to hold on to with two or three hands.

MONITOR

These handy devices let you listen to or watch your baby wherever you are. And I really do mean wherever. Some of the higher-end video monitors allow you to get real-time feeds on any Internet-enabled device (which is good if you have to go back to work but don't want to miss a second of your baby's life). If you're just going for a plain vanilla audio monitor, try hardware or sporting goods stores where you can get walkie-talkies and room monitors for quite a bit less than a similar item at traditional toy or baby-gear stores, where they call them "baby monitors."

BABY CARRIER

Whether it's a sling, a front pack, or a backpack, you'll want to get something that you can use to carry your baby around in. Make sure it's comfortable and, if you're planning to share it with your partner, adjustable.

DIAPERS

Who would have thought that diapers would become a political issue or that something so ordinary could make or break friendships? But they have.

Until just a few years ago, there were two camps: disposable and cloth. People who used disposables were evil, pumping millions of tons of human waste, plastic, and chemicals into the landfill, where they'd stay in their present form for thousands of years. (There also were some "biodegradable" diapers, which broke

Watch Out for Triboluminescence

Never heard of it? Well maybe it's time you should. In 1999 English house-wife Jill Furlough got a fright late one night when she saw green sparks shooting out of her sleeping eleven-month-old son's disposable diaper. She called the diaper manufacturers, who assured her that the sparks were the result of *triboluminescence*, a perfectly harmless buildup of energy probably caused by the friction of the baby's bottom rubbing against the inside of the diaper. It's actually exactly the same chemical reaction that produces the sparks you see when you bite down on a Wint-O-Green LifeSaver in a dark room. You can see the same thing if you strike two sugar cubes together as if striking a match or yank on a roll of tape. Unlike static electricity, tribo-luminescence doesn't generate any heat. The boy apparently slept through the entire episode, and there's no record of any injury to anyone. Just something to think about.

down after only five hundred years). People who used cloth diapers, in contrast, were the white knights, saving the earth for our children.

The reality is a bit more complicated: although cloth diapers are all natural, they're made of cotton, which is taxing on farmland. And in order to sterilize them properly (you wouldn't want to put a diaper on your baby that some other kid had worn), diaper services bleach them and wash them seven times (it's true) in near-boiling water, thereby consuming a tremendous amount of power, water, and chemical detergents. The clean diapers are then driven all over town in trucks that fill the air with toxic pollutants. Bottom line? There is no clear winner.

And it gets more confusing by the day. Regular disposables are still out there, and still playing the role of bogeyman. But you can also get a number of eco-friendly disposables that offer some or all of the following features: chlorine-free, latex-free, dye-free, fragrance-free, gel-free, made of corn-based materials, GMO (genetically modified organism)-free, hypoallergenic, organic, compostable, and flushable.

On the other side of the argument, we need to talk about "reusables" instead of cloth. My wife and I started out by using cloth diapers for our oldest daughter. But every time she filled one up, the diaper had a nasty tendency to siphon the contents away from my daughter and onto my pants—not pleasant—and that meant even more laundry! It's possible that this phenomenon was the fault of my poor diapering technique. But I was convinced that disposables, which have elastic around the leg openings, do a better job of keeping what belongs in a diaper actually in the diaper.

Today, all that's changed. Cloth diapers are no longer rectangular and held together with pins or elastic clips. Now they're hourglass shaped and hidden inside stylish washable covers that Velcro on and stretch to fit your baby. (Properly installed, these diapers can be just as leak-free as disposables.) There are also hybrid diapers, which use a washable exterior but have disposable (and sometimes flushable) liners. Kids who grow up with disposable diapers tend to become potty-trained later than those who use cloth, because the disposables do such a great job of sucking up moisture that babies have no real incentive to get out of them. If you want to see this in action, just visit someone you know who has a toddler. Chances are, he'll be running all over the house with his diaper hanging down to his knees because he's got a quart of urine in there, but he's comfortable as a fly in . . . oh, you know.

Either way, plan on going through around 3,000 diapers before you light the candle on your baby's first birthday cake, and 6,000–8,000 before your baby starts flushing the toilet. Double or triple that if you have twins or more.

Costs are all over the place, depending on the type of diaper you go with, where you live, whether or not you shop the sales, and whether or not you buy and wash your own. The best place to do all your comparison shopping is www. diapers.com.

FORMULA

You can use powdered, full-strength liquid, or liquid concentrate. But when you start checking prices, your partner may decide to keep breastfeeding a while longer. When we weaned our daughters, we put them on the powdered formula—I made a pitcher of it every morning and kept it in the refrigerator.

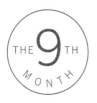

"Dear, It's Time..."

WHAT'S GOING ON WITH YOUR PARTNER

Physically

- Some change in fetal activity—the baby is so cramped that instead of kicking and punching, all she can do is squirm
- Increased sleeplessness and fatigue
- A renewed sense of energy when the baby's head "drops" into the pelvis and takes some of the pressure off the stomach and lungs
- She may have stopped gaining weight (and may even lose a pound or two), but she's still just plain miserable, with increased cramping, constipation, backache, water retention, and swelling of the feet, ankles, and face
- If her belly button was an innie before, it may have become an outie (the change isn't permanent, though)
- Little to no interest in sex (although some women's interest actually increases)

Emotionally

- More dependent on you than ever—afraid you won't love her after the baby is born (after all, she's not the same woman you married)
- Impatient: tired of being tired, frustrated with being so big, and can't wait for pregnancy to be over—or she may not want it to end
- Short-tempered: tired of answering "So when's the baby coming?" questions— especially if she's overdue
- May be afraid she won't have enough love to go around—what with loving you and all
- Fear she won't be ready for labor when it comes

- Creating endless lists of things that absolutely, positively have to be done (in most cases by you) before the baby shows up
- Increasing preoccupation with the baby and, perhaps, a sudden and unexplained interest in Martha Stewart and interior decorating

WHAT'S GOING ON WITH THE BABY

Over the course of this last month of pregnancy, your baby will be growing at a tremendous clip, putting on about a quarter to a half pound a week, although she'll stop growing a week or so before birth. Before she finally decides to leave the warm uterus, she'll weigh six to nine pounds (less if she's a twin or triplet) and be about twenty inches long—so big that there will be hardly any room for her to kick or prod your partner anymore. Her fingernails and toenails are frequently so long they have to be trimmed right after birth, and the lanugo and vernix that have been covering and protecting her little body are starting to slough off. And despite the widespread myth that babies are born blind, her sight is coming along just fine. During her last weeks in captivity, she'll practice her sucking, hand clenching, head turning, swallowing, blinking, and even breathing.

WHAT'S GOING ON WITH YOU

Confusion

Well, it's almost over. In just a few weeks, you're finally going to meet the child you've talked to and dreamed about, and whose college education you've planned. But be prepared: the last month of pregnancy is often the most confusing for expectant fathers. At times you may be almost overcome with excitement and anticipation. At other times you may be feeling so scared and trapped that you want to run away. In short, all the feelings—good and bad—that you've experienced over the last eight months are back. But now, because of the impending birth, they're more intense than before. Here are a few of the contradictory emotional states you may find yourself going through as the pregnancy winds down:

- On the one hand, you may be feeling confident about your readiness to be a father. On the other, you may be worried and unsure about whether you'll be able to handle your dual roles as husband and dad.
- You may really be looking forward to spending some time with your baby while your partner is recuperating. But you may be worried that you won't know how to do all the things that she usually does for the family. (If this last part is true, you'd better learn how to do the laundry and run the dishwasher in a hurry.)

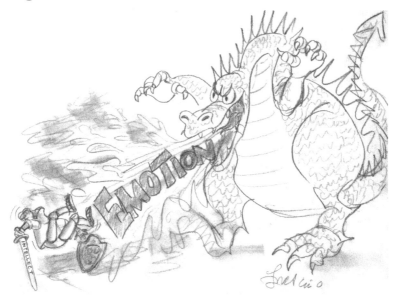

- You're looking forward to being involved, but you feel sidelined by your partner and jealous of her connection with the baby.
- If you've taken on a second job or increased responsibilities at work, all you'll probably want to do at the end of the day is go home and relax. But with your partner less and less able to handle physical tasks, you may be greeted at the door with a list of chores that need to be done.
- You may want to take a good chunk of time off after the baby comes, but you're worried about how that will affect your career, or whether your joint checking account can take the hit.
- You and your partner may be feeling an exceptionally strong emotional bond with each other. At the same time, your sex life may have completely disappeared.
- You may be horny as hell, but you saw some pretty graphic childbirth videos in your prep class and can't get those images out of your mind.
- As your partner gets more and more uncomfortable, she may feel less and less like going out with friends, so the two of you may be spending a lot more time together. This could be the last chance you have to enjoy some quiet, private time before the baby comes. But it may also be an unwelcome opportunity to get on each other's nerves.
- You may find yourself spending a lot more time with friends and family members who have small children, or you may find yourself avoiding families with kids.
- You may be practically giddy at the idea of holding your child in your arms, but petrified that you'll drop him.

Increased Dependency on Your Partner

By this time, your attention—and that of your friends and family—is focused squarely on your partner and the baby. Since you're the person she's closest to and sees most often, your partner is going to be increasingly dependent on you—not only to help her physically, but to get her through the last-month emotional ups and downs. At the same time, though, you are going to be increasingly dependent on her as you get onto the last-month roller coaster.

Your partner's increased dependency is considered a "normal" part of pregnancy. But thanks to the ridiculous, gender-specific way we socialize people in this country, men are supposed to be independent, strong, supportive, and impervious to emotional needs—especially while their partners are pregnant. So, just when you're feeling most vulnerable and least in control, your needs are swept under the rug. And what's worse, the one person you most depend on for sympathy and understanding may be too absorbed in what's going on with herself and the baby to do much for you.

This results in what Dr. Luis Zayas calls an "imbalance in interdependence," which leaves the father to satisfy his own emotional needs *and* those of his partner. In addition, in many cases this imbalance essentially becomes a kind of vicious circle that "accentuates the stress, intensifies feelings of separation, and heightens dependency needs." In other words, the less response you get to your dependency needs, the more dependent you feel.

Feeling Guilty

Especially in the last month or so of the pregnancy, many men begin to blame themselves for what they think they've been putting their partners through. Yes, you're the one who got her pregnant, and yes, she's uncomfortable as hell. But strange as it might seem to you, your partner does *not* blame you for what she's going through. She understands and accepts—as you should—that this was her idea, too, and that (at least short of surrogate motherhood or adoption) there's simply no way to have a baby without going through this. So quit torturing yourself—there are a lot more productive things you can be doing with your time during these last few weeks.

STAYING INVOLVED

Sensitivity

The bottom line is that during the last few weeks of her pregnancy, your partner is likely to be miserable and uncomfortable. Although there's not a whole lot you

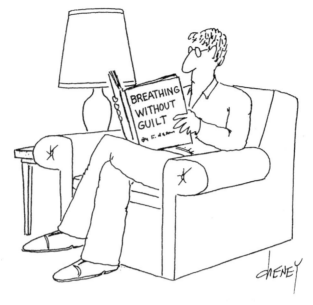

can do to ease her burden, here are a few suggestions that might make the final stretch a little more bearable—for both of you:

- Quit answering the phone. Change the outgoing message on your voice mail to something like: "Hi. No, we don't have a baby yet, and yes, Jane's fine. We'll be updating our Facebook page as soon as the baby arrives. If you're calling about anything else, please leave a message and we'll call you back." That may sound a little snotty, but believe me, it's a lot less snotty than you would be if you were really answering the same questions twenty times a day.
- Stay nearby whenever you can. Come home a little earlier from work, give away those basketball tickets, and postpone that long business trip.
- Stay in touch. A couple of quick calls, texts, or emails to her every day can make her feel loved and important. They'll also reassure her that you're all right. And never, ever go anywhere without your phone. The one time you do, she'll call and immediately panic that you've either left her or were hit by a bus.
- Stay as calm as you can. She'll be nervous enough for both of you.
- Be patient. She may do some pretty bizarre things, and the best thing you can do is bear with her. If the house has already passed the white-glove test and the car has been waxed twice, and she wants it all done over again, do it—she needs the rest.
- Review the breathing, relaxation, mirroring, and any other techniques you plan to use during labor.
- If she wants it, give her some time to herself. And if she wants time with you, make sure you're there for her.

- If she hasn't stopped working, encourage her to do so. Especially if she doesn't like her job. In a recent study of women in southern California, researchers found that those who took leave in the last month of pregnancy (starting around three to four weeks before delivery) had a C-section rate that was four times lower than women who didn't take leave. And while she's on leave, encourage her to get plenty of sleep. Exhaustion during the final weeks of the pregnancy also increases the C-section rate.

If you're running out of ideas, reread the "Ways to Show Her You Care" section on pages 96–99 and try the ones you didn't get to then, or those that got you the most mileage the first time around.

What If She's Overdue?

There's nothing more frustrating than starting the tenth month of a nine-month pregnancy. You've already given up answering the phone, afraid it's another one of those "What are you doing at home? I was sure you'd be at the hospital by now" calls. And you're sick of ending every conversation at the office with, "Now if I'm not in tomorrow, don't forget to . . ." The empty bassinet looks forlorn, and you're just dying to meet the baby face to little wrinkled face.

In most cases, however, couples who think they're late really aren't. When doctors tell a pregnant woman her due date, they often neglect to add that it's only a ballpark figure based on an assumed twenty-eight-day menstrual cycle, and there's always a window of plus or minus two weeks. If your partner's cycle is long, short, or irregular, her "official" due date could be off by as much as three weeks. And even if her cycle is like clockwork, it's nearly impossible to tell exactly when you conceived. First-trimester ultrasounds, which almost all women have, are more accurate, coming within three to four days (in either direction) of the actual due date. Second-trimester ultrasounds are less accurate, with a margin of error of around a week either way. In the third trimester, ultrasounds can be even less accurate—as much as ten to twelve days off.

There are also a number of other factors that can influence due-date accuracy. African American and Asian women, for example, tend to have shorter pregnancies (by three to five days) than Caucasian women. Younger women have shorter pregnancies than older ones, and first-time moms typically deliver as much as ten days after their due date.

The problem with this is that your partner may have been fixated on a specific due date, and when she goes past it, she's likely to be bitterly disappointed. While going past the due date by a week or so is usually not a problem, being truly overdue can have serious consequences:

She's Got More Control Than She Realizes

Women can't control when they give birth, right? Not so fast. Researchers at the Yale University School of Public Health analyzed millions of U.S. birth certificates with a focus on Valentine's Day and Halloween. They found that 5 percent more babies were born spontaneously on Valentine's Day, and 11 percent *fewer* babies were born on Halloween than on any other day in the week before or after those holidays. (Chemically induced births and elective C-section births were also higher on Valentine's Day and lower on Halloween, but those can be scheduled for any time, within reason.) Becca Levy, who led the study, speculated that pregnant women may be subconsciously avoiding Halloween because of its association with evil and death, and choosing Valentine's Day for its association with cherubs and love.

- The baby can grow so large that he or she will have problems passing through the birth canal, thus increasing the chances of a difficult delivery or a C-section.
- After a certain point the placenta gets so old that it can no longer provide adequate nourishment for the baby. This can result in the baby's losing weight in the uterus, increasing the risk of fetal distress.
- There may no longer be enough amniotic fluid to support the baby.
- There may be inadequate room for the umbilical cord to perform properly.

If your doctor feels that the baby is overdue, he or she will most likely prescribe some tests to make sure the baby is still okay. The most common are an ultrasound (to determine the level of amniotic fluid as well as to get a general idea of how the baby is doing) and a non-stress test, which monitors changes in the baby's heart rate and movement in reaction to certain stimuli.

If the baby "passes" these tests, the doctor will probably send you home, telling you to repeat the test in three to seven days, if the baby hasn't come by then. Or, he or she may suggest that you schedule a date for labor to be induced.

If all of this starts getting you down, remember the words of obstetrician J. Milton Huston of New York Hospital: "In all of my years of practice, I've never seen a baby stay in there."

What If It's a Boy?

Sadly, most people don't think about—and, consequently, never discuss—circumcising their sons until the thing is staring them in the face, so to speak. So if you and your partner haven't made up your minds about circumcision yet, now's the time to do so. Of course, if you know you're having a girl or if you and your partner have already decided what you're going to do, feel free to skip this section. But if either of you is still undecided, the pros and cons of circumcision are summarized below. If you and your partner aren't on exactly the same page, be careful: in recent years the whole circumcision debate has become extremely political, and tempers run pretty hot on both sides.

WHY YOU MIGHT WANT TO CONSIDER CIRCUMCISION

- Religious reasons. Circumcision is a traditional, ritual practice for Jews and Muslims. A few years ago, the wife of a local rabbi went to court to get an injunction preventing her husband from circumcising their newborn son. Needless to say, their marriage didn't last much longer. Other cases dealing with the same issue have ended the same way: with the couple splitting up.
- Health. A number of studies have shown that circumcision reduces a boy's (and, later, a man's) chances of getting HIV and some other sexually transmitted diseases, developing urinary tract infections (UTI) or cancer of the penis, and may reduce his future partner's chance of developing cancer of the cervix. Uncircumcised boys are ten times more likely to develop a UTI than circumcised ones (1 in 100 vs. 1 in 1,000), but the risk was very small to begin with. In addition, circumcision completely prevents phimosis, a condition in which the foreskin can't be retracted. Phimosis, which affects about 1–2 percent of uncircumcised males, can also be cured later on by circumcision, a procedure that gets a lot more painful with age. Short of that, the foreskin may be able to be loosened by gentle stretching (do not do this without proper medical supervision) or by using a topical steroid cream prescribed by your pediatrician to soften it.
- Hygiene. A circumcised penis is a lot easier to clean—both for the parents and for the boy himself.
- Conformity. If you've been circumcised, your son will probably want to look like you. Worldwide, only about 20 percent of boys are circumcised. But in the United States, it's a lot more popular, and having it done will probably make him look more like the other boys in the locker room. Nationwide, about 57 percent of boys are circumcised, but depending on where you live, the rate may be higher (67 percent in the Midwest) or lower (40 percent in the West). Those rates are probably low, since they count only circumcisions done in hospitals. Given that post-birth hospital stays are sometimes as short as twenty-four hours, there's no time to get it done.
- Pleasure. The American Academy of Pediatrics says that "Male circumcision does not appear to adversely affect penile sexual function/sensitivity or sexual

satisfaction." Millions of circumcised men around the world have perfectly delightful sex lives, and doctors have found little, if any, conclusive proof that circumcision has any negative effects on boys' or men's sexual, psychological, or emotional health. In fact, in a recent article in the journal *Urology*, Turkish researcher Temucin Senkul and his colleagues tested this hypothesis by asking uncircumcised men who were about to be circumcised for religious reasons to rate their sexual satisfaction and function before the procedure and at least twelve weeks after. The only difference between the before and the after was that it took the circumcised men a little longer to ejaculate, something many men would consider to be a good thing rather than a bad one. In other similar studies, some men actually reported an increase in pleasure.

WHY YOU MIGHT WANT TO CONSIDER *NOT* CIRCUMCISING YOUR SON

- Pain. No matter how you look at it, getting circumcised is painful. The circumcision cut will take about three days to heal fully. Until the late 1990s, most circumcisions were done without anesthetic. Today, most are done with either a numbing cream or an injection. OB/GYN Marjorie Greenfield cites research showing that babies who get some precircumcision anesthetic "cry less, have a more normal heart rate during the procedure, and are less irritable" than those who were medication-free. Younger doctors and those practicing in the western states are more likely to use pain blocks than older doctors or those anywhere else in the country. Whether the circumcision is done by the baby's doctor or the mother's depends on the doctor's medical training and where he or she is practicing.
- Other risks. Complications, while extremely rare, can occur. There is about a 1 in 500 chance of bleeding, penile injury, or local infection due to circumcision, but death is almost never a risk. In 1979, for example, there was only one circumcision-related death in the entire United States. A recent comprehensive study comparing the risks and benefits of circumcision found that the procedure prevents six urinary tract infections for every complication endured and that about two complications can be expected for every case of penile cancer prevented. "Circumcision remains a relatively safe procedure," write doctors Christakis, Harvey, Zerr, and their colleagues who conducted the study. "However, for some parents, the risks we report may outweigh the potential benefits."
- Conformity. As above, if you haven't been circumcised, your son will probably want to look like you.
- Pleasure. Some people believe that the foreskin is there for a purpose—to protect the tip of the penis—and that removing it can cause the penis to be

less sensitive, which will reduce sexual pleasure later in life. A number of anti-circumcision groups claim that penile circumcision has the same impact on boys that "female circumcision" has on girls. There is absolutely no evidence that this is true. Female circumcision (more accurately called genital mutilation) is practiced in some parts of the world and involves completely or partially removing a girl's clitoris or sewing the labia minora together. The specific purpose is to reduce the girl's sexual pleasure or ability to have intercourse before marriage, which, supposedly, will make her less likely to stray later. There is simply no comparison between the two procedures, and frankly, I think it's offensive to mention them both in the same sentence.

- Is it necessary at all? Some claim that many of the health risks thought to be reduced by circumcision may in fact be reduced simply by better hygiene—something that can be taught. The American Academy of Pediatrics and the American Urological Association have both taken fairly noncommittal positions. The AAP: "After a comprehensive review of the scientific evidence, the American Academy of Pediatrics found the health benefits of newborn male circumcision outweigh the risks, but the benefits are not great enough to recommend universal newborn circumcision." The AUA: "Neonatal circumcision has potential medical benefits and advantages as well as disadvantages and risks. Neonatal circumcision is generally a safe procedure when performed by an experienced operator. . . . When performed on healthy newborn infants as an elective procedure, the incidence of serious complications is extremely low." Bottom line? It's a personal decision that's totally up to you and your partner.

CARE OF THE CIRCUMCISED PENIS

Your son's penis will be red and sore for a few days after the circumcision. And until it's fully healed—which will take from a week to ten days—you'll need to protect the newly exposed tip and keep it from sticking to the inside of his diaper. A few tiny spots of blood on his diapers for up to two days is perfectly normal, but call your doctor if there's more blood that that, if the redness gets worse after three or four days, or if your son hasn't urinated within six to eight hours after the circumcision. How you care for your son's penis will depend on which method was used to do the circumcision, so ask the person who performed it before you do anything. The general rule is that you'll need to keep the penis dry and the tip lubricated with petroleum jelly and wrapped in gauze at every diaper change. If there's a plastic ring over the tip of the penis (it's called a Plastibell), just leave it alone and let it fall off by itself. Again, check with the person who did the procedure for specific care instructions.

CARE OF THE UNCIRCUMCISED PENIS

Even if you elect not to circumcise your son, you'll still have to spend some time taking care of his penis. Eighty-five percent of boys under six months have foreskins that don't retract (pull back to reveal the head of the penis), so don't try to force it. Fortunately, as boys get older, their foreskins retract on their own; by age one, 50 percent retract, and by age three, 80–90 percent do. The standard way to clean an uncircumcised penis is to retract the foreskin as far as it will comfortably go, and gently wash the head with mild soap and warm water. There is absolutely no need to use antiseptics, cotton swabs, or any other special cleaning measures.

Dealing with Contingencies

LABOR: REAL OR FALSE

By now, your partner has probably experienced plenty of Braxton-Hicks contractions ("false labor"), which have been warming up her uterus for the real thing. Sometimes, however, these practice contractions may be so strong that your partner may think that labor has begun. The bottom line is that when real labor starts, your partner will probably know it. (This may sound strange, especially if she is carrying her first child. Nevertheless, the majority of mothers I've spoken to have told me it's true.) But until then, you—and she—may not be sure whether the contractions and other things she's feeling are the real thing or not. So before you go rushing off to the hospital, take a few seconds to try to figure things out.

FALSE LABOR

- Contractions are not regular, or don't stay regular
- Contractions don't get stronger or more severe
- If your partner changes position (from sitting to walking, or from standing to lying down), the contractions usually stop altogether or change in frequency or intensity
- Generally, there is little or no vaginal discharge of any kind
- There may be additional pain in the abdomen

REAL LABOR

- Contractions are regular
- Contractions get stronger, longer, and closer together with time
- There may be some blood-tinged vaginal discharge
- Your partner's membranes may rupture (the famous "water" that "breaks" is really the amniotic fluid that the baby has been floating in throughout the pregnancy)
- There may be additional pain in the lower back

PLANES, TRAINS, AND AUTOMOBILES

It seems like half the births you see in the movies take place on the backseat of a speeding taxi, in a snowbound cave, in an airplane bathroom, or at the end of a bungee cord. While those sorts of images may sell movie tickets, the reality is that about 98 percent of babies are born in hospitals. (And most of the nonhospital births were *planned* that way.) Nevertheless, at some point, just about every pregnant couple—okay, it's really more of a guy thing—starts worrying about giving birth unexpectedly.

EMERGENCY BIRTHS

Emergency births fall into two general categories: either you have a lot of time before the actual birth (you're snowed in, trapped in your basement because of an earthquake, or shipwrecked, and you know you're not going to get to a hospital for a while), or you have little or no time before the birth (you're caught in traffic, you're parachuting to safety, or your partner's labor was extremely short). Either way, there's not a whole lot you can do to prepare.

Of course, your first step should be to call 911 (assuming that's even possible). If you have some time, try to make sure that your partner is in the most sheltered area of wherever you happen to be, and that she's comfortable, which, given her condition, is a relative term. If you have facilities available, get yourself some clean towels or sheets and boil a piece of string or a shoelace and a pair of scissors or a knife. Then, just sit tight and let nature take its course.

If you don't have time, try to stay cool. Handling a birth is not as difficult as you might think. Doctors who do it for a living, in fact, usually show up just a few minutes before the birth and are there primarily in case any complications arise. The truth is that most of the time babies pretty much deliver themselves when they're good and ready. The ones who seem to be in a hurry usually come out without any complications.

Whether you have time to prepare or not, once the baby starts to come, the procedure for performing a delivery is the same. And you'll know the process has started when:
- Your partner can't resist pushing.
- The baby's head—or any other body part—is visible.

For the rest of this chapter, we'll describe what you should do if there's no way to avoid delivering the baby yourself. The information isn't intended to replace the years of training your doctor or midwife has. So don't try this at home—unless there's no other option.

STEP ONE: PREPARATION.

Call for help if you have reception. Try to keep your partner focused on the breathing and relaxation techniques. Put a pillow or some clothing under her buttocks in order to keep the baby's head and shoulders from hitting a hard surface.

STEP TWO: THE HEAD.

When the head begins to appear, don't pull on it. Instead, support it and let it come out by itself. If the umbilical cord is wrapped around the baby's neck, slowly and gently glide it over the head. Once the head is out, try to remove any mucus from the baby's nose and mouth (although the baby's passage through the birth canal is usually enough to do the trick).

STEP THREE: THE REST OF THE BODY.

Holding the baby's head, encourage your partner to push as the baby's shoulders appear. After the head has emerged, the rest of the baby's body should slide out pretty easily. Support the body as well as the head as it slides out. Despite what you may have seen or heard, you don't have to slap the baby's bottom to make him cry: he'll take care of that—and the associated breathing—all by himself. Of course, if he's blue or not breathing at all, you'll need to make use of those baby CPR skills you hopefully learned a month or two ago.

Place the baby on your partner's chest and encourage her to begin breast-feeding right away. (Breastfeeding makes the uterus contract, which helps expel the placenta and reduces the chances of excessive bleeding.) And don't worry—the umbilical cord is generally long enough to allow the baby to nurse while still attached. Dry the baby off immediately and cover mom and baby to keep them as warm as possible.

STEP FOUR: CUTTING THE CORD.

Using the clamp or the shoelace or piece of string you boiled a while ago, tie a tight knot around the cord three or four inches away from the baby. If you know

Things to Remember During an Emergency Birth

- Call for help as soon as possible.
- Try to relax. Do everything carefully, thoughtfully, and slowly.
- Keep the area where the baby will be delivered as clean as possible.
- Baby CPR. If you haven't taken a baby CPR class already, you should really consider it—just in case.

An Emergency Kit

It's extremely unlikely that your partner will give birth anywhere but in the hospital. However, if you want to make absolutely sure all the bases are covered, here's a list of supplies to keep at home, in the car, or anyplace else you and your partner are likely to be spending a lot of time during the last month or so of the pregnancy. Please keep in mind, though, that this list is for emergencies only. If you're planning a home birth, you'll need a lot more supplies.

- Chux pads (large, sterile pads) for absorbing blood, amniotic fluid, and so forth. They're available at medical supply stores. If you can't find any, newspapers are fine—don't worry, a little ink won't hurt anything.
- Nonlatex gloves.
- A suction bulb, so you can Hoover out the baby's nose and mouth.
- A clamp for clamping off the umbilical cord. You can get these at any hospital supply store. If you can't find one, you can do the job with a clean string or shoelace.
- A plastic zipper bag to store the placenta.
- Clean scissors or knife for cutting the cord, if necessary (see below).
- Some towels to warm the baby and mother after the birth.

you can get to a hospital within two hours, don't cut the cord yet. If you're not going to make it by then, tie a second tight knot in the cord about two inches farther away from the baby and cut the cord between the knots with your knife or scissors. Don't worry about the cord stump that's still attached to the baby: it will fall off by itself in a week or so.

STEP FIVE: THE PLACENTA.

Don't think your delivery job is over as soon as the baby's out. Anywhere from five minutes to half an hour after the baby is born the placenta will arrive. Do not pull on the cord to "help" things along; in most cases the placenta, which is surprisingly large and meaty (it kind of reminds me of a hefty chunk of liver), will slip out on its own with a soft "plop." When it does, wrap it up in something clean or drop it into a plastic bag—but don't throw it away; your doctor will want to take a look at it as soon as possible.

After the placenta is out, gently massage your partner's lower abdomen every few minutes. This causes contractions, which limit blood loss and start the process of returning her uterus back to its original shape, or at least close to it.

Labor and Delivery

WHAT'S GOING ON WITH YOUR PARTNER

The entire labor process typically lasts twelve to twenty hours—toward the high end for first babies and the low end for subsequent ones—but there are no hard and fast rules. Labor is generally divided into three stages. The first stage consists of three phases.

Stage 1

PHASE 1 (EARLY OR LATENT LABOR) is the longest part of labor, lasting anywhere from a few hours to a few days (but the average is about eight hours). Fortunately, you'll be at home for most of it. At the beginning of this phase, your partner may not be able to feel the contractions. Even if she can, she'll probably tell you that they're fairly manageable. Contractions will generally last from thirty to forty-five seconds and come as much as twenty minutes apart. Over the next few hours they'll gradually get longer (as long as a minute), stronger, and closer together (perhaps as little as five minutes apart).

Every woman will have a slightly different early labor experience. My wife, for example, had from six to twelve hours of fairly long, fairly regular (three to five minutes apart) contractions almost every day for a week before our second daughter was born. Your partner may have "bloody show" (a blood-tinged vaginal discharge), backaches, and diarrhea.

PHASE 2 (ACTIVE LABOR) is generally shorter—from three to five hours—but far more intense than the first phase. It's likely to last as much as ten minutes longer if you're having a boy than if you're having a girl. If you aren't already there, it's time to head off to the hospital. In the early part of this phase, your partner will still be able to talk through the contractions. They'll keep getting closer together (two to three minutes apart now), longer, and stronger. As this stage progresses, she'll start feeling some real pain. The bloody show will increase and get redder, and your partner will become less and less chatty as she begins to focus on the contractions.

PHASE 3 (TRANSITION) usually lasts one or two hours. And once it starts, you can stop wondering why they call it "labor." Your partner's contractions may be almost relentless, each lasting as long as ninety seconds. And with just two or three minutes from the beginning of one until the beginning of the next one, there's barely any time to recover in between. The pain is intense, and if your partner is going to ask for some drugs, this is probably when she'll do it. She's tired, sweating, her muscles may be so exhausted that they're trembling, and she may be vomiting.

Stage 2 (Pushing and Birth)

This is by far the most intense part of the process—and fortunately for your partner, it lasts only about two hours ("only" being a term that's used by anyone who's not in labor. Your partner would probably prefer "for-friggin'-ever"). Your partner's contractions are still long (more than sixty seconds) but are further apart. The difference is that during the contractions, she'll be overcome with a desire to push—similar to the feeling of having to make a bowel movement. She may feel some unpleasant pressure and stinging as the baby's head "crowns" (starts coming through the vagina), but this will be followed by a huge sense of relief when the baby finally pops out.

Stage 3 (After the Birth: Delivering the Placenta)

Less than twenty minutes after the baby is born, the placenta will separate from the wall of the uterus. Your partner will continue to have contractions as her uterus tries to eject the placenta and stop the bleeding. See "The Placenta" on pages 225–27, 230 for more.

WHAT'S GOING ON WITH YOU

Starting labor is no picnic, for her or for you. She, of course, is experiencing—or soon will be—a lot of physical pain. You, in the meantime, are very likely to feel a heavy dose of psychological pain.

I couldn't possibly count the number of times—only in my dreams, thankfully—I've heroically defended my home and family from armies of murderers and thieves. But even when I'm awake, I know I wouldn't hesitate before diving in front of a speeding car if it meant being able to save my wife or my children. And I know I would submit to the most painful ordeal to keep any one of them from suffering. This instinct perhaps explains the adrenaline rush you'll probably feel. A team of Scandinavian researchers took fathers' pulses during the birth of their children and found that they went from an average of 72 beats/minute to 115 beats/minute just before the birth. But helping your partner through labor is not the same as deciding to rescue a child from a burning building.

The most important thing to remember about this final stage of pregnancy is that the pain—yours and hers—is finite. After a while it ends, and you get to hold your new baby. Ironically, however, her pain will probably end sooner than yours. She'll be sore for a few weeks or so, but by the time the baby is six months old, your partner will hardly remember it. If women *could* remember the pain, I can't imagine that any of them would have more than one child. But for six months, a year, even two years after our first daughter was born, my wife's pain remained fresh in my mind. And when we began planning our second pregnancy, the thought of her having to go through even a remotely similar experience frightened me.

STAYING INVOLVED

Being There—Mentally and Physically

Despite your fears and worries, this is one time when your partner's needs—and they aren't all physical—come first. But before we get into how you can best help her through labor and delivery, it's important to get a firm idea of how to tell when she's actually gone into labor, and what stage she's in once she's there.

STAGE 1

PHASE 1 (EARLY OR LATENT LABOR) Although the contractions are fairly mild at this point, you should do everything you can to make your partner as comfortable as possible (back rubs, massages, and so forth). Some women may tell you exactly what they want you to do; others may feel a little shy about making any demands. Either way, ask her regularly what you can do to help. And when she tells you, do it. If taking a walk makes her feel better, go with her. If doing headstands in the living room is what she wants to do (fairly unlikely at this point), go ahead and spot her.

The easiest way to tell whether she's really in labor is to watch the contractions. If they're getting longer, stronger, and closer together, it's the real deal. If

Checking Things Out When You're Checking In

Here's what Sarah McMoyler recommends to her students. "On the day you check into the hospital, take a few minutes to survey the room and the labor and delivery unit. You're going to be in that room for hours and hours, go ahead and open up the cabinets to see where they keep the washcloths, gowns, bath blankets, extra pillows. While you're at it, try to find out where the wheeled stool is (for you to sit on), the shower, the nurse call button, and the controls for the electronic bed. Most of the time the nurse will get these for you, but if she's also busy caring for other patients, understand that she may not be able to get them as quickly as you need them."

While you're getting the lay of the land, be sure to locate the ice chip maker, the snack bar, and the place where they keep those warmed-up blankets. And make a special point of introducing yourself to the nursing staff. Let them know about any special concerns your partner might have. Does she have any allergies? Did she have a bad pregnancy experience sometime in the past? Is she afraid of needles? And tell them about your goals—in particular, your desire to be as involved as possible—while also letting them know that you'd love their input and advice. This is a great time to ask questions. They really are on your side, and they know a ton about labor and delivery. The warmer your relationship with the medical team, the smoother the whole experience will go.

---

not, take it easy. You should be recording the contractions anyway, because when you call her practitioner to ask whether to head off to the hospital, he'll want to know what's been going on.

During early labor, it's important for your partner to keep her strength up, so many OBs will recommend light eating—salads, soups, and so on. And drinking water during early labor is crucial. No matter what your partner does, *you* should eat and drink something. You need to keep your energy level up too, and you're not going to want to try to make a dash to the snack bar between contractions. Finally, try to get some rest—and encourage her to do the same. Don't be fooled by the adrenaline rush that will hit you when your partner finally goes into labor. You'll be so excited that you'll feel you can last forever. But you can't. She's got some hormones (and pain) to keep her going; you don't.

PHASE 2 (ACTIVE LABOR) One of the symptoms of second-phase labor is that your partner may seem to be losing interest in just about everything—including

221

arguing with you about when to call the doctor. After my wife's contractions had been two to three minutes apart for a few hours, I was encouraging her to call. She refused. Many women, it seems, "just know" when it's time to go. So chances are, if she tells you "it's time," you should grab your car keys. That said, you're going to be in regular contact with your partner's practitioner, and if he or she thinks it's time to come in, that trumps your partner's desires to stay home.

One of the biggest hints that your partner is in active labor is whether she can walk and talk through the contractions. If not, she most likely is. If you're still not sure that the second phase has started, here's a pretty typical scenario that may help you decide:

YOU: Honey, these contractions have been going on like this for three hours. I think we should head off to the hospital.

HER: Okay.

YOU: Great. Let's get dressed, okay?

HER: I don't want to get dressed.

YOU: But you're only wearing a nightgown. How about at least putting on some shoes and socks?

HER: I don't want any shoes and socks.

YOU: But it's cold out there. How about a jacket?

HER: I don't want a jacket.

Get the point?

Another common symptom of second-phase labor is an uncharacteristic loss of modesty. A number of nurses, midwives, and doulas have told me that they can always tell what stage of labor a woman is in just by looking at the sheet on the bed (when the pregnant woman is in it). If she's in phase one, she'll be covered up to her neck; in phase two, the sheet is halfway down; by phase three (see below), the sheet's all the way off.

Once active labor has started, your partner shouldn't eat anything unless her doctor specifically says that it's okay (she probably won't be allowed to eat anything after getting admitted to the hospital). If she ends up needing any medication or even a Cesarean, food in her stomach could complicate matters.

PHASE 3 (TRANSITION) Whenever laboring women are portrayed in TV shows, they almost always seem to be snapping at their husband or boyfriend, yelling things like "Don't touch me!" or "Leave me alone, you're the one who did this to me." I think I'd internalized those stereotypes, and by the time we got to the hospital I was really afraid that my wife would behave the same way when she got to the transition stage, blame me for the pain, and push me away. Fortunately, it never happened. The closest we ever came was when my wife was in labor with our second daughter. The only place she could be comfortable was in the shower, and for a while I was in there with her, trying to talk her through the contractions as I massaged her aching back. Then she asked me to leave the bathroom for a while. Sure, that stung for a minute—I felt I should be there with her—but it was clear that she had no intention of hurting me.

Unfortunately, not every laboring woman manages to be as graceful under pressure. If your partner happens to say something nasty to you or throws you unceremoniously out of the room for a while, you need to imagine that while she's in labor her mind is being taken over by an angry rush-hour mob, all trying to push and shove their way onto an overcrowded subway train. Quite often, the pain she's experiencing is so intense and overwhelming that the only way she can make it through the contractions is to concentrate completely on them. Something as simple and well-meaning as a word or a loving caress can be terribly distracting.

So what *can* you do? Whatever she wants. Fast. If she doesn't want you to touch her, don't insist. Offer to feed her some ice chips instead. If she wants you to get out of the room, go. But tell her that you'll be right outside in case she needs you. If the room is pitch black and she tells you it's too bright, agree with her and find something to turn off. If she wants to listen to the twenty-four-hour Elvis station, turn it on. But whatever you do, don't argue with her, don't try to reason with her, and above all, don't pout if she swears at you or calls you names. She really doesn't mean to, and the last thing she needs to deal with at this moment of crisis is your wounded pride.

STAGE 2: PUSHING

Up until the pushing stage, I thought I was completely prepared for dealing with my wife's labor and delivery. I was calm, and, despite my occasional feelings of inadequacy, I knew what to expect almost every step of the way. The hospital staff was supportive of my wanting to be with my wife through every contraction. But when the time came to start pushing, they changed. All of a sudden, they were in control. The doctor was called, extra nurses magically appeared, and the room began to fill up with equipment—a scale, a bassinet, a tray of sterilized medical instruments, a washbasin, diapers, towels. (We happened to be in a combination labor/birthing room; if, in the middle of the pushing stage, you find yourself chasing after your wife, who's being rushed down the hall to a separate delivery room, don't be alarmed. It may feel like an emergency, but it probably isn't.)

The nurses told my wife what to do, how to do it, and when. All I could do was watch—and I must admit that at first I felt a little cheated. After all, *I* was the one who had been there right from the beginning. *My* baby was about to be born. But when the most important part finally arrived, it looked like I wasn't going to be anything more than a spectator. And unless you're a professional birthing coach or a trained labor and delivery nurse, chances are you're going to feel like a spectator, too. Useless and out of control.

As I watched the nurses do their stuff, I quickly realized that simply holding your partner's legs and saying, "Push, honey: that's great!" isn't always enough. Recognizing a good, productive push, and, more important, being able to explain how to do one—"Raise your butt…lower your legs…keep your head back…curl up around your baby like a shrimp…"—are skills that come from years of experience.

But just because you *feel* like a spectator doesn't mean you actually have to be one. Your partner needs you to be there, to support her, to encourage her—not in another corner of the room or hiding behind a camera, but right there with her. If you back away at this critical time, she may feel abandoned—even though she's surrounded by professionals. So let the medical team take the lead, but hang in there and ask them how you can be involved (this is a question you should have asked when you first got to the hospital; see "Checking Things Out When You're Checking In" on page 221 for more).

STAGE 2: BIRTH

Intellectually, I knew my wife was pregnant. I'd been to all the appointments and I'd heard the heartbeat, seen the ultrasound, and felt the baby kicking. Still, there was something intangible about the whole process. And it wasn't until our baby started "crowning" (peeking her hairy little head out of my wife's vagina) that all the pieces finally came together.

At just about the same moment, I also realized that there was one major advantage to my having been displaced during the pushing stage: I had both hands free to "catch" the baby as she came out—and believe me, holding my daughter's hot, slimy, bloody little body and placing her gently at my wife's breast was easily the highlight of the whole occasion.

If you think you might want to do this, make sure you've worked out the choreography with your doctor and the nurses before the baby starts crowning. (See "Birth Plans" on pages 180–85 for more information.)

Your partner, unfortunately, is in the worst possible position to see the baby being born. Most hospitals, however, have tried to remedy this situation by making mirrors available. Still, many women are concentrating so hard on the pushing that they may not be interested in looking in the mirror.

If you were expecting your newborn to look like the Gerber baby, you may be in for a bit of a shock. Babies are generally born covered with a whitish coating called vernix. They're sometimes blue, and frequently covered with blood and mucus. Their eyes may be puffy, their genitals swollen, and their backs and shoulders may be covered with fine hair. In addition, the trip through the birth canal has probably left your baby with a cone-shaped head. All in all, it's the most beautiful sight in the world.

The Placenta

Before our first child was born, it had simply never occurred to me (or to my wife, for that matter) that labor and delivery wouldn't end when the baby was born. While you and your partner are admiring your new family member, the placenta—which has been your baby's life support system for the past five months or so—still must be delivered. Your partner may continue to have mild contractions for anywhere from five minutes to about an hour until this happens. The strange thing about this stage of the delivery is that neither you nor your partner will probably even know it's happening—you'll be much too involved with your new baby.

Once the placenta is out, however, you need to decide what to do with it. In this country, most people never even see it, and those who do just leave it at the hospital, where it will either be incinerated as medical waste or, more likely, used for biomedical research or sold to a cosmetics company (there are actually a surprising number of placenta-based beauty products). But in many other cultures, the placenta is considered to have a permanent, almost magical bond with the child it nourished in the womb, and disposal is handled with a great deal more reverence. In fact, most cultures that have placenta rituals believe that if it is not properly buried, the child—or the parents, or even the entire village—will suffer some terrible consequences.

In rural Peru, for example, immediately after the birth of a child, the father is required to go to a far-off location and bury the placenta deep enough so that no animals or people will accidentally discover it. Otherwise, the placenta may become "jealous" of the attention paid to the baby and may take revenge by causing an epidemic.

In some South American Indian cultures, people believe that a child's life can be influenced by objects that are buried with its placenta. According to anthropologist J. R. Davidson, parents in the Qolla tribe "bury miniature implements copied after the ones used in adult life with the placenta, in the hopes of assuring that the infant will be a good worker. Boys' placentas are frequently buried with a shovel or a pick, and girls' are buried with a loom or a hoe." In the Philippines, some mothers bury the placenta with books as a way of ensuring intelligence.

But placentas are not always buried. In ancient Egypt, pharaohs' placentas were wrapped in special containers to keep them from harm. Sometimes a placenta

Helping Her Cope

Throughout labor and delivery, your focus should be on your partner. But because childbirth is such a female-intensive thing, a lot of guys don't really understand how important they are to the process. The reality is that you're absolutely indispensable. Yes, there are doctors and nurses and midwives running around all over the place, but your partner is really counting on *you* most of all to help get her through this. Your being there—and being actively involved—can make a big, big difference. Women whose partners are supportive during labor and delivery tend to have shorter labors and report experiencing less pain. They also have a more positive attitude toward motherhood.

Here are a number of ways you can help your partner cope throughout the labor and delivery. Some of these are drawn from *The Best Birth*, which I wrote with childbirth educator Sarah McMoyler (see page 163 for more about her approach).

- Remind her to slow her breathing down. Just taking in long, deep breaths—inhale for five seconds, exhale for five seconds—can be very calming.
- Encourage her to moan during the contractions and rest in between. Screaming isn't very effective in coping with pain, and neither is the patterned breathing taught in many childbirth prep systems. Instead, go for low, growly, guttural sounds—deep and loud—the kind of sounds you'd make if you tried to lift a car. This is no time to be dainty or to worry about what the people in the next room—or on the next floor—will think. They're probably making plenty of noises of their own.
- Help her relax. People coping with pain often clench their jaws, make fists, tense their shoulders, or hold their breath. None of this helps. In fact, it does more harm than good.

would be used as a stand-in for the pharaoh at public events, according to researcher Anne Glausser. Some historians believe that the smallest pyramids were actually built as tombs for pharaohs' placentas. And a wealthy Inca in Ecuador built a solid-gold statue of his mother—complete with his placenta in "her" womb.

Even today, the people of many cultures believe that placentas have special powers. A lot of women—including a growing number of Hollywood celebrities—believe that *placentophagy* (ingesting cooked or dried placenta) can reduce or eliminate postpartum depression or help keep their skin looking youthful. In parts of Peru placentas are burned, the ashes are mixed with water, and the mixture is then fed to the babies as a remedy for a variety of childhood illnesses.

- Get in her face and be direct. This may seem a little aggressive, but it really does work. In early labor, lock eyes with her and tell her what to do: unclench your jaw, un-fist your hands, drop your shoulders, breeeeeeathe . . . As labor progresses, skip the words and just show her what you want her to do by letting your body melt, unclenching, and moaning. Doing this is especially important between contractions. Staying tense—or tensing up in anticipation of the next uterus-wrenching contraction—will make it harder for her to recover during those all-too-brief breaks.
- Offer sips of water, ice chips, and cold compresses.
- Offer a massage. Back, hands, feet, or whatever she'd like (if she wants anything at all). Sometimes, when massage is annoying, sustained counterpressure can be just the ticket. Ask her which helps more: high or low on the back, or closer to the tailbone.
- Verbal anesthesia. Tell her she's doing a great job—it means a lot more coming from you than from a nurse she doesn't know. Simple things like "Great job!" or "Stay with it" are remarkably effective.
- Make sure she hits the bathroom at least once every hour. If she's not peeing that often, she's not drinking enough.
- Get her up and moving around. Being upright, if at all possible, makes gravity kick in and help the baby descend. Walking around keeps her body in motion and maximizes the effect that relaxin (a hormone that does just that) can have on the pelvic joints. You may be able to do this during the contractions in early labor. But once she's deep into active labor, do it between contractions.

Traditional Vietnamese medicine uses placentas to combat sterility and senility, and in India, touching a placenta is supposed to help a childless woman conceive a healthy baby of her own. In China, some believe that breastfeeding mothers can improve the quality of their milk by drinking a broth made of boiled placenta, or speed up labor by eating a piece of it dried.

This sort of placenta usage isn't limited to non-Western cultures. In medieval Europe, if a child was born with a caul (with the amniotic membranes over his head), the placenta would be saved, dried, and fed to the child on his tenth birthday. If it wasn't done, it was believed that the child might become a vampire after death.

The Three Stages of Labor and Delivery

STAGE	WHAT'S HAPPENING	WHAT SHE'S FEELING
Stage 1/ Phase 1 (early or latent labor)	• Her cervix is effacing (thinning out) and dilating (opening up) to about 3 centimeters • Her water may break	• She may be excited but not totally sure that "this is really it" • She may be anxious, restless, and wondering whether she'll remember anything from the childbirth prep class you took • She may not feel like doing much of anything • She may have diarrhea
Stage 1/ Phase 2 (active labor)	• She's increasingly uncomfortable • Her cervix continues to efface and will dilate to 7 or 8 centimeters • Her water may break (if it hasn't already) or may have to be broken	• She's getting serious and impatient about the pain • She's beginning to concentrate fully on the contractions and on the labor of labor • Bye-bye, sense of humor
Stage 1/ Phase 3 (transition)	• Her cervix is now fully dilated (if not, the baby may have to descend a bit before she'll be allowed to push) • She may feel the urge to push • She may be nauseated, and may cry—from pain, fear, or both	• She may be confused, frustrated, and scared • She may announce that she can't take it anymore and is going home
Stage 2 (pushing and birth)	• Increase in bloody discharge • The baby is moving through the birth canal • Doctor may have to do an episiotomy	• She's feeling confident that she can finish the job • She may have gotten her second wind • She may be very worried that she'll poop while she's pushing. And there's a good chance she's right.
Stage 3 (after the birth)	• The placenta is separating from the wall of the uterus • Episiotomy or tearing (if any) will be repaired	• RELIEF • Euphoria • Talkative • Strong, heroic • Hungry, thirsty • Empty (of the baby) • Desire to cuddle with her baby (and her partner)

WHAT YOU CAN DO

- Reassure her
- Tell jokes, take a walk, go out for your last romantic prebaby dinner, or rent a movie—anything to distract her
- Keep her hydrated—and make sure she hits the bathroom regularly
- Record the contractions—how long they last and how often they come
- If it's nighttime, encourage her to try to sleep; active labor will wake her up, but any rest she can get now will really pay off later on
- While she's napping, double-check that your bags are packed, that you've got your phone, and that you've made arrangements for someone to feed the dog until you get home

- Call the doctor before you leave to make sure it's okay to head to the hospital
- Don't bother with conversation. She's not going to be able to keep up her end. So keep communication short and to the point.
- Reassure and encourage her
- Help her take one contraction at a time
- Feed her ice chips
- Praise her for her progress
- Massage, massage, massage

- Do whatever she wants you to do
- Try to help her resist pushing until the doctor tells her she should
- Mop her brow with a wet cloth
- Feed her ice chips
- Massage her (if she wants it)

- Continue to reassure and comfort her
- Encourage her to push when she's supposed to and tell her how great she's doing
- Encourage her to watch the baby come out (if she wants to and if there's a mirror around)
- Let the professionals do their job

- Praise her
- Put the baby on her stomach
- Encourage her to relax
- Encourage her to start nursing the baby, if she feels ready
- Bond with her and the baby

Whatever you and your partner decide to do, it's probably best to keep it a secret—at least from the hospital staff. Some states try to regulate what you can do with a placenta and may even prohibit you from taking it home (although if you really want to, you can probably find a sympathetic nurse who will pack it up for you). We deliberately left our first daughter's placenta at the hospital. But we stored the second one's in our freezer for a year before burying it, along with the placentas of some of our friends' children, and planting an apple tree above them. Twelve years later, at her bat mitzvah, we ate some of the apples from that tree. And yes, they tasted perfectly fine.

Dealing with Contingencies

Unfortunately, not all labors and deliveries proceed exactly as planned. In fact, most don't. As we'll discuss in the next chapter, nearly a third of babies in the U.S. are born by Cesarean section. And 60–80 percent of mothers who deliver vaginally are medicated in some way, usually with an epidural (we'll talk about that in detail below). As with so many other aspects of your pregnancy experience, having good, clear information about what's really going on and what the options are during labor and delivery will help you make informed, intelligent decisions about how to handle the unexpected or the unplanned. The key to getting the information you need is to ask questions—and to keep on asking until you're completely satisfied. Find out about the risks, the benefits, and the effects on your partner, as well as on the baby. The only exception to this rule is when there's a clear medical emergency. In that case, save your questions for later.

Here are a few of the contingencies that can come up during the birth and how they might affect you, your partner, and the baby.

PAIN

If you've taken a traditional Lamaze or Bradley childbirth class or read many pregnancy books (and even if you haven't), you and your partner may be planning to have a "natural" (medication-free) childbirth. Unfortunately, natural childbirth often sounds better—and less painful—than it actually turns out to be. According to Marci Lobel, Ph.D., director of the Stony Brook Pregnancy Project at Stony Brook University, "Popular books written for pregnant women often understate the degree of pain experienced during birth, and may overstate the effectiveness of childbirth preparation in reducing pain." And think about all those childbirth images you've seen in movies and on TV. The pain looks unbearable, but it never lasts any more than a few minutes.

Because your partner is the one who is experiencing the physical pain, defer to her judgment when considering ways to manage it. This doesn't mean, however, that you don't have anything to say about the issue. As labor progresses, your partner will become less rational and less able to make big decisions. So it's up to you to be her advocate, to make sure she has the kind of birth she wants (or at least as close to it as you can get). That's why I strongly suggest that the two of you have some thorough discussions about her attitude toward medication *before* she goes into labor, so you know whether she'd want you to suggest it when you get concerned or wait until she requests it. You might also want to come up with a code word that means "I really want drugs NOW." Some women may scream for the doctor (or you) to "do something about the pain" but not really want drugs.

If you do end up having a discussion about medication sometime *during* labor, make sure you do it in the most supportive possible way. It's painful to have to watch the one you love suffer, but starting an argument when she's in the middle of a contraction isn't a smart idea (and you're not going to resolve anything anyway). Despite the fact that most women get some kind of chemical pain relief, many feel that taking medication is a sign of weakness, or that they've failed—as women and as mothers. It's as if having an unmedicated childbirth is part of the transition to womanhood. In addition, some childbirth preparation methods view medication as the first step along a path that ultimately leads to birth complications and/or Cesarean section. Neither of these scenarios is, by any stretch of the imagination, the rule. If you check into the hospital with a pregnant partner and leave a few days later with a no-longer-pregnant partner and a healthy baby, you win. It shouldn't matter at all how it happened, as long as the medication or the procedure was medically necessary (and it almost always is).

I'm not suggesting that your partner should use—or that she'll even need—pain medication. But whatever you do, knowing a little about your options is always a good idea (see "Whew! That's a Relief" on pages 232–34).

EXHAUSTION

Pain isn't the only reason your partner might need some chemical intervention. In some cases, labor is progressing so slowly (or has been stalled for so long) that your partner's practitioner may become concerned that she'll be too exhausted by the time she needs to push. This was exactly what happened during the birth of my middle daughter. After twenty hours of labor and only four centimeters of dilation, our doctor suggested *pitocin* (a drug that stimulates contractions) together with an epidural (see pages 232–33). This chemical cocktail removed the pain of labor while allowing my wife's cervix to dilate fully and quickly. I'm convinced that this approach actually prevented a C-section by giving my wife a well-deserved breather before she started pushing.

Whew! That's a Relief

FOR THE BABY

There is, as Sarah McMoyler puts it, "a big difference between coping and suffering." Despite all the emphasis on natural (unmedicated) childbirth these days, more and more women seem to be opting for some kind of chemical pain relief during labor and childbirth. Actually, there's evidence that women have been searching for alternatives to natural birth ever since they were first introduced in the 1840s, says obstetric anesthesiologist Donald Caton, author of *What a Blessing She Had Chloroform: The Medical and Social Response to the Pain of Childbirth from 1800 to the Present.*

Women today have literally dozens of options that fall into to two basic categories: *regionals*, which reduce or eliminate pain only in certain parts of her body, and *systemics*, which will relax her whole body.

REGIONALS

These medications work only on specific regions of the body, hence the name. The most common of all regionals (and of all childbirth-related pain medication, for that matter) is the epidural, which is usually administered during active labor (the second phase of the first stage), when the pain is greatest. Your partner will have to lean over or curl up on her side while an anesthesiologist numbs her lower back, inserts a medication-carrying catheter into the "epidural space" that surrounds the spinal cord, and tapes it to her back.

According to the American Pregnancy Association, "The goal of an epidural is to provide analgesia, or pain relief, rather than anesthesia which leads to total lack of feeling." Epidurals are widely considered the safest and most effective labor painkiller available. They kick in within a few minutes and will block the pain of your partner's contractions while still leaving her awake and alert. Perhaps most important, they don't "cross the placenta" (affect the baby).

Until just a few years ago, epidurals carried the risk of decreasing maternal blood pressure or reducing the woman's ability to feel when to push (which could slow down the course of labor), as well as causing headaches and nausea. And a lot of people thought that epidurals increased the risk of a Cesarean or instrument birth. But today, anesthesiologists are better able to fine-tune the dose, greatly reducing these risks. A growing body of research shows that women who have epidurals aren't any more likely to have a C-section or instrument birth. In fact, epidurals may actually move labor along more quickly. By blocking the pain, the woman can get a well-deserved break (sometimes even a nap), so when it's time to push, she'll be refreshed and strong.

Another problem with epidurals used to be that, since they numb the lower body, women were confined to their beds for the duration. But the combined spinal epidural (CSE), or "walking epidural," offers the same pain relief and allows at least some mobility (although, despite the name, your partner probably won't be able to walk). Walking epidurals aren't available everywhere, so ask your partner's practitioner whether it's available at your hospital.

Epidurals aren't perfect—for about 10 percent of women, the epidural doesn't completely block the pain, and sometimes it can affect one side of the body more than the other. And there may be side effects, but they're rare. These include shivering, nausea, itching, and a drop in blood pressure.

You might also check with the hospital to see whether PCEA (patient-controlled epidural anesthesia) is a possibility. The way it works is that the anesthesiologist gets the epidural up and running and then allows the patient to adjust the amount of medication she gets (within reason). As with any kind of patient-controlled medication, patients don't use nearly as much as a doctor would have given them. Seems that just knowing relief is a button-push away decreases the need.

Other less common regional options include the pudendal block (an injection given into each side of the vagina that deadens the vaginal opening) and the spinal block (an injection into the fluid around the spinal cord in the lower back—it's similar to an epidural but doesn't last as long and carries a slightly greater risk of complications).

SYSTEMICS

This type of whole-body pain relief includes sedatives, tranquilizers, and narcotics such as Demerol and fentanyl, which are usually given as injections or added to existing intravenous (IV) lines. It also includes general anesthesia, which knocks the recipient out completely and is rarely used, except when performing an emergency Cesarean.

Besides taking the edge off the contractions almost immediately, one of the major advantages to systemic medications is that your partner can use them from the very beginning of labor. They may relieve a lot of her anxiety and won't usually have much of an impact on her ability to push or sense her contractions.

Whew! That's a Relief *continued*

On the downside, though, these medications affect your partner's entire body and can cause a wide variety of side effects, including drowsiness, dizziness, and nausea. In some ways, these drugs do less to remove the pain than to make your partner simply stop caring about it. Even worse, since they go right into your partner's bloodstream, they also "cross the placenta," meaning that at birth, the baby could be drowsy, unable to suck properly for a short while, or, in rare cases, unable to breathe without assistance. Fortunately, those symptoms go away pretty quickly on their own. There's also a drug, Narcan (naloxone), that can reverse these side effects.

Interestingly, your partner's use—or nonuse—of pain medication may have an impact on you as well. For most expectant dads, anything that makes our partners more comfortable and hurt less is great. But besides that, medication can also reduce the stress and make the whole experience more pleasant for us. In a study of how a laboring woman's use of epidurals affects her partner, Italian researchers Giorgio Capogna and Michela Camorcia found that "fathers whose partners did not receive epidural analgesia felt their presence as troublesome and unnecessary." On the other hand, when the mom did have an epidural, fathers felt three times more helpful and involved and were less anxious and stressed than dads whose partners went med-free.

For other guys, though, reducing her pain may be a source of disappointment—in a twisted, yet understandable, sort of way. We're supposed to be there to help her through the pain, the thinking goes, but if she doesn't need us to do that, maybe she doesn't need us at all. In other words, reducing the pain may also reduce the father's sense of usefulness and importance. A word of advice: if your partner wants some pain medication, support her. There are plenty of other ways to be helpful.

INDUCED LABOR

Anytime after forty weeks of pregnancy, your baby is officially fully baked. They don't always get this piece of news, though, and are sometimes reluctant to come out. There are all sorts of supposedly surefire ways to bring on labor, and you'll start hearing every one of them as soon as you mention that the baby is late: eat certain kinds of salad dressings or vinegars, eat spicy food, go on long walks, drink cod-liver oil, and more. There is actually some research suggesting that sex may help: nipple stimulation and your partner's orgasm may trigger some contractions, plus semen has prostaglandin in it, which is similar to the gel or pill that's used to induce labor. And, as Lissa Rankin puts it, "Messing around with the cervix can trigger contractions and get things started." But before you try any kind of home remedy, check with your practitioner to make sure it's safe.

If your partner's due date is long past, your practitioner may decide that things have gone on long enough (this will happen about two months after your partner reached the same conclusion), and he'll suggest jump-starting the labor with pitocin (a chemical version of oxytocin) or Cytotec (a type of prostaglandin). Some people claim that pitocin results in more painful labors and increases the Cesarean rate, but just as many disagree, saying that all it does is jump-start normal labor.

Other Common Birth Contingencies

FORCEPS OR VACUUM

If your partner's cervix is completely dilated and she's been pushing for a while, but the baby refuses to budge, her practitioner may suggest using forceps—long tongs with scoops on the end (imagine salad tongs that are big enough to pick up a coconut)—to help things along. It used to be that the very word *forceps* struck fear into every expectant parent's heart. But today they're used only to gently grasp the baby's head to guide it through the birth canal. Some forceps deliveries will leave the baby with bruises in the temple or jawline area for a few days or a week. In very rare instances, permanent scarring or other damage can occur. In addition, your partner will need additional medication and may require a larger-than-normal episiotomy (see page 236).

In an increasing number of cases, instead of forceps, doctors are using a vacuum-type suction device that attaches to the top of the baby's head, to move the baby around in the same way. Vacuum extractors may leave some swelling or bruising on your baby's scalp. But your partner won't need as much pain medication as she would have with forceps.

The doctor may also suggest using forceps or vacuum if the baby is in distress and a vaginal birth needs to be sped up, or if your partner is too exhausted (or medicated) to push effectively. Keep in mind that most OB/GYNs are trained in either forceps (typically, older docs) or vacuum extraction (younger docs), not both. Used appropriately, one and/or the other can sometimes prevent the need for a C-section.

Not So Fast There, Little Lady

If your partner's or your baby's health is genuinely at risk, her doctor may want to induce labor before the thirty-ninth or fortieth week. It seems that an increasing number of women are trying to give birth early. They give all sorts of nonmedical reasons. Some are afraid of giving birth to a baby who's too big, some want to make sure they deliver on a day their doc will be on call or maybe before she goes on vacation. Some want to have their baby born on a specific day (a relative's or friend's birthday, a particularly auspicious day, or the last day of the year to get the tax deduction), and others want to make sure a particular person can be there for the birth (close friend, relative, *People* magazine paparazzi). And some are just sick and tired of being pregnant.

Hopefully, your partner's provider won't go along with any nonmedical preterm induction requests. But if she does, try to talk her and your partner out of it. New research from the National Child & Maternal Health Education Program (NCMHEP) has found that even a few weeks can make a big difference. The NCMHEP considers full-term to be thirty-nine to forty weeks. Babies born earlier, they say, are "at risk for problems with breathing, feeding, and controlling their temperature." They're also more likely to be admitted to the neonatal intensive care unit and develop infections. Catherine Spong, deputy director of the National Institute of Child Health and Human Development (www.nichd.nih.gov), adds, "The baby's brain almost doubles in size in the last several weeks of pregnancy. And the brain is forming all of the connections that are going to be important for coordination, for movement, and for learning." 'Nuf said?

EPISIOTOMY

An episiotomy involves making a small cut in the perineum (the area between the vagina and the anus) to enlarge the vaginal opening and allow for easier passage of the baby's head. (Did you just wince? I sure as hell did.) Only a decade or so ago, the episiotomy rate for first-time mothers under an obstetrician's care was 70–90 percent. The thought was that a controlled cut would help women avoid bowel, urinary, and sexual problems after delivery. But recent research has shown that episiotomy may actually increase the risk of those problems. Today, the episiotomy rate is under 20 percent. Overall, about 70 percent of first-time moms will have a small, spontaneous tear. The phrase "spontaneous tear" sounds absolutely frightening to me, but it turns out that with an episiotomy, the flesh can tear even more. So as contradictory as it might seem, those natural tears are preferable (and less painful) than a routine episiotomy. But the procedure may be legitimately indicated if:

- The baby is extremely large, and squeezing through the vagina might harm the baby or your partner.
- Forceps are used.
- The baby is breech (see below).
- The practitioner can see that numerous tears are going to happen.

BREECH PRESENTATION

If a baby is breech, it means that the head is up and the butt or feet are pointing down (only 3–4 percent of single babies are born this way, but about a third of all twins are). Actually, there are several different types of breech births: Frank breech means that the baby's feet are straight up next to his head and the baby will come out butt first. Complete breech means that the butt is down and the baby is "sitting" cross-legged. Footling breech means that one or both feet are pointing down. There's little you can do to prevent your baby from getting into any position he or she wants to. But most doctors in the United States will not deliver breech babies vaginally. This means that if the baby can't be turned, usually through a nonsurgical process called "external version," it's going to be delivered by C-section.

ELECTRONIC FETAL MONITORING (EFM)

EFMs have been around since the early 1970s, and today they're used in 85 percent of births. They come in two flavors: external and internal.

The external variety is a rather complicated-looking machine—complete with graphs, digital outputs, and high-tech beeping. Two belts are connected to the machine and get strapped to your partner's abdomen. One monitors your baby's heartbeat, the other monitors your partner's contractions.

Fetal monitors are really pretty cool. Properly hooked up, they are so accurate that by watching the digital display, you'll be able to tell when your partner's contractions are starting—even before *she* feels them—and if she has an IUPC (intrauterine pressure catheter, which is a tube that lies next to the baby and measures contraction strength), you'll actually be able to tell how intense they'll be. In one fascinating study, researchers Kristi Williams and Debra Umberson found that most expectant fathers like fetal monitors—partly because by getting information, we feel like we're really involved. "By observing and communicating the changing intensity of the contractions, these men believed that they were able to provide valuable information to their wives," they wrote. "This creates a role for husbands to play in labor and delivery that is, from their perspective, more important than merely providing support and encouragement."

Notice the use of the phrases "these men believed" and "from their perspective." Williams and Umberson also found that women often perceived the monitors as a nuisance and the information they provided not particularly helpful. After all, they're getting the same information anyway, but in a slightly different way: it hurts like hell. And the monitors don't always reflect reality. The contraction may look like it's over on the screen, but it can be far from over for her.

So be careful. These monitors may help you guide your partner through the contraction. But think long and hard before saying something like "Ready, honey? Here it comes—looks like a big one" (unfortunately, I know whereof I speak).

In many hospitals, laboring women are routinely hooked up to external fetal monitors as soon as they check in—despite the fact that the American College of Obstetricians and Gynecologists doesn't recommend it for low-risk pregnancies. If your partner doesn't have an epidural and is still walking, she may be able to get intermittent monitoring (done with a stethoscope or a hand-held Doppler like the one you heard your baby's heartbeat through in the doc's office all those months ago). Another option is portable monitoring: she'll still have the belts strapped on, but they'll wirelessly broadcast heartbeat and contraction data to the medical team. If, however, she has an epidural or is on pitocin, continuous monitoring is usually non-negotiable. Ditto when it comes time to push.

Internal fetal monitors come in two varieties: an electrode attached to the baby's scalp, and the IUPC mentioned above. If your practitioner feels that it's important to keep closer tabs on the baby's heart rate, your partner will get one or both of these internal monitors.

Unless there's some compelling reason why your partner needs continuous monitoring (if there have been signs of fetal distress, for example), you and she will be a lot better off with as little of it as possible. Here's why:

- There's too much room for misinterpreting the results. One study had four doctors interpret fifty different tracings (the printouts generated by the monitor). The four concurred only 22 percent of the time. Worse yet, two months later, when the same docs were asked to evaluate the same tracings, they interpreted more than 20 percent of them differently.
- It can scare the hell out of you. When my wife was hooked up to a fetal monitor during her first labor, we were comforted by the sound of the baby's steady, 140-beats-per-minute heartbeat. But at one point the heart rate dropped to 120, then 100, then 80, then 60. Nothing was wrong—the doctor was just trying to change the baby's position—but hearing her little heart slow down that much nearly gave my wife and me heart attacks. If your partner's practitioner believes

that monitoring is medically necessary, turn the volume down (better yet, all the way off).

- It's not clear that it works. Fetal monitoring was originally implemented in the hope that it would prevent cerebral palsy. But despite the very best of intentions, it has led to an increase in C-sections and instrument deliveries. And, ironically, it didn't do anything for cerebral palsy either—the rate has stayed the same for the past fifty years. The moral of the story is that continuous monitoring can sometimes generate too much information: the doctor might see something happen to the baby on the monitor, get worried, and operate. In a lot of cases, what looks like fetal distress on the tracing ends up going away on its own.

After the Birth: Hey, Baby!

One of the first contacts you'll have with your baby is cutting his or her umbilical cord. With a vaginal birth, you'll actually be disconnecting your baby from mom. With a C-section, the surgeons will do the actual removal and you'll do a ceremonial snip. Either way, there's something amazing about the way it makes you feel connected to (ironic, isn't it?) the baby.

Researchers Sónia Brandão and Bárbara Figueiredo found that fathers who cut their baby's cord were more emotionally involved with the baby a month after the birth than those dads who didn't make the cut.

Your baby's first few minutes outside the womb are a time of intense physical and emotional release for you and your partner. At long last, you get to meet the unique little person you created together. Your partner may want to try nursing the baby (although most newborns aren't hungry for the first twelve hours or so), and you will probably want to stroke his or her brand-new skin and marvel at his or her tiny fingernails. But depending on the hospital, the conditions of the birth, and whether or not you've been perfectly clear about your preferences, your

Seeing the Baby

Some hospitals have very rigid rules regarding parent/infant contact—feeding may be highly regulated and the hours you can visit your child may be limited. Others are more flexible. The hospitals where all three of my children were born no longer have a nursery (except for babies with serious health problems). Healthy babies are expected to stay in the mother's room for their entire hospital stay. And many hospitals allow the new father to spend the night with mom and baby. Check with the staff of your hospital to find out their policy.

baby's first few minutes could be spent being poked and prodded by doctors and nurses instead of being held and cuddled by you.

One minute after birth, your baby will be given an APGAR test to allow the medical staff a quick take on your baby's overall condition. Created in 1953 by Dr. Virginia Apgar, the test measures your baby's Appearance (skin color), Pulse, Grimace (reflexes), Activity, and Respiration. A nurse or midwife will score each category on a scale of 0 to 2. (A bluish or pale baby might get a 0 for color while a very pink one would get 2; a baby who's breathing irregularly or shallowly might get a 0 for respiration, while one who's breathing well, or crying loudly, would get a 2.) Most babies score in the 7–9 range (just on principle, almost no one gets a 10—unless it's the child of someone the medical team knows). The test will be repeated at five minutes after birth.

Shortly after the birth, your baby will need to be weighed, measured, given an ID bracelet, bathed, diapered, footprinted, and wrapped in a blanket. Some hospitals also photograph each newborn. After that, most hospitals (frequently as required by law) apply silver nitrate drops or an antibiotic ointment to your baby's eyes as a protection against gonorrhea. Although these procedures should be done within one hour of birth, ask the staff if they can hold off for a few minutes while you and your partner get acquainted with your baby.

If, however, your baby was delivered by C-section, or if there were any other complications, the baby will be rushed off to have his or her little lungs suctioned before returning for the rest of the cleanup routine (see pages 243–44 for more on this).

Cesarean Section

All things being equal, most parents would prefer to bring their babies into the world "normally." And most of the time that's what happens. But childbirth is one of those uncontrollable, unpredictable events, and things don't always go exactly the way they're supposed to. In the United States, in fact, more than 30 percent of all children born in hospitals are delivered by C-section.

WHAT'S GOING ON WITH YOUR PARTNER

Most childbirth preparation classes (see pages 160–65) put a great deal of emphasis on natural, unmedicated deliveries. As we discussed earlier, many women, therefore, feel a tremendous amount of pressure to deliver vaginally and may actually consider themselves "failures" if they don't—especially after they've invested hours and hours in a painful labor.

In addition, recovering from a Cesarean is much different from recovering from a vaginal birth (see page 249 for more details). My wife (and I) spent three nights in the hospital after the C-section delivery of our first daughter. But after our second daughter was born (vaginally), we stayed in the hospital for only five hours. (Okay, we rushed it a little; most people stay twenty-four to forty-eight hours after a vaginal birth, but my wife really wanted to leave.)

WHAT'S GOING ON WITH YOU

Your take on the C-section is undoubtedly going to be quite different from your partner's. Researcher Katharyn May found that only 8 percent of men whose partners delivered by C-section objected to the operation; 92 percent were "greatly relieved." Although I didn't participate in this study, it accurately reflects my own experience. It simply had never occurred to me that my wife might somehow have "failed." On the contrary, I remember feeling incredibly thankful that her suffering would finally end. And seeing how quickly and painlessly the baby was delivered made me wonder why we hadn't done it sooner.

Despite the relief a father may feel on his partner's behalf, a C-section can be a trying experience for him. As a rule, he's separated from his wife while she's being prepped for surgery and usually isn't given any information about what's happening. I remember being left in the hall outside the operating room, trying to keep an eye on my wife through a tiny window. Besides being terribly scared, I felt completely helpless—and useless—as the doctors, nurses, and assistants scurried around, blocking my view, getting dressed, washing, opening packages of scalpels, tubes, and who knows what else. Only one person—the pediatrician who ended up attending the delivery—took a minute to pat me on the shoulder, call me by name, and tell me that everything would be all right. I've never felt more grateful to another person in my life.

When they finally let me into the operating room (wearing a fashionable set of scrubs and a mask that I still have), I was told—no discussion allowed—to sit by my wife's head. There was a curtain across her chest that prevented me from seeing what the surgeons were doing. I was ready to put some gloves on and help out with the operation, but whenever I stood up to get a better view, the anesthesiologist shoved me back down into my seat. I was too exhausted to argue, but a friend of mine whose partner had a C-section in the same hospital a few years later did argue and was able to go around to the "business end" of the operation.

I've heard from several OBs that part of the reason they often try to keep dads up by the mom's head is that if there's ever a time when dads pass out, this is it. And the anesthesiologists simply don't want to have to deal with two patients at the same time. As OB Lissa Rankin puts it, "It's not personal. I'm happy to have dads at the business end, but they sometimes end up on the floor."

STAYING INVOLVED

My friend and I may be among the lucky ones; in some hospitals men aren't allowed into the operating room at all. Others permit them in only if they've taken a special C-section class (which most people wouldn't do unless they were planning for one). Hopefully, even before you check in, you and your partner will have already told your OB exactly what your preferences are should there be a C-section, and you'll be familiar with any relevant hospital policies. (See pages 20-21 for other things to discuss with your OB.)

Don't forget that although a C-section is a fairly commonplace operation—American doctors do about 1.5 million every year—it's still major surgery. And after the operation, your partner will need some extra special care.

First of all, as strange as it may sound, after having a C-section your partner may feel terribly left out. She will probably have been fully awake during the operation and will be anxious to meet the new baby. But whereas after a vaginal birth the mother gets to see and touch the baby immediately, after a C-section the baby is usually quickly whisked away to have his or her lungs suctioned out. Sometimes the suctioning may happen even before the baby has been fully delivered. (Babies born vaginally have most of the amniotic fluid and other gunk in their lungs squeezed out on the way through the birth canal. But with C-section babies, it often has to be removed manually.)

You may get to make a "ceremonial" umbilical cord cut (the surgeons will have already cut the cord during the delivery). If the baby is being cared for right in the delivery room, make sure to tell your partner exactly what's happening—she'll want to know (although, depending on what the anesthesiologist used, she may be too drugged up to care very much, so take plenty of pictures). In some hospitals, C-section babies are removed from the delivery room immediately after the birth and taken straight to the nursery, where they're washed, examined, and put through basically the same procedures as vaginal birth babies (see the preceding chapter). This whole process can take anywhere from a few minutes to a few hours.

Although you might want to remain with your partner and comfort her immediately after the delivery, ask the doctor whether you can stay with your baby instead. It's bad enough for a newborn to be deprived of snuggling with one of his parents right away, but it would be worse if the baby couldn't be with either of you. Staying with our daughter also eased my paranoia that she might be switched in the nursery (a highly unlikely occurrence, given the rather elaborate security measures in place in most hospitals). But don't get too upset if the doctor says no—a lot of C-section babies are not medically stable at birth (not in danger, just requiring a little extra attention), and the medical staff won't want you hovering around, getting in the way.

When you finally do get to the nursery, start getting undressed. Not completely—just take off your shirt. Some skin-to-skin contact with your baby can have wonderful effects. "After births with complications, mothers are often not available to their babies for contact," writes Swedish researcher Kerstin Erlandsson. "Babies who do not have that contact take longer to settle and may lag in learning to breastfeed." According to Erlandsson, the dad's skin-to-skin contact with his baby after a C-section is just as comforting and calming as the

Common Medical Reasons for a Cesarean Section

Although some C-sections are planned, most happen when a vaginal birth could be dangerous to the mom, baby, or both. Here are some of those reasons:

- The mother's pelvis is too small to allow the baby's head to pass through the birth canal (although there's no way to tell whether this is true until she tries to deliver vaginally).
- Failure of the labor to progress. After hours of labor, the woman may be too exhausted to push the baby out. Or, her cervix stops opening after active labor has begun.
- The baby is distressed in some way. Her heartbeat has dropped too far, the heartbeat pattern is worrisome, or there are other problems.
- You're about to have more than one baby.
- Your partner has a medical condition that puts her at risk, including a heart condition, diabetes, high blood pressure, an active case of genital herpes, or obesity.
- Placenta problems. Abrupto placenta (separation of the placenta from the uterine wall before labor begins) causes bleeding and can threaten the lives of both mother and baby. Placenta previa (the placenta is fully or partially blocking the opening of the cervix) causes hemorrhaging and prevents the baby from leaving the uterus.
- Position of the baby. Under certain circumstances, if the baby is breech (coming out butt or feet first) or transverse (lying sideways instead of head down), a C-section is more likely.
- Previous C-section birth(s). Until the 1980s, the prevailing wisdom was, "once a C-section, always a C-section." Then, in response to an increasing C-section rate, many OB/GYNs proposed VBAC (vaginal birth after Cesarean) as a way of reducing that rate. The VBAC rate increased steadily until the '90s. But as more women opted for VBAC, the number of cases of uterine

mother's—and it's a lot better than leaving the baby alone in a bassinet in the nursery. C-section babies stop crying within 15 minutes of being put on dad's chest, and they become drowsy within an hour after birth, compared to 110 minutes for those in bassinets.

Your Partner's Emotional Recovery

Having an unplanned C-section can trigger a whole host of conflicting emotions in your partner. She, like you, may feel greatly relieved that the pain is over and rupture increased (percentage-wise, the risk was still very low). Still, just to be safe, many OBs started recommending against VBAC, and some hospitals have banned them entirely. But recent research has found that many women who've had a C-section are good candidates for VBAC (typically that means she's under thirty-five, hasn't had any pregnancy complications, isn't overdue, and isn't carrying an especially big baby). About 75 percent of women who attempt a VBAC are successful. If your partner has had a C-section with a previous birth, ask her practitioner to explain the risks and benefits of VBAC vs. a scheduled, repeat C-section, and make the decision that's best for your growing family.

- Your doctor thinks the baby is too big. The American College of Obstetricians and Gynecologists defines "too big" as anything over 4,500 grams (about 9 pounds, 4 ounces). With babies this size there's an increased chance of shoulder dystocia—when the head delivers but the shoulders get stuck. (This definition goes down to 4,000 grams/8½ pounds if mom is a diabetic.)
- Your partner's age. The older she is, the greater her chance of needing a C-section. Laurie Green, a San Francisco OB/GYN who delivered my youngest, puts it this way: "The uterus is a muscle, and like any other muscle, its strength decreases with age. A woman whose uterus struggles to force a baby out when she's forty-two, might very well have been able to deliver the same size baby with no problem when she was twenty-two."
- Suspected abnormality of the baby. If the baby is expected to have a birth defect or other abnormality that might make vaginal delivery risky, the doctor might recommend a C-section, not just to minimize birth trauma but to make sure all the right specialists can be on hand to give your baby the best shot at thriving.

the baby is safe. At the same time, it's very natural for her to second-guess herself and the decisions she made, to start wondering whether there was anything she could have done to avoid the operation, or to believe she's failed because she didn't deliver vaginally. These feelings are especially common when the C-section was performed because labor "failed to progress" (meaning that the cervix wasn't dilating as quickly as the doctors may have thought it should, or stopped dilating altogether despite adequate contractions).

Some of the Most Common Nonmedical Reasons for a Cesarean Section

As cynical as it sounds, sometimes C-sections aren't really necessary.

- It's easier. Some OBs consider C-sections safer than vaginal deliveries.
- Demographics. Although the national C-section rate is nearly 33 percent, the actual number varies widely. In some states—Florida, New Jersey, and Louisiana—the rate is close to 40 percent; in others—New Mexico, Utah, Alaska—it's under 25 percent. Married women and those with insurance are more likely to have a Cesarean than women without—34 percent vs. 25 percent. And women over forty are about twice as likely as women under twenty-five—50 percent vs. 25 percent. High C-section rates aren't limited to the United States. In Thailand and Vietnam, for example, the rate is over 35 percent. In Paraguay and Ecuador, it's over 40 percent; in China, it's close to 50 percent; and in Brazil, where it's considered "low class" to give birth vaginally, it's 70 percent (80–90 percent or more in private hospitals).
- Your partner may just want one. Picking the exact delivery date may enable a woman to have the baby at a time that's particularly convenient for her or her family. Then there's the "too posh to push" idea that's been driven by Hollywood. Quite a few celebrity moms have opted for a C-section because they're worried about the pain of a vaginal delivery or the impact that a natural birth could have on their sexual or urinary function. "Cesarean section prior to advanced labor is virtually 100 percent effective at eliminating these problems," writes OB and researcher Brent Bost. Dr. Bost has also found that "healthy women who undergo elective Cesarean section experience a relatively low rate of short-term complications. And long-term complications are rare." On the other hand, Sarah McMoyler says, "Consider the tradeoff: Several hours of pain—most of which can be eliminated with an epidural— vs. six weeks of not being able to go up and down the stairs, hold your baby

If you sense that your partner is experiencing any of these negative emotions, it's important that you help her get past them. Some doctors believe that, left unchecked, these feelings can escalate and contribute to postpartum depression. She really needs to know that no one could have done more, or been stronger or braver than she was; that she didn't give in to the pain too soon; that she tried everything she could have to jump-start a stalled labor; that another few hours of labor wouldn't have done anyone any good; and that the decision she made (or at least agreed to) was the best one—both for the baby and for herself.

without hurting, or drive." I guess if you have a chauffeur and servants, that's not much of an issue.

- Culture. In Chinese, Hindu, and other cultures, the calendar is filled with auspicious and non-auspicious days, and some people feel that the right birthday can make a huge difference in a child's life.
- Fear of lawsuits. If something goes wrong with the birth—fetal or maternal distress, or even a birth defect that a lawyer might attribute to something that happened during delivery—the obstetrician is likely to be blamed for having let the labor go on too long. In some cases (but by no means all), OBs perform a C-section to minimize risk and speed things up.
- Finances. The vast majority of medical professionals perform C-sections only when they're medically necessary. But sometimes money creeps into the equation—usually subconsciously. Researchers Marit Rehavi (University of British Columbia) and Erin Johnson (MIT) found that in hospitals where there are financial incentives to perform C-sections (usually higher insurance reimbursements to both doctor and hospital), the C-section rates are higher. Clearly, some of those C-sections aren't truly necessary. Mothers who are physicians—and who would presumably be less likely to go along with an unnecessary procedure—are 7–9 percent less likely to have "emergency" C-sections than "other highly educated patients."
- Convenience. Your partner may want a guarantee that a specific doctor will be available to do the delivery. You may plan a C-section to make sure you have child care lined up or to meet school entry cut-off dates. Or your partner may have a personal or professional deadline she must meet. (In Lissa Rankin's case, she desperately wanted her father, who was dying of cancer, to meet his granddaughter.)

Some of these thoughts might seem obvious to you—so obvious that you might think they don't need to be said at all. But they do—especially by you. You were there with her, and you know better than anyone else exactly what she went through. So, being comforted and praised by you will mean a lot more to her than hearing the same words from a well-meaning relative, nurse, or even her own doctor. Having a baby isn't some kind of competition. As author Vicki Iovene writes, "It is not designed for your personal enjoyment and fulfillment. It is not an opportunity to demonstrate your abilities or fitness. It is designed to perpetuate

Equal Opportunity Trauma

Life-threatening emergencies during labor and birth are relatively rare, but they do happen. And when they do, there's no question that they're traumatic to the mother. But what about dad? One of expectant fathers' most common fears is that their partner will die in childbirth. And seeing her go through a "near-miss" event brings that fear to the forefront.

Marian Knight and her team at Oxford University found that the combination of not knowing what's going on, not knowing whether their partner and baby are alive or dead, and feeling powerless to do anything to help, leaves some dads with post-traumatic stress disorder (PTSD). The results can affect everyone in the family. The men themselves rarely seek help because they don't want to be perceived as weak, they fear people will make fun of them, or they think they should ignore their own needs and focus 100 percent on their partner and baby. As a result, they feel more isolated and depressed as time goes on. That plus the flashbacks associated with PTSD can make it hard for dads to bond with their baby. It also makes it hard for them to be there to support the new mom. Women whose partners were involved during labor have better health outcomes than those with less involved partners. And the dad's involvement after the birth increases the likelihood that the mom will breastfeed.

Communication with the medical staff during the emergency is key to helping dads cope. No question, their priority is—and should be—the mom and baby. But even the smallest things can make a huge difference, like the shoulder pat and reassuring words I got from one of the docs before my wife's emergency C-section.

the species and nothing more." Not the most romantic way of looking at having a baby, but quite accurate.

An Important Warning

Never, never, never suggest to your pregnant partner that she have a C-section—let your doctor make the first move. When my wife was pregnant with our second daughter, the pain she had been through during her first labor and delivery was still fresh in my mind. At one point I told her that I was really upset by the thought that she might have to endure another horrible labor, and I suggested that she consider a C-section.

Facts to Remember about Recovery from a Cesarean Section

- Your partner's incision will be tender or downright painful for at least several days. Fortunately, she'll undoubtedly be receiving some intravenous (IV) pain medication.
- The nursing staff will visit quite frequently to make sure that your partner's uterus is getting firm and returning to its proper place, to see whether she's producing enough urine, and to check her bandages.
- Your partner will have an IV until her bowels start functioning again (usually within twenty-four hours after delivery). After the IV is removed, she'll start on a liquid diet, then add a few soft foods, and finally return to her normal diet (although some doctors will have their patients skip the liquid diet and go straight to real food—well, as real as hospital food can be).
- Your partner will need to get up and move around. Despite the fact that a C-section is major abdominal surgery, less than twenty-four hours after the delivery the nurses will probably encourage—and help—your partner to get out of bed and take a couple of rather painful-looking steps.
- The whole thing resembles a kindergarten art project. Besides stitches, your partner's incision may well be closed up with tape, glue, and/or staples. Yes, staples. Until I heard the clink as the doctor dropped them into a jar, I'd just assumed that my wife had been sewn up. But staples may be on the way out. Dhanya Mackeen, a researcher at Pennsylvania's Geisinger Health System, recently found that women whose Cesarean incisions are closed with sutures are 80 percent less likely to have their wound reopen, and 57 percent less likely to have postoperative complications than those who get stapled. The downside is that it takes eight or nine minutes longer to close the incision with sutures, but it's not like your partner has anyplace else she needs to be.

I had no idea that someone could get so furious so quickly. Even though I had the very best intentions and was sincerely thinking only of her and how to minimize her pain, she thought I was being completely insensitive. Clearly, I had underestimated how incredibly important giving birth vaginally—especially after already having had one C-section—was to her.

Many of the men I've talked to have had similar thoughts about making the C-section suggestion to their partners. Most of them were wise enough not to act on their impulse. And hopefully, you won't either. Telling your partner how you're feeling and what you're going through is, in most cases, the right thing to do. But when it comes to C-sections, really and truly, it's an issue that's just too hot to handle.

One Final Thought

As mentioned, about a third of babies in the U.S. are born by C-section—that's up from 20.7 percent in 1996 and 4.5 percent in 1965. But is that too high? Unfortunately, there's no clear answer because there are a number of complicating factors, and one of the biggest, so to speak, is obesity. According to the American College of Obstetricians and Gynecologists (ACOG) more than half of pregnant women are overweight or obese. The C-section rate for normal-weight women is 20.7 percent. For overweight women, it's 33.8 percent, and for obese women, it's 47.4 percent. Obese and overweight women also have higher rates of diabetes and hypertension and are more likely to be carrying a baby with congenital abnormalities—all of which raise the C-section rate even further. When you control for all those factors, the actual C-section rate in the U.S. is very much in line with the rates in other industrialized countries.

Regardless of where you stand on the issue, Cesareans are here to stay. Noted OB/GYN and fertility specialist Elan Simckes believes that in a few hundred years, almost all babies will be born this way. Why? To start with, says Dr. Simckes, the human pelvis is shrinking over time. And thanks to a diet that consists more and more of sugar, carbs, and fat, babies are getting bigger. In 1965, the average baby born in the United States weighed about six and a half pounds. Today, the average is more than seven and a half pounds. Bigger baby + smaller pelvis = more Cesareans. It's inevitable.

Gee Honey,
Now What Do We Do?

WHAT'S GOING ON WITH YOUR PARTNER

Physically

- Vaginal discharge (called lochia) that will gradually change from bloody to pink to brown to yellow over the next six weeks or so
- Major discomfort if there is an episiotomy or C-section incision (the pain will disappear over the next six weeks)
- Constipation and hemorrhoids—hopefully not at the same time
- Breast discomfort starting about the third day after the birth (when her breasts become engorged with milk); if she's breastfeeding, her nipples may be sore for about two weeks
- Gradual weight loss
- Exhaustion—especially if her labor was long and difficult
- Continued contractions—especially while breastfeeding—but these will disappear over the next several days
- Hair loss (most women stop losing hair while they're pregnant, but when the pregnancy's over, so are all those great hair days)

Emotionally

- Relief that it's finally over
- Excitement, depression, or both (see pages 252–54)
- Worried about how she'll perform as a mother, and whether she'll be able to breastfeed (but over the next few weeks, her confidence will build and these worries should disappear)
- A deep need to get to know the baby

- Impatience at her lack of mobility
- An odd sense of grief or loss—at no longer being the center of attention, at the undeniable fact that, as everyone you've ever met has told you 18 million times, life will never be the same
- Decreased sex drive, assuming she had any left before the baby came anyway

Postpartum Blues and Depression

Anywhere from 50 to 80 percent of new mothers get what a lot of people call "baby blues"—periods of mild sadness, weepiness, mood swings, exhaustion or lack of energy, loss of appetite, difficulty concentrating or making decisions, irritability, or anxiety after the baby is born. (This shouldn't come as much of a surprise, when you think about the sleepless nights, lack of physical intimacy, worries about not being able to cope with her new responsibilities, and feelings of isolation that many new moms experience.) Many believe that the baby blues are caused by dramatic hormonal shifts in a new mother's body. Others say the cause is lack of sleep. Anthropologist Edward Hagen, however, believes that postpartum blues have little, if anything, to do with hormones. Instead, he says, it's connected to low levels of social support—especially from the father. And it could be the new mother's way of "negotiating" for more involvement.

Whatever the cause, the symptoms of baby blues won't really be severe enough to affect your partner's life too much. They typically start a day or two after the delivery, peak four or five days later, and in most cases, disappear on their own within a few weeks.

If you notice that your partner is experiencing any of these symptoms, be as supportive and involved as possible. Take on more of the child-care responsibilities, encourage her to rest if she can or to get out of the house for a while, do as much of the nighttime duty as you can without jeopardizing your career, and see to it that she's eating well. Again, most of this is completely normal and nothing to worry about. So be patient, and don't expect her to bounce back immediately. And don't demand that she "snap out of it."

For about 10–20 percent of new moms, postpartum blues can develop into postpartum depression, which is more serious. Symptoms include:
- Postpartum blues that don't go away after two weeks, or feelings of depression or anger that surface a month or two after the birth
- Feelings of sadness, doubt, guilt (that she's not loving every second of motherhood), helplessness, shame (if she didn't perform as she wanted to during the labor and delivery), or hopelessness that begin to disrupt your partner's normal functioning
- Inability to take pleasure in activities she used to enjoy

- Inability to sleep when tired, or sleeping most of the time, even when the baby is awake
- Marked changes in appetite
- Extreme concern and worry about—or lack of interest in—the baby and/or other members of the family
- Worries that she'll harm the baby or herself

Pay close attention to her behavior and her attitude. If you're really concerned—and since you know her better than anyone, you'll have a good sense of whether she's behaving abnormally or not—encourage your partner to talk with you about what she's feeling and to see her doctor or a therapist. If she doesn't want to go (and many women who have postpartum depression will deny that anything is wrong), take her yourself.

Sadly, a lot of moms who have postpartum depression don't get the assistance they need—they feel embarrassed to admit to anyone else what they're feeling. Untreated, these symptoms can last for years. In some cases antidepressants may be required.

You can play a major role in helping your wife get through her postpartum depression. Here are a few ways you can help:

- Remind her that the depression is not her fault, that you love her, that the baby loves her, that she's doing a great job, and that the two of you will get through this together.
- Do as much of the housework and child care as you can so she won't have to worry about not being able to get everything done herself.
- Encourage her to take breaks—regularly and frequently.
- Take over enough of the nighttime baby duties that your partner can get at least five hours of uninterrupted sleep.
- Get regular breaks to relieve your own stress. Yes, she's relying on you to help her, but if you're falling apart yourself, you can't be an effective caregiver.

A very, very important note. There's a good chance that you're going to be hearing stories about Carol Coronado, Inakesha Armour, Deanna Laney, Andrea Yates, and other new mothers who killed their children. You'll also hear—usually from reporters or TV anchors who really should know better—that these women were suffering from postpartum depression. They absolutely were not. Women with postpartum depression do not harm their children. What these women had was *postpartum psychosis*—a condition that affects only one or two mothers in a thousand.

Symptoms usually start right after the birth and should be immediately recognizable by anyone. They include wild mood swings, hallucinations, being out of touch with reality, and making crazy or delirious statements. Postpartum psychosis is treatable—often with powerful antipsychotic drugs—but women who have it need help and they need it fast. Fortunately, despite the media hype, the majority of women with postpartum psychosis don't hurt their babies or anyone else.

WHAT'S GOING ON WITH THE BABY

For thousands of years, most people believed that newborn infants were capable only of eating, sleeping, crying, and looking around. But if you pay attention, you'll see that your new baby has an incredible arsenal of talents.

Just a few hours out of the womb, your baby is already trying to communicate with you and everyone else around him. He can imitate your facial expressions, has some control over his body, can express preferences (most prefer patterned objects to plain objects and curved lines to straight ones), and has a remarkable memory. Marshall Klaus told me about a game he played with an eight-hour-old girl in which he asked one colleague (who was a stranger to the baby—who isn't at that age?) to hold her and slowly stick out her tongue. After a few seconds, the baby imitated the woman. Then Dr. Klaus took the baby and passed her around to twelve other doctors and nurses who were participating in the game, all of whom were told not to stick their tongues out. When the baby finally came back to the first doctor, she—without any prompting—immediately stuck out her tongue again. Even at just a few hours old, she had obviously remembered her "friend."

If you want your baby to respond to and play with you, the time to do it is when she is active and alert. (During the first few months infants are particularly responsive to high contrast, so black-and-white toys and patterns are often a big hit.) But be patient. Infants are incredibly bright little creatures, but they also have minds of their own. This means that despite your best efforts, your baby may not be interested in performing like a trained seal whenever you wish.

WHAT'S GOING ON WITH YOU

Unconditional Love

Sooner or later, almost every writer takes a crack at trying to describe love. And for the most part, we fall short. But there's a line in Maurice Sendak's classic children's book *Where the Wild Things Are* that captures the feeling of loving one's own child exactly: "Please don't go—we'll eat you up—we love you so." As crazy as it may sound, that's precisely what my love for my daughters feels like to me. Whether we're playing, reading a book, telling each other about our days, or I'm just gazing at their smooth, peaceful faces as they sleep, all of a sudden I'll be overcome with the desire to pick them up, mush them into tiny balls, and pop them in my mouth. If you don't already know what I mean, believe me, you will soon. Just you wait.

One of my biggest fears during my wife's second pregnancy was that I wouldn't be able to love our second child as much as the first—that there wouldn't be enough of the consuming, overpowering love I felt for our first daughter to share with the new baby. But I really had nothing to worry about. Three seconds after my second daughter was born, I already wanted to eat her up too. Same with the third.

Feeling, Well, Paternal

Despite all the excitement, you may be filled with a sense of calm and peaceful-ness. You may feel less like going to work and more like hanging out with the new family. If so, you certainly aren't alone. Canadian researcher Anne Storey found that new fathers' testosterone levels often drop by as much as a third right after the birth of their children. Storey speculates that this kind of testosterone reduc-tion would make a man feel more parental or more like "settling down."

Awe at What the Female Body Can Do

Watching your partner go through labor is truly a humbling experience; chances are, your own physical courage, strength, and resolve have rarely (if ever) been put to that kind of test. But there's nothing like seeing a baby come out of a vagina to convince you that women are *really* different from men.

I know that vaginal birth has been around for millions of years and that that's the way babies are supposed to be born. Yet in a strange way, there's something almost unnatural about the whole process—the baby seems so big and the exit so small (it kind of reminds me of the ship-in-a-bottle conundrum). Ironically, a C-section somehow seems more "normal" and humane: when the fetus is full-grown, cut an appropriately sized exit and let the baby out. Seems simple enough to me. You'd think that with all the technological advances we've made in other areas, we'd have invented a quicker, easier, less painful way to have children.

Jealousy

"The single emotion that can be the most destructive and disruptive to your expe-rience of fatherhood is jealousy," writes Dr. Martin Greenberg in *The Birth of a Father*. There's certainly plenty to be jealous about, but the real question is, Whom are you jealous of? Your partner for being able to breastfeed and for her close rela-tionship with the baby, or the baby for taking up more than his or her fair share of your partner's attention, and for having full access to your partner's breasts while you aren't even supposed to touch them? The answer is, Both.

Now that the baby's born, communication with your partner is even more important than before. Jealousy's "potential for destruction," writes Greenberg, "lies not in having the feelings but in burying them." So if you're feeling jealous, tell her about it. But if you can't bring yourself to discuss your feelings on this issue with your partner, take them up with a male friend or relative. You'll be surprised at how common these feelings are.

Feeling Pushed Away or Left Out

Almost every new father in my research (and there have been more than a thousand) has talked about feeling pushed away or excluded from the new parenting experience. "The mother plays a critical role," writes Pamela Jordan. "She can bring her mate into the spotlight or keep him in the wings. The most promoting mothers...brought their mates into the experience by frequently and openly sharing their physical sensations and emotional responses. They actively encouraged their mates to share the experience of becoming and being a father."

While it's easy to give in to your feelings, throw up your hands, and leave the parenting to your partner, don't do it. Encourage her to talk about what she's feeling and thinking, and ask her specifically to involve you as much as possible.

A good way to cut down on your potential feelings of jealousy or of being pushed away is to start getting to know your baby right away—even before you leave the hospital. Change as many diapers as you can (if you've never changed one before, get one of the nurses to show you how), give the baby a sponge bath, or take him or her out for a walk while your partner rests.

Be prepared, though. When you get home, you may find yourself feeling pushed away by your baby. Here's a typical scene: You're home, having a perfectly delightful time with the baby, when she starts fussing and then crying. Hard. You try everything you can to resolve the issue, but after a few minutes it's clear that she's hungry and wants Mom. Now. So you turn her over to your partner and then spend the next twenty minutes feeling inadequate, useless, and completely superfluous.

Having been there many times, I guarantee that it's going to hurt. It's perfectly natural to want to distance yourself from anyone or anything that's causing you pain. But try not to take it personally. The baby isn't expressing a preference for your partner over you or saying that you're a lousy dad; it's just that Mom happens to be her favorite restaurant. So instead of withdrawing, try to focus on other ways to build your own, independent relationship with your child, one that's completely separate from your partner and is based on activities that don't involve feeding.

Amazement at How Being a Parent Changes Your Life

It's virtually impossible to try to explain the myriad ways becoming a parent will change your life. You already know you'll be responsible for the safety and well-being of a completely helpless person. You've heard that you'll lose a little sleep (all right, a lot) and even more privacy. And you've prepared yourself for not being able to read as many books or see as many movies or go to as many concerts as you did before. These are some of the big, obvious changes, but it's the tiny details that will make you realize just how different your new life is from your old one.

The best way I can describe it is this: sometimes one of my daughters would put food into her mouth, and after a few chews change her mind, take it out, and hand it to me. Most of the time I'd take the offering and pop it into my mouth without a second thought. You probably will too. Even more bizarre, since becoming a father, I have actually had serious discussions with my friends about the color and consistency of the contents of children's diapers. So will you.

Bonding with the Baby

No one knows exactly where or when it started, but one of the most widespread—and most enduring—myths about child rearing is that women are somehow more nurturing than men and are therefore better suited to parenting. In one of the earliest studies of father-infant interaction, my colleague, pioneering researcher Ross Parke, made a discovery that came as a shock to the traditionalists: fathers were just as caring about, interested in, and involved with their infants as the mothers were, and they held, touched, kissed, rocked, and cooed at their new babies with at least the same frequency as the mothers did. Several years later, Martin Greenberg coined a term, *engrossment*, to describe "a father's sense of absorption, preoccupation, and interest in his baby."

Parke and a number of other researchers over the years have repeatedly confirmed these findings about father-infant interaction, and have concluded that what triggers engrossment in men is the same thing that prompts similar nurturing feelings in women: early infant contact. The more time you spend with your baby, the stronger those feelings will be. Not surprisingly, Parke and others have found that men who attended their baby's birth bonded slightly more quickly than those who didn't. But if you weren't able to be there for the birth, don't worry. "Early contact at birth is not a magic pill," writes Ellen Galinsky, author of *The Six Stages of Parenthood*. "It does not guarantee attachment. Neither does lack of contact prevent bonding."

But What If I Don't Fall in Love Right Away?

Although we've spent a lot of time talking about the joys of loving your child and how important it is to bond with the infant as soon as possible, a lot of new

Postpartum Depression for Dads? Yep.

According to Will Courtenay, a psychotherapist specializing in male postpartum depression, as many as one in four new dads experience the kinds of depression symptoms mentioned earlier in the days, weeks, and even months after the birth of a child. Unfortunately, men rarely discuss their feelings or ask for help, especially during a time when they're supposed to "be there" for the new mom. One big problem is that men and women express depression differently. Women tend to get tearful and sad; men get angry or withdraw from their family and retreat to the office. Because depression—including the postpartum kind—is usually seen as affecting women more than men, many mental health professionals don't recognize the symptoms, or write them off as normal adjustment to the challenges of new parenthood. If the symptoms aren't recognized, there's no possibility of treatment, which explains why so many fathers are still showing signs of depression nine months after the baby arrives. And, of course, the fact that the whole not-asking-for-help thing just makes it worse.

The symptoms usually crop up a week or two after the birth and can include feelings of stress, irritability, or discouragement; aversion to hearing the baby cry; resentment of the baby and all the attention he gets; exhaustion; and disappointment with how you're doing as a new dad. There's been a lot of research on the negative effects of new mothers' depression on their baby. Research on the effects of dads' depression is sparse, but what there is doesn't paint a very pretty picture. As you might expect, depressed new dads

fathers (and mothers, for that matter) don't feel particularly close to the new baby immediately after the birth. Very few people—especially mothers—will come right out and say, in public, that they feel nothing for their baby. It sounds kind of creepy, doesn't it? But in private, the truth comes out. Psychiatrists Kay Robson and Ramesh Kumar found that 25–40 percent of mothers and fathers admit that their first response to their baby was "indifference." Putting things in slightly stronger terms, researcher Katharyn May says, "This bonding business is nonsense. We've sold parents a bill of goods. They believe that if they don't have skin-to-skin contact within the first fifteen minutes, they won't bond. Science just doesn't show that."

I have to admit that, in a way, this makes a lot more sense than the love-at-first-sight kind of bonding you hear so much about. After all, you don't even know this new little person. He or she may look a lot different than you'd expected. And have trouble bonding with their baby. And children whose dads suffered from postpartum depression are about twice as likely to have behavioral, emotional, and social problems, as well as delays in language acquisition, than kids whose dads weren't depressed.

While no one knows exactly what causes postpartum depression, some groups of men are more susceptible than others. The clearest risk factors are a partner who is depressed herself or has a personal history of depression. Other factors include financial problems, a poor relationship with your partner or parents, being unmarried, or a pregnancy that had been unplanned or unwanted. Postpartum depression doesn't discriminate based on socioeconomic level or ethnicity. It typically affects first-time parents, but can occur after subsequent births even if there were no symptoms after the first child.

If you suspect you may be experiencing postpartum depression, understand that it's not a sign of weakness. It doesn't make you a bad dad or mean that you don't love your child. It's a recognized medical condition that affects hundreds of thousands of fathers, and you shouldn't have to suffer when treatment is available. If you aren't sure, Courtenay's website, www.postpartummen.com, offers an anonymous survey that can clarify the issues, and a listing of good resources for getting help. Whatever you do, don't sweep your feelings under the rug. Depression—regardless of what triggers it—is nothing to be ashamed of, and getting treatment is important. Don't let depression rob you of the joys a new baby brings, ruin your relationships, or destroy your family.

if your partner's labor and delivery were long and painful—or possibly even life threatening—you may unconsciously be blaming the baby for the difficulties or may simply be too exhausted to fully appreciate the new arrival. He seems to do nothing but cry, eat, and fill diapers. That's on a good day. And the kid never, ever laughs at your jokes. It's downright demoralizing. And anyway, with all the extra work involved in being a new parent, who's got time to fall in love with a baby?

Let me assure you that if you haven't whipped yourself up into a frenzy of love for your baby, there's absolutely nothing wrong with you. More important, there's no evidence whatsoever that your relationship with or feelings for your child will be any less loving than if you'd fallen head over heels in love in the first second. Just take your time, don't pressure yourself, and don't think for a second that you've failed as a father. Almost all new dads get that bonding feeling within two months.

There's a lot of evidence that parent-child bonding comes as a result of physical closeness. So if you'd like to speed up the process, try carrying the baby every chance you get, taking him with you whenever you can, and taking care of as many of his basic needs as possible.

The whole bonding thing is probably going to be a lot tougher if you've got twins (or more). Because they tend to be born somewhat more prematurely than single babies, multiples may have to stay in the hospital nursery for a few days or even weeks, which can limit the amount of time you can spend with them—separately or together. Things can get even more complicated if one of the babies comes home with you and the other(s) stay behind. You're going to feel torn between spending time with the baby in the hospital, the other baby, and your partner. Unfortunately, there's no magic formula for how much time each of them gets. Just do the best you can and spend a lot of time talking with your partner about how you're both feeling and what each of you needs.

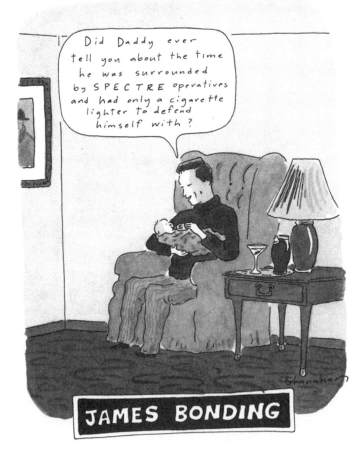

Gee, This Isn't at All What I Expected...

Despite everything you've heard about how gorgeous babies are, you may have a slightly different opinion—at least for the first week or so after your baby is born. If your baby was born vaginally, the trip through the birth canal may have flattened his nose and made him look a little cone headed. Calm down. His nose will pop out and his head will get rounder over the next few months.

Do those green, tarlike bowel movements make you think there's something wrong with the baby's intestines? There isn't. Those first few loads are normal and will be replaced by a much more pleasant-looking concoction as your baby starts breastfeeding. Is the baby's skin splotchy—especially on the neck and the eyelids—and does she have strange-looking birth marks or tiny pimples? Relax. Just keep her clean—no scrubbing or zit popping—and she'll be fine. Does your infant seem a little cross-eyed? It's fine. As soon as his eye muscles get a bit more developed and coordinated, he'll be able to look you straight in the eye. Do his hairy back and shoulders have you worrying about what'll happen to him when the moon is full? Don't. That fuzz is called *lanugo* and it'll fall out pretty soon. I'm mentioning all this because there's a strong connection between depression and unmet expectations.

STAYING INVOLVED

The First Few Days

In the first few days you're going to have to learn to juggle a lot of roles. You're still a lover and friend to your partner, and, of course, you're a father. But for now, your most important role is that of support person to your partner. Besides her physical recovery (which we'll talk more about below), she's going to need time to get to know the baby and to learn (if she chooses to) how to breastfeed.

When our first daughter was born (by C-section), the three of us spent four days in the hospital (which meant three uncomfortable nights on a crooked, lumpy cot for me). But when our second daughter was born (vaginally), we all checked out less than half a day after the birth. In both cases, though, my first few days at home were mighty busy—cooking, shopping, doing laundry, fixing up the baby's room, getting the word out, screening phone calls and visitors, and making sure everyone got plenty of rest. For the rest of this chapter, we'll be talking about issues you're likely to face in the first week or two of fatherhood. We go into much more detail—and cover a lot more ground—in the sequel to this book, *The New Father: A Dad's Guide to the First Year*.

Coming Home...and Beyond

Within a few minutes after we'd brought our first daughter home from the hospital, my wife and I looked at each other and almost simultaneously asked, "Well, now what are we supposed to do?" An important question, no doubt, and one that seems to come up time and time again.

A NOTE ON RECOVERY

As far as the baby is concerned, there's not much to do in the beginning besides feeding, changing, and admiring. But your partner is a different story. Despite everything you've heard about women giving birth in the fields and returning to work a few minutes later, that's not the way things usually happen. Having a baby is a major shock to a woman's system. And, contrary to popular belief, the recovery period after a vaginal birth is not necessarily any shorter than the recovery period after a C-section (although most women who have had both say that vaginal birth recovery is easier).

Whatever kind of delivery your partner has, she'll need some time—probably more than either of you think—to recover fully. According to a recent study, more than 40 percent of new mothers experience fatigue and breast soreness in the first month after giving birth. In addition, vaginal discomfort, hemorrhoids, poor appetite, constipation, increased perspiration, acne, hand numbness or tingling, dizziness, and hot flashes are common for a month after delivery. And between 10 and 40 percent of women feel pain during sexual intercourse, have respiratory infections, and lose hair for three to six months. Aren't you glad you can't have a baby?

Here are some things you can do to make the recovery process as easy as possible and to start parenting off on the right foot.

- Help your partner resist the urge to do too much too soon.
- Take over the household chores or ask someone else to help. If the house is a mess, don't blame each other.
- Be flexible. Expecting to maintain your normal, prefatherhood schedule is unrealistic—especially for the first six weeks after the birth.
- Don't allow your relationship with your partner to be based solely on your child. If she's up to it, go on a date with your partner and leave the baby with a relative or friend.
- Be patient with yourself, your partner, and the baby. You're all new at this.
- Be sensitive to your partner's emotions. Recovery has an emotional component as well as a physical one.
- Make sure to get some time alone with the baby. You can do this while your partner is sleeping or while she's out for a walk.

Adoptive and ART Dads Bond Too

Plenty of adoptive parents—particularly if they adopted because of infertility—feel a little insecure or inadequate. And a lot of ART parents feel the same way—especially if they aren't the baby's biological parents (due to donor eggs or sperm). They often believe that the process of bonding and forming an attachment to the baby comes more naturally to birth or biological parents than to them. They're wrong.

Studies of adoptive and ART parents have shown that a majority feel some kind of love for their children right from the very first contact; it doesn't matter whether it's when they go to pick up the baby, when they first look at a picture that arrived months before, or right at the birth, if they're lucky enough to be there. At the same time, though, just like biological parents, a good percentage of adoptive parents or parents who are only partially biologically related to their child don't feel anything particularly parental when meeting their child for the first time.

If you're adopting a newborn, it's going to be a little easier to establish a bond. But a lot of adoptions aren't finalized until the babies are a few months older. Realistically, this makes the bonding process tougher for all concerned, as babies and parents take a little time to get used to each other. But it's by no means an impossible task. "Being a first-time parent, whether by birth or adoption, evokes a variety of feelings," writes Marshall Klaus. "And although many parents feel attached to their baby at first contact, many others find that it takes a week or longer to feel the baby is theirs." If you aren't consumed with paternal feelings right away, the first thing to do is take a look at the "But What If I Don't Fall in Love Right Away?" section on pages 257–60.

In the long run, the news is good. According to researcher Susan Golombok and her colleagues, "Fathers of assisted reproduction children were found to interact more with their children and to contribute more to parenting than fathers with naturally conceived children."

- Control the visiting hours and the number of people who can come at any given time. Dealing with visitors takes a lot more energy than you might think. And being poked, prodded, and passed around won't make the baby very happy. Also, for the first month or so, ask anyone who wants to touch the baby to wash his or her hands first.
- Keep your sense of humor.

Welcome Home, GI Dad

Coming home to a baby who was born while you were deployed can be both exciting and terrifying. Of course, if this is your second or third or fourth child, you've already got a pretty good handle on what to expect and what you need to do. But if this is baby number one, you'll be stepping into a home that may look nothing like the one you left, and you may have no clue what to expect, what your wife will want from you, and how you'll react to the whole thing.

One of the first things you'll probably feel is a conflict between wanting to jump in immediately and take care of your wife and wanting to run away as fast as you can. No question, it hasn't been easy for your wife to make it through the pregnancy and birth without you. But at least she had nine months to prepare. Your world is going to change in an instant. Military man one minute, daddy the next. Different uniforms, similar responsibilities.

Next, you'll start feeling guilty—in part for even thinking about running away, but mostly for not having been there for Mom and baby during the pregnancy and the birth. Get over it! The two of you knew that your being deployed was a distinct possibility, and there was absolutely nothing you could have done to change the situation. You may also feel some jealousy at the closeness of the connection between Mom and baby (see pages 255–56 for more on this). Try to let that one go too. There's not much you can do about it, and you wouldn't want to even if you could. Your only option is to jump in as soon as

HELPING OLDER KIDS ADJUST TO THEIR NEW SIBLING

Handling your older children's reactions to their new baby brother or sister requires an extra touch of gentleness and sensitivity. Kids often start out wildly excited at their new status as big brother or big sister, but most will have some adjustment problems later on—as soon as they realize that the new kid is more than just a temporary visitor.

Some react with anger and jealousy. Who wouldn't? For the past few years he had you and Mom all to himself. Then, without even consulting him, you bring in someone who steals all your attention. Worse yet, the instant playmate he was hoping for turns out to be a blobby baby who does nothing but sleep, cry, eat, cry, poop, and cry some more. And to top it off, with everyone ooohing and aaahing over the new baby, your older child is feeling unwanted and unloved. As a result, new older siblings may shed a few tears themselves, have tantrums, and even try possible. Your wife will appreciate your being there to take on some of the parenting load. More important, you'll have a chance to start bonding with your baby.

But don't put a lot of pressure on yourself to start bonding right away, and don't worry about trying to make up for lost time—there's no such thing. Just do as much as you can: hug, bathe, change, feed, play, relax, read the "Staying Involved" section of this chapter, and just marvel at all the cool things babies can do. And remember, (a) it's never too late to start, (b) the sooner you get involved, the stronger your relationship with your child, and (c) you're going to make a ton of mistakes. That's another fun part of being a new daddy.

The first few weeks, however, are going to be a little less fun. Even if your partner showed the baby your picture every day and played the YouTube videos you made of yourself reading bedtime stories, it's going to take a while for your baby to get used to having you around. When you hold her, she may cry, fuss, pull away from you, or cling to your wife or another more familiar caregiver. And boy, is that going to hurt. You may be the toughest, most combat-hardened vet on earth, but that tiny infant of yours will be able to reduce you to Jell-O in seconds. For a lot more about the special concerns of deployed dads, you may want to pick up a copy of my book *The Military Father: A Hands-on Guide for Deployed Dads*.

to hit the baby. They need to know immediately and in no uncertain terms that you understand how they feel and that it's okay to be mad and talk about how mad they are. It's even okay to draw hateful pictures or beat up a doll. But it's absolutely not okay to do anything to hurt the baby.

Others may react by regressing. My oldest daughter, for example, was completely potty trained before her sister was born, but began wetting her bed again a few weeks after we brought the new baby home. Some kids suddenly start talking baby talk again, need more bedtime stories and cuddling, or make demands for attention that you may not be able to satisfy.

So what can you do to help your older child cope with those inevitable feelings of jealousy?

- If your older child comes to the hospital, keep the visit short. It won't take long for the initial excitement to wear off. And be sure to let him spend some time visiting with Mom too. He may have been worried about her, and seeing her in a hospital bed, possibly with IV tubes hanging out of her arms, can be a scary sight. Having a chance to hug her and be reassured that she's okay is important.

- Tell him—often—that you and Mom love him very much and that those feelings will never change. I remember having a similar conversation with my oldest when her younger sister was born. She was afraid that if I loved the baby I couldn't love her as much. I lit a candle and asked her to imagine that the flame was my love for her. Then I took a second candle and lit it with the flame from the first one. The second candle burned as brightly as the first, which wasn't diminished in any way. It's the same with love.

- Keep a few small presents around in case your older child feels left out when people bring gifts for the baby but not for him. It doesn't have to be a big deal, just a little something to let him know he's special too. If you have an album or a scrapbook of him as a baby, show him the photos and tell him about the presents he received when he was born.

- Stress the perks of being a big kid. For example, the baby is too little to play with big-kid toys or eat food that big kids do.

- Start fostering a relationship between your older child and the new baby by teaching big bro or sis to gently interact with the baby. Letting the older sibling help diaper, bathe, feed, and clothe the new baby is a great idea; it helps bring him into the process by making him feel that the baby is "his." But don't force the older child to get too involved. It can make him feel as though you want him around only to wait on the more important new baby, which can make him resent the little interloper even more.

- Model good behavior. Show your older kids the right ways to hold and behave with a new baby. Practicing with a doll is a great, risk-free way to get the hang of it—particularly the all-important head-supporting part. If you're bottle feeding, show the older kids the right way to hold a bottle and how to recognize when the baby's had enough. Never, ever leave the baby unattended with an older sibling (unless you've got a teenager—and if you do have a teen around, he or she will expect to get paid, so make sure you have plenty of cash on hand). Make sure the older child is always sitting down when holding the baby, and don't forget to praise loving, gentle behavior whenever you see it.

- Try to carve out some one-on-one time with your older child, doing all the activities you used to do before the baby's arrival—reading, going for walks, drawing, talking, seeing movies, or just hanging out. He may be an older sibling now, but he still needs your time, presence, and attention as much as ever. And make sure the big kid gets to spend some private time with Mom too.

A Note on Dressing Children

Getting a baby dressed is not an easy task; their heads always seem too big to go through the appropriate openings in their shirts, and their hands regularly refuse to come out of the sleeves. There are a few things you can do to make dressing a little easier:

- Reach through the sleeve and pull your baby's hands through—it's a lot easier than trying to shove from the other side.
- Buy pants or overalls with legs that snap open. Some manufacturers make baby clothes that are absolutely beautiful but impossible to put on or take off. The snap-open legs also make diaper changing much easier—you don't have to remove the whole outfit to access the diaper. Clothing legs that don't have snaps all the way to the ankles are a big pain—elasticized cuffs aren't so easy to maneuver when the kid is squirming on the changing table!

Also, don't overdress your baby. For some strange reason, people tend to bundle their children up in all sorts of blankets, sweaters, hats, and gloves—even in the summer. But unless you're Eskimos, there's no reason to dress your children like one. A basic rule of thumb is to have the baby wear the same kind of clothes you do, plus a hat. Layering clothing is sometimes a good way to go—if the baby gets too hot, you can remove a layer. Finally, I mentioned this earlier, but it's worth repeating: if they can't walk, they don't need shoes. It's not only a waste of money, but confining a baby's growing feet in a hard pair of shoes all day long can actually damage the bones.

Immediate Concerns...with Long-Term Impact

FEEDING THE BABY: BREAST VS. BOTTLE

When you were a baby, breastfeeding was probably out of style, and there's a pretty good chance that your mom's doctors gave her a wide variety of reasons not to breastfeed. But starting in the 1970s, breasts came back big time—so much so that it's pretty hard these days to find anyone who doesn't advocate breastfeeding. Even in the medical community, there's general agreement that breastfeeding is just about the best thing you can do for your child. The American Academy of Pediatrics recommends that new babies get nothing but breast milk for the first six months, and that breast milk should then be phased out and solid food phased in over the next six.

If you and your partner haven't already decided to breastfeed, here are the reasons why you should (besides the fact that you'll get a lot of nasty looks from people if you don't):

A Special Note on Breastfeeding

As natural as breastfeeding is, your partner and the baby may need any-where from a few days to a few weeks to get the hang of it. The baby may not immediately know how to latch on to the breast properly, and your partner—never having done this before—won't know exactly what to do either. This initial period, in which cracked and even bloody nipples are not uncommon, may be quite painful for your partner. And with the baby feeding six or seven times a day, it may take as long as two weeks for your partner's nipples to get sufficiently toughened up.

Surprisingly, she won't begin producing any real milk until two to five days after the baby is born. But there's no need to worry that the baby isn't getting enough food. Babies don't eat much in the first day or two, and the sucking they do is almost purely for practice. Whatever nutritional needs your baby has will be fully satisfied by the tiny amounts of *colostrum* your partner pro-duces. (Colostrum is a kind of premilk that helps the baby's immature diges-tive system get warmed up for the task of dealing with the real stuff later.)

Overall, the first few weeks of breastfeeding can be very stressful for your partner. If this is the case, don't be tempted to suggest switching to bottles. Instead, be supportive, praise her for the great job she's doing, bring her something to eat or drink while she's feeding, and encourage her to keep trying. You also might want to ask your pediatrician for the name of a local lactation consultant—yes, there really is such a thing. Many hospitals have them on staff and they'll stop by your room to give your partner some coaching before you head back home. To give you a sense of how much of an on-the-job-training activity breastfeeding is, the lactation consultant the hospital sent to our room was a male nurse. Despite not having breasts, he was actually able to show my wife how to do it. Your support is particularly important. Research shows that women whose husbands are supportive and encouraging breastfeed longer and are happier with the decision—an outcome that's good for everyone.

Feeding Twins

Although there's no question that breastfeeding is best, nursing two infants at the same time often presents some real complications. First of all, for the first weeks or so each of them is going to want to eat every two or three hours. Sometimes they'll be hungry at the same time, sometimes not. Ideally, you'll be able to get them both on the same feeding schedule. That's not always easy, though, because typically one will want to eat more often than the other. If that's the case for you, a lot of nursing moms find it easier to start serving both babies whenever the hungrier one wants it. Either way, by the time the feedings are over and the diapers are changed it'll be just about time to start again, which will leave your partner feeling something like a 24-hour drive-through milk bar. In a valiant attempt to give themselves some downtime, a lot of new mothers of twins opt for a mix of breast- and bottle feeding. The bottles can be filled either with breast milk (which can be pumped out faster than a baby can suck it out) or formula. Either way, if you've got twins, you're really going to have to be a lot more involved in feeding them than you otherwise might have been.

FOR THE BABY

- Breast milk provides exactly the right balance of nutrients needed by your newborn. In addition, breast milk contains several essential fatty acids that are not found in baby formula.
- Breast milk adapts, as if by magic, to your baby's changing nutritional needs. None of my children had a single sip of anything but breast milk for the first six or seven months of life, and they're all incredibly healthy kids.
- Breastfeeding greatly reduces the chance that your baby will develop food allergies. If your family (or your partner's) has a history of food allergies, your pediatrician may advise you to withhold solid foods for a few more months.
- Breastfed babies are less likely to become obese as adults than formula-fed babies. This may be because with the breast, it's the baby—not the parent—who decides when to quit eating.
- Breastfed babies have a lower risk of developing asthma, stomach problems, diabetes, cavities, pneumonia, ear infections, childhood leukemia, and sudden infant death syndrome (SIDS).

- Breastfeeding is thought to transmit to the infant the mother's immunity to certain diseases. This is especially important for the first few months, until the baby's immune system matures.
- Breastfed babies may have higher IQs than their non-breastfed buddies.

FOR YOU AND YOUR PARTNER
- It's convenient—no preparation, no heating, no bottles or dishes to wash...
- It's free. Formula can cost a lot of money.
- It gives your partner a wonderful opportunity to bond with the baby. In addition, breastfeeding will help get your partner's uterus back into shape and may reduce her risk of ovarian and breast cancer, type 2 diabetes, and postpartum depression.
- In most cases there's always as much as you need, and never any waste.
- Your baby's diapers won't stink. It's true. Breastfed babies produce stool that—at least compared to "real food" stools—doesn't smell half bad.

A NOTE ON SIDS

Sudden infant death syndrome, which affects otherwise healthy babies, is one of the scariest issues confronting new parents—and there's good reason: every year SIDS claims between 2,000 and 4,000 lives. It's the most common cause of death of children between one week and one year old, striking about one of every thousand babies. Despite all the millions of dollars spent on researching and fighting SIDS, no one's quite sure what, exactly, causes it. And there's no medical test to determine which babies are at the greatest risk. That said, here's what we do know:
- It's most likely to strike infants two to four months old.
- Ninety percent of deaths happen by six months.
- It's more likely to happen to boys than girls; to preemies, multiple-birth babies, babies whose mothers are under eighteen, African American, or Native American; and in families in which a parent or caretaker smokes.
- It's more common in cold weather, when respiratory infections and overheating are more prevalent.
- It is not caused by vaccinations.

Since two-thirds of SIDS babies don't fall into any of the highest-risk categories, there are a few things you can do to minimize the risk:
- Put your baby to sleep on his back. Experts used to think that babies who slept on their backs would choke on their vomit if they spit up. Turns out that's not true—babies are smart enough to turn their heads. People also preferred to put

their babies on their tummies as a way to avoid getting a bald or flat spot on the back of the head. Now we know that tummy sleeping may double or triple the risk. Since the Back to Sleep campaign began, SIDS deaths have dropped 43 percent. One thing, though: babies who sleep on their backs don't get to exercise their arms as much and take longer to learn to push themselves up and roll over. So make sure your baby spends plenty of his awake time on his belly working out that upper body.

- Don't smoke, and don't let anyone who does near your baby. While it's not possible to say that smoking directly increases SIDS risk, there does seem to be a connection.
- Don't overdress the baby (see page 267).
- Put the baby to sleep on a firm mattress: no pillows, fluffy blankets, plush sofas, waterbeds, shag carpets, or beanbags. The crib mattress should fit snugly into

Do You Really Want Your Mother-in-Law to Move in with You Right after the Birth?

Be careful about having people stay over to help with the newborn—especially parents (yours or hers). The new grandparents may have more traditional attitudes toward parenting and may not be supportive of your involvement with your child. They may also have very different ideas about how babies should be fed, dressed, carried, played with, and so on. If you do have someone stay with you to help out after the birth, make sure he or she understands that you and your wife are the parents and that what you say ultimately goes.

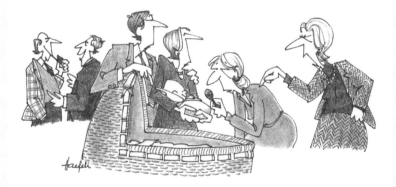

"Not so fast. I want to be called 'Nana.'"

the crib so the baby can't slip in between it and the frame. And take out any-thing else, such as stuffed animals or extra blankets that might accidentally cover the baby.

- Breastfeed. As with not smoking, while there's no definitive proof that breast-feeding actually reduces the risk, there seems to be a connection.

- Give your baby a pacifier. No one is sure why, but there's a lot of evidence that pacifiers reduce the risk. Wait until breastfeeding is well established before starting with the pacifier. And if it falls out of the baby's mouth, leave it alone—there's no need to try to jam it back in there.

- Don't panic. Although losing a child to SIDS is a devastating, horrible experi-ence for any parent, remember that 999 out of 1,000 babies don't die of it.

Hands-on Tips for Dads of Preemies

If your baby was born before about 35–36 weeks, he may have to spend some time in an incubator bulking up to at least four or five pounds before you can take him home.

One of the things you can do to make that happen a little sooner is to massage your baby. Tiffany Field, director of the Touch Research Institute at the University of Miami School of Medicine, found that preemies who had three fifteen-minute periods of gentle massage every day in addition to their normal treatment grew almost 50 percent more than those who didn't get the massage. Hospital stays were shortened by almost a week, and the bills were correspondingly lower as well. On their first birthdays, premature babies who'd been massaged were bigger and better developed than similarly premature kids who didn't get massaged. Pretty neat, eh?

SEX AFTER THE BABY: DON'T GET YOUR HOPES— OR ANYTHING ELSE—UP

Most doctors advise women to refrain from intercourse for at least six weeks after giving birth to give the cervix time to close and the bleeding time to stop. But before you mark that date on your calendar, remember that the six-week rule is only a guideline. For some couples, it takes a lot longer than that; others jump back in the saddle sooner. The stereotypical image people have of postpartum sex is that the moms don't want to and the dads are getting blue balls. Turns out that's not true. That same drop in testosterone that Anne Storey identified leaves many new dads less interested in sex. And sometimes those birth images are hard to shake. But according to University of Michigan researcher Sari van Anders,

"Is There Anything We Can Do?"

One of the most common questions you'll hear from people is whether they can help out in any way. Some people are serious, others are just being polite—what they mean by "Can I help?" is, "Can I hold the baby for a little while, then give her back?" You can tell one group from the other by keeping a list of chores that need to be done and asking them to take their pick. Laundry, grocery shopping, rotate the tires, file your taxes, paint the living room, whatever.

When my two oldest were born, a group of our friends got together and, taking turns, brought us meals every day for more than a week. Not having to cook or shop gave us a lot more time to spend together and let us get some rest. And of course, when our friends had their children, we were there with our spinach lasagna and a bottle of wine.

When baby number three arrived, my wife's sister came out and stayed with us for a couple of weeks. At least I think she was there. I saw her only a few times. But before she left, she'd made us enough frozen meals to last several months.

couples' lack of sexual desire wasn't necessarily related to what she eloquently calls "messy vaginas." In fact, the most common reasons for low sexual desire are fatigue, stress, not having enough time, and the baby's sleeping habits.

CRYING

Let's face it, babies cry; it's their job. The fact is that 80–90 percent of all babies have periods of crying that can last from twenty minutes to an hour every day. Still, there's nothing like holding an inconsolably crying child to make even the most seasoned parent feel inadequate.

I think fathers tend to feel this sense of inadequacy more acutely than mothers, perhaps because most men have been socialized to view themselves as less than fully equipped to care for children and therefore have less than complete confidence in their parenting abilities.

When (not if) your child starts to cry, resist the urge to hand him or her to your partner. She knows nothing more about crying babies than you do (or will soon enough). To start with, however, here are a few things you can do to reduce the amount of time your child will spend crying:

• Respond immediately. It is absolutely impossible to spoil an infant by picking her up when she's crying. At the very least you'll be teaching your baby that she's safe and that you're there for her. At the same time, when you pick her up and the crying stops, you'll get a jolt of much-needed self-confidence.

- Take note of what your partner eats while breastfeeding. After several horrible, agonizing evenings of inexplicable crying from our usually happy baby and a frantic call to the doctor, we discovered that the broccoli my wife had eaten for dinner was the culprit. There's also a possibility that your baby could be reacting to the milk in your partner's diet. If so, the pediatrician may suggest that she cut dairy out of her diet for a few days to see what happens.
- Have your partner nurse more often. The baby could be literally crying out for more intimacy. Besides that, smaller, more frequent meals may be easier on the baby's newly operating digestive system.
- Know your baby. Within just a few days after birth, your baby will develop distinct cries: "I'm tired," "Feed me now," "Change my diaper," "I'm uncomfortable as hell," "I'm bored in this car seat," and "I'm crying because I'm mad and I'm not going to stop no matter what you do." Once you learn to recognize these cries, you'll be able to respond appropriately and keep your baby happy. It's also important to know your child's routine—some babies like to thrash around and cry a little (or a lot) before going to sleep; others don't.
- Carry your baby more. Some studies show that the more babies are held (even when they're not crying), the less they cry.
- Watch the calendar. Your baby's cries will be pretty manageable for the first week or two. After that, she'll cry more and more, peaking at six to eight weeks before tapering back down to manageable again.

Colic

Starting at about two weeks of age, some 20 percent of babies develop colic—crying spells that, unlike "ordinary" crying, can last for hours at a time, sometimes even all day or all night. The duration and intensity of crying spells peaks at around six weeks and usually disappears entirely within three months.

Since there's no real agreement on what causes colic or on what to do about it, your pediatrician probably won't be able to offer a quick cure. Some parents, however, have been able to relieve (partially or completely) their colicky infants with an over-the-counter gas remedy for adults. Talk to your doctor about whether he or she thinks taking this medication would benefit your child.

A Note on Crying in Public

Dealing with a crying child in public was particularly stressful for me. It wasn't that I didn't think I could handle things; rather, I was embarrassed by and afraid of how other people would react. Would they think I was hurting the baby? Would they call the police? If they did, how could I possibly prove that the baby was mine? Fortunately, no one ever called the police, but there was no shortage of comments, which ranged from the seemingly helpful ("Sounds like that baby is hungry") to the blatantly sexist and infuriating ("Better get that baby home to her mother").

Although my fears about my children crying in public may sound a little paranoid (okay, a lot), I know I'm not alone. Just about every father I've spoken to has had similar thoughts in similar situations. I have to admit, however, that most of the women I've mentioned this to (including my dear wife) think I'm completely nuts on this point.

COPING WITH CRYING

If you've tried everything you can think of to stop the baby from crying, but to no avail, here are some things that may help you cope:

- Tag-team crying duty. There's no reason why both you and your partner have to suffer together through what Martin Greenberg calls "the tyranny of crying." Spelling each other in twenty-minute or half-hour shifts will do you both a world of good. Getting a little exercise during your "time off" will also calm your nerves before your next shift starts.

- Get some help. Dealing with a crying child for even a few minutes can provoke incredible rage and frustration. And if the screams go on for hours, it can become truly difficult to maintain your sanity, let alone control your temper. (To make things worse, the baby will pick up on your tension and anger and will be even harder to soothe than before.) If you find yourself concerned that you might lash out (other than verbally) at your child, call someone: your partner, pediatrician, parents, babysitter, friends, neighbors, clergyperson, or even a parental stress hotline. If your baby is a real crier, keep these numbers handy. You may find some comfort in the fact that this is something that affects every parent. If anyone tells you that they haven't felt like throwing their crying baby out a window, they're lying to you (or they don't have children).

- Let the baby "cry it out." Sort of. If the crying goes on for more than twenty minutes or so, try putting the baby down in the crib and letting him or her cry.

If the screaming doesn't stop after five or ten minutes, pick the baby up and try a different approach from the section above for another five or ten minutes or so. Repeat as necessary. Note: don't let your baby cry it out until you've tried everything else. Ordinarily, you should respond promptly and lovingly to your baby's cries. Several studies show that babies who are responded to this way learn that someone will be there to help them if they need it. This ultimately makes them cry less and helps them grow up more confidently.

- Don't take it personally. Your baby isn't deliberately trying to antagonize you—really. It's all too easy to let your frustration at this temporary situation permanently interfere with the way you treat your child.

PLAYING WITH YOUR BABY

You might not think that you can play with your newborn, but you can—and should. Playing with your child is one of the most important things you can do with him or her. Kids learn just about everything they need to know from playing. And to top it off, it's fun for you too. In general, babies love physical play, and by the time they're just a few days old, they've already learned which of their parents will play with them which way—and they'll react accordingly. Here are some important things to keep in mind about playing:

- As a rule, men and women have different play styles. Women tend to stress the social and emotional type of play, while men are much more physical and high-energy. Neither kind of parent-child interaction is truly better than the other—each is different and indispensable, and there's no point in trying to compare or rate them. Ross Parke and others have found that playful dads seem to have smarter kids than dads who don't play with their kids as much—they're better at math and score higher on intelligence tests. Physical play—particularly the dad kind—helps encourage kids' independence. Both boys and girls who are exposed to high levels of physical play are more popular among their peers and more assertive (in a good way) in their interactions later in life. They also do a better job of reading others' emotional cues and regulating their own emotions than kids who don't get as much chance to play.
- Pay attention. Even though your baby is nowhere near being able to catch a fly ball, sink a jumper, or even hold on to a rattle, you can still have fun together. Take all that wild arm and leg flailing. Surprisingly, it has a real purpose, as do many of the baby's other natural reflexes. The arm swinging, for example, may be a protective device designed to push dangerous things away. And you've probably noticed that your baby starts sucking the second anything—finger, nipple, thumb—gets in her mouth. This reflex helps ensure that they get nourishment in the days and weeks before they learn how to control their sucking

muscles. We talk extensively about reflexes and how you can have fun with them in the sequel to this book, *The New Father: A Dad's Guide to the First Year.*

- Use moderation. It's perfectly fine to play with a baby as young as a few days old, but restrict each session to five minutes or so. Too much playing can make your child fussy or irritable.
- Start simple. Imitation games are a good beginning. Stick your tongue out or make an O with your mouth, hold it for a few seconds, and see if the baby will do the same.
- Take your cues from the baby. If you pay attention, your baby will give you some pretty strong hints about whether he's interested in playing or would rather not. If he tries to raise his head, turns to look at you, or his eyes and face look bright, this is a good time to interact together. If he cries, squirms a lot, looks away from you, seems bored, or his face and eyes look glazed over, stop what you're doing and take a break.
- Put on some music. Doesn't matter what kind, but try to expose the baby to a nice variety. Baby ears are pretty sensitive to noise, so keep the volume low, particularly if you have a preemie.
- Schedule your fun. The best time for physical play is when the baby is active and alert; reading and other calmer activities are best when the baby is quietly alert. Choose a time when your full attention can be devoted to the baby—no

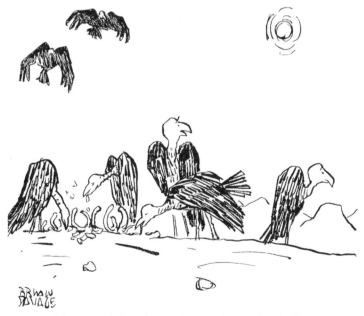

"I'm worried about him. He's not picking at his food."

phone calls or other distractions. Finally, don't play too vigorously with the baby immediately after feeding. Believe me—I learned the hard way.

- Get comfortable. Find a place where you can get down to the baby's level—preferably on your back or stomach on the floor or bed.
- Be patient. As mentioned above, your baby is not a trained seal—don't expect too much too soon. And certainly don't expect him to perform on cue.
- Be encouraging. Use lots of facial and verbal encouragement—smiles, laughter. Although the baby can't understand the words, he or she definitely understands the feelings. Even at only a few days old, your baby will want to please you, and lots of encouragement will build his or her self-confidence.
- Be gentle—especially with the baby's head. Because babies' heads are relatively large (one-quarter of their body size at birth vs. one-seventh by the time they're adults) and their neck muscles aren't very well developed yet, their heads tend to be floppy for the first few months. Be sure to support the head—from behind—at all times, and avoid sudden or jerky motions.

A COUPLE OF WARNINGS

- Never shake your child. This can make their little brains rattle around inside their skulls, causing bruises or permanent injuries (commonly referred to as Shaken Baby syndrome).
- Never throw the baby up in the air. Yes, your father may have done it to you, but he shouldn't have. It looks like fun but can be extremely dangerous and just isn't worth the risk. Even small bumps can cause concussions, which we now know can have serious, negative long-term consequences.

THE DIFFERENCES BETWEEN BOYS AND GIRLS

Back in the 1970s and 1980s, all the politically correct people insisted that there were no real differences between boys and girls—except for the obvious anatomical ones, of course. Any behavioral differences were supposedly the result of socialization, and were imposed on children by their parents and their environment. But in the past few years, researchers have started questioning this theory, and their answers are confirming what most parents have always known: boys and girls are just not the same. And the differences may even be present in our children's brains before they're born. Here's what we know:

- Within hours of birth, girls are much more interested in people and faces, while boys seem just as happy looking at an object dangled in front of them, says Ann Moir, Ph.D., author of *Brain Sex*. At only four months, girls can tell the difference between photographs of people they know from those of strangers; boys can't.

- The same applies to toys. When given a choice of two objects to look at—a doll or a toy truck—three-month-old girls tend to prefer the doll and boys prefer the truck, according to researcher Germaine Alexander. At a year old, boys prefer mechanical motion over human, choosing to watch windshield wipers going back and forth over people talking. Girls choose just the opposite.
- Infant boys and girls are hardwired to imitate adults. But even at three hours old, girls are better mimics than boys.
- Boys tend to take in less sensory data than girls, according to gender roles researcher Carole Beal. They're generally less discriminating when it comes to food, and less sensitive to touch and pain. They also hear worse in one ear than the other, meaning they don't pick up background noises as well as girls can, which may explain why your parents always thought you were ignoring them when you were little. It may also account for why girls typically learn to speak before boys do, usually by a month or two.

Despite all this, the distinctions between boys and girls during the first eighteen months of life are so slight that when babies are dressed in nothing but diapers, most adults can't tell a boy from a girl. But that doesn't stop us from treating them quite differently.

In one of the first studies of its kind, two Cornell University researchers, John and Sandra Condry, showed two hundred adults a videotape of a nine-month-old baby playing with various toys, including a jack-in-the-box. Half were told that they were watching a boy, the other half that they were watching a girl. Although everyone was actually viewing the same tape, the descriptions the two groups gave of the baby's behavior were incredibly different. The "boy" group overwhelmingly perceived the child's startled reaction when the jack-in-the-box popped up as anger. The "girl" group saw the reaction as fear.

Parents not only perceive their boys and girls differently but often treat them differently as well (your reaction to an angry child would be much different than to a frightened one). Mothers, for example, respond more quickly to crying girls than to crying boys and breastfeed them longer, according to psychologist Michael Gurian. And when girls have a difficult disposition, mothers tend to increase their level of affection, holding and comforting the child. But when a boy is similarly fussy, they generally back off. (This kind of behavior can have some serious, long-term consequences. In one study, researcher Laura Allen found that boys who received more cuddling had higher IQs than boys who received less.)

When playing with their children, dads tend to be more rough-and-tumble with boys but treat their daughters more gingerly. And when babies are just starting to take their first steps, both parents tend to let their sons fall repeatedly but will step in and pick up their daughters even before they hit the ground.

The upside of this kind of thing is that it encourages boys to be independent and teaches them to learn to solve their own problems without adult intervention. The downside, though, is that they often end up with less supervision and, as a result, are more likely to be injured than girls. In addition, "parents who step in to rescue their daughter before she is truly 'stuck,'" writes psychologist Katherine Karraker, "not only deprive her of a chance to overcome obstacles through her own efforts, but may also be sending the message that they have no faith in her ability to do so."

So what can you do to keep from falling into these traps? Start with this:

- Don't let your own prejudices and preconceived notions get in the way.
- Make an effort. If you have a son, there's no reason why you can't cuddle with him—it's a perfectly masculine thing to do. If you have a daughter, there's no reason why—a few months from now—you can't wrestle with her. She'll love it and so will you.
- Give your child a broad range of things to play with. Most girls end up playing with dolls, but some would be just as happy with a fire truck, if they only got the chance (although there's a better than average chance that she'll wrap it in a blanket and sing it a lullaby). And while most boys will end up biting their toast into the shape of a gun, some might have a lot of fun playing with a doll.

Fathering Today

For the first weeks and months after the birth of your child, you'll be spending a lot of your time in the role of support person for your partner. But after a while, you'll settle into a more "normal" life—one and/or both of you will go back to work, and you might feel like taking in a movie or visiting some friends. And gradually, you'll figure out exactly what it means to be a father and how involved you intend to be in your child's life. Do you want to be someone he runs to when hurt or sad? Will you know her shoe size or whether she likes pants that zip up or slip on? Will you schedule his medical appointments or playdates, or will you leave all that to your partner?

Whatever you decide, it won't take long before you come face-to-face with the fact that being a father in America—especially an involved one—isn't easy. The responsibilities of the job itself are difficult and at times frustrating, but the biggest obstacles you'll face—ones you've probably never even thought about before—are societal.

According to one stereotype, men haven't taken an active role in family life because they haven't wanted to. But is this true today? Hardly. More and more of us are figuring out that the traditional measures of success are not all they're cracked up to be, and we are committed to being a major presence in our children's lives, physically and emotionally. In study after study, the overwhelming majority of men aged twenty to forty-five say that having a work schedule that lets them spend more time with their family is more important than doing challenging work or even earning a high salary. And most of these men would gladly give up pay for more family time. The hitch is that society (and by this I mean all of us) not only won't support us but actively discourages us. Quite simply, Americans don't value fatherhood nearly as much as motherhood. (Even the words conjure up very different images:

motherhood is equated with caring, nurturing, and love, while *fatherhood* doesn't seem to be much more than a biological relationship.) As a result, men are rarely accepted if they assume a different role than the one they are "supposed" to assume.

The emphasis on traditional roles starts early. Even before they can walk, children of both sexes are bombarded with the message that fathers are basically superfluous. Just think of the books your parents read to you, and that you'll probably read to your own children. Have you ever noticed that there aren't any fathers in *The Cat in the Hat*; *Babar*; *Where the Wild Things Are*; *Are You My Mother?*; *Goodnight Moon*; *The Runaway Bunny*; or *Peter Rabbit*?

The very first article I ever had published appeared in *Newsweek* and was called "Not All Men Are Sly Foxes." It was all about what I perceived to be the negative stereotyping of fathers in children's literature. I spent an entire day in the children's section of my local library talking to the librarians and reading children's books, and found that dads were almost completely absent. In the vast majority of children's books, a mom is the only parent, while the dad—if he appears at all—was much less loving and caring than Mom, coming home late after work and bouncing baby around for five minutes before putting her to bed. The library had (and still has) a special listing of children's books with positive female characters—heroines *and* mothers. As the father of a daughter, I thought that was great. But as a father who was sharing the child-care responsibilities equally, I found it incredibly frustrating and annoying that they didn't have a listing (or even many books) with positive *male* role models. Even my three-year-old wanted to know why there weren't more daddies in the books we read.

You'll find the same negative portrayals of fathers in the majority of children's classics. Take *Babar*. Every once in a while someone will complain about the book's colonialist slant (you know, little jungle dweller finds happiness in the big city and brings civilization—and fine clothes—to his backward elephant village). But no one seems to find it strange that after his mother is killed by the evil hunter, Babar is an "orphan." Why can he find comfort only in the arms of another female? Why do Arthur and Celeste's mothers come alone to the city to fetch their children? Don't the fathers care? Do they even have fathers?

Today, we routinely refer to "firefighters" and "mail carriers" (instead of firemen and mailmen), and most new children's books make a conscious effort to take female characters out of the kitchen and the nursery and give them professional jobs and responsibilities. We've eliminated negative stereotypes (*Little Black Sambo*, for example, has all but disappeared from library and bookstore shelves), and there are dozens of books that feature positive portrayals of the disabled, minorities, and people from other religions and cultures. Only the portrayals of fathers have stayed the same, as three researchers from the University of Brighton

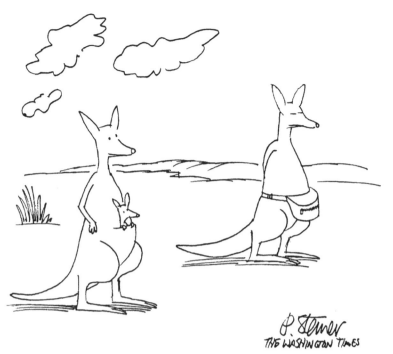

P. Steiner
THE WASHINGTON TIMES

(in the U.K.) found in their recent study of much newer books. According to Matthew Adams, Carl Walker, and Paul O'Connell, "Fathers were significantly less likely to appear than mothers, to be mentioned by characters or narrators, to appear with their children, to appear in or around the home, to be involved in physical contact with them, to be portrayed as expressing any emotion, or to be involved in any kind of domestic activity."

If books were the only place children got messages about the way the world is supposed to be, you might be able to edit out the negative messages. But sooner or later your kids are going to find themselves in front of some kind of screen. Did you know that the average six-month-old spends about an hour a day in front of a television? Within just a few years that'll be up to more than four hours a day! (That doesn't include time spent playing computer or console games or watching movies streamed from Netflix or Hulu). And much of that time they'll be bombarded by the same stereotypes: if dads are there at all, they're usually fairly useless. If only because of the sheer number of hours involved, these images have the potential to do a lot more damage than the ones they get from books.

Study after study has found that fathers are eight times more likely than mothers to be portrayed negatively. In fact, if you just think of the most prominent television dads, you'll find that most of them are outwitted or shown up by their wives, ridiculed by their children, and portrayed as complete incompetents in every way. Of course these dads love their kids, but good intentions aside, they can't handle even the simplest child-related tasks without detailed instruction from Mom, and need a Hazmat suit to change a diaper.

Portrayals of fathers (and men in general) in commercials are pretty much the same: they're not only dumber than everyone else but also almost completely oblivious to the needs of their children. Mothers, it seems, are the only ones who care. In fairness, I should point out that some advertisers are portraying dads in a nurturing, caring, nonmoronic kind of way. Jif peanut butter, for example, sometimes replaces their decades-old tagline "Choosy moms choose Jif" with "Choosy moms and dads choose Jif." But there are still holdouts. For example, hundreds of ads running during the three or four most recent Olympics tell us over and over that Procter & Gamble is the "Proud Sponsor of Moms." Nothing against mothers, but dads are usually the ones who encourage their kids to get involved in sports, who coach their teams, and who play catch, shoot hoops, or ski moguls with them. Ignoring their contribution is just plain insulting.

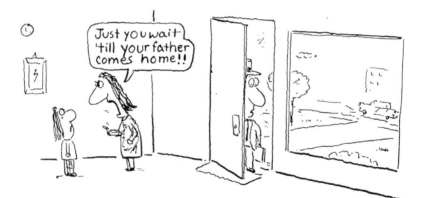

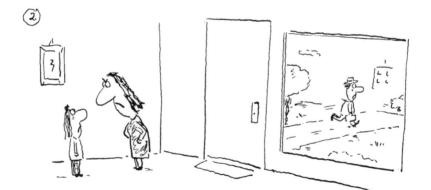

SIPRESS

So what does all this mean? Plenty. We know that repeated exposure to media violence contributes to violent behavior. And we know that being bombarded with images of stick-figure models contributes to eating disorders in girls and young women, and that being bombarded with images of muscle-bound superheroes contributes to "manorexia" (a compulsive need to get bigger and bigger) in boys and young men. So it follows that the negative portrayals of fathers (and husbands and men in general) in the media have a profound effect on children's (and adults') attitudes and beliefs about fatherhood. Those same portrayals contribute to "a decrease in men wanting to assume those roles in society, and creates the impression among others that men need not assume such roles anyways, that such simply aren't important," says Matt Campbell, with www.mensactivism.org.

As far as I'm concerned, we've already lost the current generation of parents. But what makes me especially sad is that we're producing yet another generation of girls who've been raised on dad-as-idiot images and think they'd be better off bringing up kids on their own, and another generation of boys who think there's no sense being an involved dad because everyone will make fun of them.

None of this, of course, is meant to imply that men are just hapless victims, or that all the obstacles fathers face are someone else's fault. In fact, some of the most significant barriers have been erected by men themselves. In the workplace, for example, where men still occupy the majority of positions of power, men who try to take time off from work to be with their families—either as paternity leave or by reducing their work schedules—find that their employers abuse them, treat them like wimps, and question how serious they are about their jobs (see pages 136–44 for more on this).

Despite the many obstacles, some of us have risked our careers and jeopardized our finances to try to break through the "other glass ceiling" that keeps us at work and away from our families. But in many cases, when we finally get home, we run smack into another barrier—this one imposed by none other than our partners.

Although most mothers feel that fathers should play an important role in the kids' lives, research has shown that they want that role to be "not quite as important as Mom's." In fact, researchers in one nationwide study found that two out of three women seem threatened by equal participation and may themselves be "subtly putting a damper on men's involvement with their children because they are so possessive of their role as primary nurturer." Bottom line? As I've said before, like it or not, you'll be as involved with your children as your partner will let you be. The more encouraging and supportive she is, the more you'll do.

It may sound as though all these obstacles are almost too numerous to overcome. Well, there may be a lot of them, and they may be quite ingrained, but if you're willing to put in the time and effort, you'll be able to have—and maintain—an active, involved relationship with your children. Here are some things you can do:

- Get off your butt. If you don't start taking the initiative, you'll never be able to assume the child-rearing responsibilities you want—and that your kids deserve. So instead of letting your partner pluck a crying or smelly baby from your arms, try saying something like, "No, honey, I can handle this," or "That's okay; I really need the practice." There's nothing wrong with asking her for advice if you need it—you both have insights that the other could benefit from. But have her tell you instead of doing it for you.

- Get some practice. Don't assume that your partner magically knows more than you do. Whatever she knows about raising kids, she's learned by doing—just like anything else. And the way you're going to get better is by doing things too. Research has shown, for example, that lack of opportunity may be one of the biggest obstacles to fathers' being more affectionate with their children. Once they get to hold them, fathers are at least as affectionate with their children—cooing at, looking at, holding, rocking, and soothing them—as their partners are. (So much for the stereotype about men being emotionally distant by nature.)

- Don't devalue the things you like doing with the kids. As discussed in the preceding chapter, men and women generally have different ways of interacting with their children; both are equally important to your child's development. So don't let anyone tell you that wrestling, playing "monster," or other "guy things" are somehow not as important as the "girl things" your partner may do (or want you to do).

- Get involved in the day-to-day decisions that affect your kids' lives. This means making a special effort to share with your partner such responsibilities as meal planning, cooking, food and clothes shopping, taking the kiddies to the library or bookstore, getting to know their friends' parents, and planning playdates. Not doing these things can give the impression that you don't think they're important or that you're not interested in being an active parent. And by doing them, you make it more likely that your partner will feel comfortable and confident in sharing the nurturing role with you. But try to log some private, "quality" time with the kids too. Sure, somebody has to schlep the kids all over town—to doctor appointments, ballet lessons, or soccer practice—but that shouldn't be the only contact you have with them.

- Keep communicating. If you don't like the status quo, let your partner know. But be gentle. If at first she seems reluctant to share the role of parent with you, don't take it too personally. Men aren't the only ones whom society has done a bad job of socializing. Many women have been raised to believe that if they aren't the primary caregivers (even if they work outside the home as

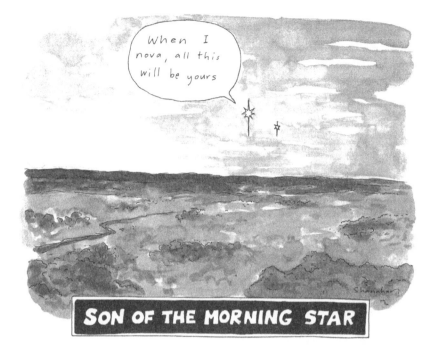

SON OF THE MORNING STAR

well), they've somehow failed as mothers. A 2010 study done at the University of Texas at Austin found that the more involved dads are with their children, the lower the mother's self-esteem. "We believe that employed mothers suffer from self-competence losses when their husbands are involved and skillful because those mothers may consider that it is a failure to fulfill cultural expectations," said Takayuki Sasaki, the lead researcher. If your partner works outside the home, you might want to remind her of what the late Karen DeCrow, a former president of the National Organization for Women (NOW), once told me: "Until men are valued as parents, the burden of child-rearing will fall primarily to women and frustrate their efforts to gain equality in the workplace."

- If you're in a position to do something for other men, do it. All things being equal, try hiring a male babysitter once in a while. Or consider asking a male friend instead of the usual women friends to do some babysitting when you and your wife want a night out. If you need to ease yourself into it, try the responsible teenage son of some friends. Continuing not to trust men and boys will keep men and boys thinking of themselves as untrustworthy and will make it difficult for them to be comfortable enough in their role as parent to take on as much responsibility as they—and their partners—would like.

- Get your partner to be your publicist. Pamela Jordan writes that "men tend not to be perceived as parents in their own right by their mates, co-workers, friends or family. They are viewed as helpmates or breadwinners." The cure? "The mother can mitigate the exclusion of the father by others by including the father in the pregnancy and parenting experiences and actively demonstrating her recognition of him as a key player," Jordan says.

- Get some support. Even before your baby is born, you're likely to become aware of the vast number of support groups for new mothers. It won't take you long to realize, however, that there are few, if any, groups for new fathers. And if you find one, it will probably be geared toward men whose contact with their kids is limited to five minutes before bedtime.

Having read this book, you know that men have just as many pregnancy, birth, and parenting questions as their partners. So if you can't find a new fathers' support group in your own neighborhood, why not be a trailblazer and start one of your own? Get the ball rolling with male friends who already have kids, talk on the phone, go for walks with the kids, meet in a park for lunch. Who knows—if you do a good enough job publicizing your new fathers' group, you might even be able to turn it into a real business. Don't laugh: plenty of people are making money on mothers' groups.

A FINAL WORD

Throughout this book we've talked about the benefits—both to you and to your children—of your being an active, involved father, and about how fatherhood actually begins long before your first child is born. What we haven't touched on, though, is the positive effect your fatherhood role can have on your relationship with your partner.

Back in the 3rd month chapter, I mentioned that in the first year after the birth of a baby, 90 percent of new parents suffer a major drop in the quantity and quality of their communication, and that half the time, it's permanent. One way to make sure you don't fall into the wrong half is for you, the dad, to get and stay involved, meaning that you're engaged with your children, you help maintain your household, and you and your partner are committed to raising your children together.

Sociologist Pepper Schwartz has found that couples who worked together to raise their children "seemed to create a more intimate and stable relationship. They did more together. They talked on the phone together much more and spent more child-related time together. Wives in the study said they believed that raising children together created a more intimate adult relationship." Parenting together can also help both of you cope if you happen to have a difficult child. "When couples with a supportive marital relationship have a difficult baby, they tend to rise to the challenge," says Ohio State University professor Sarah Schoppe-Sullivan.

Aside from all that, when you're actively involved, your partner will be less stressed, less depressed, and generally happier in her relationship with you. Not surprisingly, a number of studies have shown that fathers who are actively involved with their children have a much lower divorce rate than those who aren't.

So it's in everyone's best interests for you to do everything you possibly can to jump in and get involved right now. And stay that way for the rest of your life. It's not easy, but the rewards—for you, your children, and your partner—are incalculable.

THE PROCESS CONTINUES

We'll, we've reached the end of *The Expectant Father*. I hope you've enjoyed it as much as I've enjoyed bringing it to you. But don't think that just because you've got a baby now means you can stop learning. Not a chance. In fact, your journey is just beginning; being an involved father takes work, patience, and a lot of understanding. If you're interested in learning more—and I hope you are—I've written a number of other books to help you along the way. *The New Father: A Dad's Guide to the First Year* covers, as you might guess, your baby's first year. *Fathering Your Toddler* continues though your child's third birthday. *Fathering Your School-Age Child* picks up there and goes through age nine. All of these books continue and expand on the process we started here: getting to know yourself and what you're going through, how your child is developing, what's going on with your partner, and how to be the kind of father you want to be and your family needs you to be.

Now get out there and be a great dad!

Appendixes

Infertility: When Things Don't Go As Planned

Among couples who consciously try to get pregnant (or at least consciously stop trying *not* to get pregnant), about 25 percent conceive naturally in the first month. About 50–60 percent get it done within six months, 60–75 percent within nine, and 80 percent within a year. But that 80 percent statistic means very different things to different couples. A number of studies estimate that if you and your partner are in the 20–24 age group, your chances of conceiving naturally within a year are 86 percent; if you're 25–29, it's 78 percent; if you're 30–34, the odds go down to down to 63 percent; and if you're in the 35–39 group, it's only 52 percent. If you haven't conceived within a year (six months if your partner is thirty-five or older), you'll slip into the mysterious category called *infertility*, and you may need some outside intervention to have that baby you've been working so hard to get.

Despite what you may have heard, infertility is not just a female problem. About 35–40 percent of the time, the problem can be traced to the woman and approximately the same percentage to the man. For 20 percent of couples, it's a mix of his and her issues. Some of these reasons are listed in the chart on page 295. The rest of the time, there's simply no explanation.

Diagnosing a fertility problem can be a long and expensive process. Actually *treating* the problem will take even more time and money, which, most likely, won't be covered by your insurance. Technology is getting better all the time, and though fertility treatments definitely improve the odds for many couples—sometimes to as high as 50 percent—there's no guarantee that it will actually have the desired effect. Ever.

The doctors will start the diagnostic process by taking, from both of you, a complete medical history designed to investigate the cause of the infertility. You'll both also have a physical exam. In yours, the doctor will manhandle and squeeze your testicles. He may also order a semen analysis (see "Give Yourself a Hand" on page 301).

Here's the good news. Around 90 percent of couples seeking help with fertility get pregnant after relatively benign treatments such as lifestyle changes (diet, exercise, changing medication that may prevent fertility, timing of intercourse), drugs (to stimulate ovulation, increase sperm volume, or prevent miscarriage), artificial insemination (with either the male partner's sperm or a donor's), and minor surgery (to bypass obstructions, remove tumors or cysts, clear scar tissue, or correct other physical issues that are causing problems).

Only 3–5 percent of fertility patients need any of the high-tech options such as IVF, egg donation, ICSI, PGD, and a few others (see pages 298–99 for definitions of these and other helpful terms). For those who don't conceive after all that, the remaining options are surrogacy or adoption.

LIFE ON PLANET INFERTILITY

Ready for an understatement? Dealing with infertility—especially if you're among the minority that's undergoing expensive, time-consuming procedures—is not easy. To start with, there's the physical part: the semen samples, egg retrieval, blood tests, medication and hormone injections and the associated side effects, intrusive physical exams, and mad dashes to have sex at exactly the right time. All that, by itself, would be hard enough. But throw in the psychological toll of infertility, and you're in for a rough ride.

WHAT'S GOING ON WITH YOUR PARTNER

Most women in our society have grown up assuming that they will be mothers. So when that assumption—and the dreams that go with it—is shattered, it can bring up all sorts of feelings. Some experts believe that women take infertility harder than men. (In one study, 49 percent of women going through treatment said that being infertile was "the most upsetting event of their lives," compared to 15 percent of men.) Your partner has monthly reminders of her fertility, or lack thereof. And since she's the one who will carry the baby, society, family, friends, and maybe even her religion put more pressure on her to reproduce than on you. As she goes through the infertility process, she may experience some of the following:
- Anxiety and depression. A recent study cited in the Harvard Mental Health Letter found that "women with infertility felt as anxious or depressed as those diagnosed with cancer, hypertension, or recovering from a heart attack."
- Grief and sorrow. At the loss of her dreams.

- Shame and inadequacy. At being unable to fulfill her biological role.
- Guilt. Especially if the infertility is "her fault."
- Anger. Especially if the infertility is "your fault."
- Protectiveness. Again, if it's "your fault." She may want to keep you from feeling bad about yourself or your masculinity. Sometimes this plays out as wanting to have sex with you more often, as if to say that she still finds you sexually attractive—even if you have a low sperm count.
- Resentful. Nearly a third of women going through infertility treatment don't feel that their partner shares "the same level of commitment and dedication to getting pregnant," according to a study conducted by Organon, a manufacturer of fertility products. In the same study, 40 percent of women said that someone other than their partner was "their greatest source of support," and 26 percent felt their partner "could have been more supportive."
- A lack of intimacy. As one fertility doc told me, couples undergoing fertility treatment can either have sex or make love. Not both. Having sex on a schedule can become a real chore and will suck all the romance right out of it.

WHAT'S GOING ON WITH YOU

In my view, one of the reasons that the study above found that more women than men rate infertility as the most upsetting event in their lives is that people take men's silence and withdrawal as an indication that they aren't suffering. Nothing could be further from the truth. Here's what you may be feeling:
- Discomfort and embarrassment. Those physical exams can be really unpleasant.
- Inadequacy. We try to convince ourselves that size doesn't matter, but most guys want to know how they stack up to others. Hearing that the average sperm count is 50 million per milliliter but that yours is only 10 million, or that there's some other reason you can't impregnate your partner, can come as a real blow to your masculinity.
- Anger. At yourself, if the infertility is on your end. At your partner, if it's on hers.
- Lack of control. We're supposed to be the provider/protectors, the guys with all the answers. But on Planet Infertility, there's little or nothing that we can do to change things.
- Grief and depression. If you lost a baby to miscarriage, you have something a bit more tangible to grieve about. But even if you didn't get that far, you can still mourn the loss of potential, of the future, of being able to pass on the family name and genes, of being able to be a dad.
- Loneliness. A lot of guys in infertile couples have no one to talk to—or at least they think they don't. You don't want to talk to your partner because you know

Causes of Infertility

Because infertility is such a complex subject, there's no way I can do it justice here. Fortunately, the fertility doctor or clinic you work with will have tons of great resources for you, and they can explore every issue with you in great detail. What they probably won't have, though, is much information on how the ups and downs, and the ins and outs, of infertility will affect you, your partner, and your relationship with each other. So after a brief look at what you might be in for, that's exactly what we'll focus on. Let's start with what might cause infertility.

YOURS
- Low sperm count or damaged/irregular sperm shape and movement. These can be caused by:
  - Smoking
  - Drugs
  - Alcohol
  - Environmental toxins such as fertilizers, aluminum, and hazardous materials
  - Medication, including testosterone replacement, steroids, and ulcer drugs
  - Medical conditions such as diabetes, chromosome defects, genital infection, obesity, prostate problems, sexually transmitted disease, trauma to the testicles, testicular tumors
  - Radiation you may have received as part of chemotherapy
  - Tight underwear or keeping the testicles too warm
- Testosterone deficiency
- Having had mumps after puberty
- Having a mother or grandmother who took DES, a medication designed to prevent miscarriage and other pregnancy complications (it was prescribed as recently as the 1970s)
- Undescended testicle
- Varicocele, which is the swelling of a vein in the scrotum that may keep the testicle from cooling off
- Age (see "That Clock You Hear Ticking May Not Be Hers" on pages 296–97)
- Prolonged bicycling
- Stress

HERS
- Damaged or blocked fallopian tubes and/or ovaries
- Ovulation problems
- Hormone imbalance
- Many of the same factors that could affect you:
  - Smoking
  - Drugs
  - Alcohol
  - Medication
  - Environmental toxins (pesticides, heavy metals, air pollution)
  - STDs
  - Radiation
  - Poor diet
  - Lack of exercise
  - Being significantly over- or underweight
- Uterine problems, including endometriosis, cysts, fibroids, and scar tissue
- Having a mother or grandmother who took DES during pregnancy
- Exposure to environmental toxins while her mother was pregnant with her
- Age
- Stress

That Clock You Hear Ticking May Not Be Hers

The average age of first-time mothers and fathers keeps rising. The birth rate for mothers over thirty-five today is more than 40 percent higher than it was in 1970; for mothers over forty, it's nearly 50 percent higher. And although most people know about the difficulties that women over thirty-five have in getting pregnant, and the increased risk of miscarriage, preterm birth, and birth defects they face, we rarely hear anything about the effects of "older" fatherhood. In fact, having a child later in life is considered kind of cool and a confirmation of one's masculinity. (Alec Baldwin, David Bowie, Mick Jagger, Jack Nicholson, David Letterman, and Eric Clapton all became dads in their fifties. Pablo Picasso, Van Morrison, Larry King, Steve Martin, and Clint Eastwood were in their sixties. Charlie Chaplin became a dad at seventy-three, Julio Iglesias Sr. was eighty-nine, and there are plenty more.) While there's no question that being an older dad can indeed be cool and masculinity affirming, there are some risks that you should be aware of. Here's a quick overview:

- Researchers at Bristol University in the U.K. found that men's fertility begins to decrease starting at around age twenty-four. Other studies say the beginning of the end starts at thirty-five or forty. But regardless of when the decrease starts, most experts agree that the odds of conceiving within six months of trying go down 2 percent per year after that age.

- Sperm count decreases with age, and the little guys gradually lose their speed and accuracy, meaning fewer of them will make it all the way to the egg, and those that do will take a lot longer to get there.

- Sperm quality also decreases, meaning that the ones that reach the egg are less able to fertilize it. According to French researcher Stephanie Belloc, men over thirty-five are less likely to impregnate their partners; men over forty are significantly less likely. And even if they do, the resulting pregnancies have a slightly increased risk of ending in miscarriage.

- A number of very rare health risks and genetic conditions are associated with older dads. For example, research shows that compared to men under thirty, dads over forty have a higher risk of fathering children with schizophrenia, dwarfism, heart defects, facial abnormalities, autism, epilepsy, and some childhood cancers. Advanced paternal age may also be associated with children's lower IQ scores, increased risk of developing breast cancer, and shortened life span (for women born to dads forty-five and over). But again, these conditions are rare. And the connection between a dad's age and elevated risks is small. Still, the American Society for Reproductive Medicine has set forty as the upper limit for sperm donations, and many clinics have even lower limits. Just something to keep in mind.

- As your kids get older, you may not like it when people assume you're the grandfather instead of the dad.
- As you get older, it may be a bit harder for you to do some of the physical things young dads do, such as skateboarding, giving piggyback rides, and just crawling around on the floor.

On the other hand, being an older dad has its advantages. And in many people's eyes, those advantages far outweigh the disadvantages.

- Older dads are generally more financially secure, less worried about saving up for a down payment or making partner, and better able to provide for their families.
- Research indicates that older dads are more likely to share responsibility for taking care of their children and tend to be more actively involved with them.
- Older dads may also be warmer, more nurturing, and more focused on their children than younger dads.
- Older dads rate themselves as being more patient, more mature, and calmer than the young bucks.
- There is some indication that children with older dads do better in school. That's probably at least partly due to some of the factors above.

you're supposed to be strong for her, you want to protect her, and you don't want her to have to take care of your needs in addition to her own. And it's hard to imagine talking about something as sensitive and personal as infertility over a beer with the guys.

- Withdrawal. Because infertility can make you question your self-image and your masculinity, a lot of guys pull away from their partner and begin spending more time at work or hanging out with their friends—places where they feel more in control and can get some praise for doing a good job.
- Guilt. At not being able to fulfill your partner's desires to be a mom.
- Fear. The intensity of your partner's reactions to the situation may expose a side of her that you never knew existed. You may wonder whether she loves you anymore or whether your relationship will survive all of this.
- Frustration. The things you used to do to comfort your partner may not work anymore.

A Few Helpful Terms

Baby-making, like any other science, has a vocabulary all its own. Here are a few of the most common terms you're likely to come across.

- ART (Assisted or Artificial Reproductive Technology). Refers to any non-sexual method of producing a pregnancy. Includes IVF, donor eggs, donor sperm, PGD, and surrogates (see below for definitions).

- AI (Artificial Insemination—also referred to as IUI, for intrauterine insemination). The process of inserting sperm directly into a woman's uterus. This is the lowest-tech ART.

- Donor eggs. If your partner's eggs are not viable or healthy, or there's a significant risk of passing on a genetic disorder, doctors can use eggs harvested from another woman. Donor eggs will be combined with sperm—yours or a donor's—in IVF.

- Donor sperm. If your sperm is damaged or otherwise unhealthy, doctors can use sperm collected from someone other than you. This sperm will be combined with eggs—your partner's or a donor's—in IVF.

- ICSI (Intracytoplasmic Sperm Injection). Unlike regular IVF procedures, in which the lab puts the egg and millions of sperm together and gives them some privacy to do their thing, in this procedure, the doctor or embryologist injects a single sperm into the egg. This expensive procedure is sometimes used if AI has failed and the man's sperm count and motility are extremely low. The sperm can be collected the usual way (via masturbation) or through one of two amazing processes, called Testicular Sperm Extraction (TESE) and Microsurgical Epididymal Sperm Aspiration (MESA), both of which remove sperm directly from the testicle. With IVF, there's a 75 percent chance of the egg being fertilized. With ICSI, fertilization is guaranteed.

- IVA (In Vitro Activation). This is a new technique to help women with "primary ovarian insufficiency" or "diminishing ovarian reserve." It involves stimulating the ovaries outside the body to produce eggs, then re-implanting them in the fallopian tube.

- IVF (In Vitro Fertilization, meaning "fertilization in glass"). This involves collecting a woman's eggs and a man's sperm and mixing them in a dish or tube. A few days after conception, anywhere from two to five healthy-looking (under a microscope) embryos will be implanted in the woman's uterus.

- Ovulation. The release of the egg from the ovary, which typically happens twelve to fourteen days before a woman's period starts. The egg moves down the fallopian tubes to the uterus, where it hopes to be fertilized by sperm.

- PGD (Preimplantation Genetic Diagnosis). The main reason why many embryos don't result in a pregnancy is that they have some kind of chromosomal abnormality. The PGD process allows doctors to genetically analyze each embryo to determine whether it's normal or not (they can actually screen for about four hundred diseases or abnormalities). Since only the healthiest embryos are implanted, they're more likely to result in a viable pregnancy, and the rates of miscarriage or birth defects are significantly lowered.

- Semen. The whitish, sticky fluid that carries the sperm (see below). Semen protects the sperm and helps them swim toward the egg.

- Sperm. The cells containing the man's DNA that do the actual impregnating of the egg. Sperm are tiny—there are as many as 300 million in a single drop of semen—and look like tadpoles, with a big head and a long tail. Average sperm count is around fifty million per milliliter, which is down from about one hundred million just fifty years ago.

- Surrogate. Essentially a womb for rent. If a woman is unable to carry a pregnancy to term, it's possible to "commission" another woman who can. In some cases, the surrogate mother and the commissioning father may be the genetic parents of the child. In others, the surrogate mother may not be genetically related at all, and is simply carrying the biological product of the commissioning couple. And given where IVF technology is today, it's even possible that the surrogate mother, the genetic mother, and the commissioning mother are all different. Pretty crazy.

- Protectiveness. You'll be amazed at the level of insensitivity that people—most of whom probably mean well—will display. You'll get all sorts of suggestions on how to get pregnant, hear horror stories about fertility treatments, and suffer through tons of anecdotes about people who got pregnant within fifteen seconds of trying. You'll do everything you can to protect your partner from hearing these things, but some of it's bound to get through.

- Oversexed. At one point in your life, the idea of having sex every day may have seemed like a dream. But when you're dealing with infertility, the sex can very quickly move from hot and steamy to routine and boring. And there's no one to talk to about this. Who's going to believe a guy who complains about having sex too often?

Coping with Infertility

Infertility can take a real toll on your relationship with your partner. But being aware of the potential pitfalls, and having some strategies in place to deal with rough spots, will make the whole process more tolerable.

- Stick together. The two of you may be experiencing different things at different times, but you're in this together. Be patient with each other and support each other every way you can. This may include coming up with some snappy responses to the inevitable questions from family and friends about when you're going to have children. And in fact, besides your relationship with your partner, infertility can affect your relationships with other family members and friends. Understanding this—and recognizing that each of you is the other's closest ally—is critical.

- No second-guessing or self-blame. It's very easy to slip into "shoulda, woulda, coulda" mode. Okay, maybe you shouldn't have waited so long to begin trying to start a family. Maybe your partner shouldn't have had an abortion years ago. Maybe you should have lost weight or quit smoking a long time ago, or whatever. But there's nothing you can do about any of that now, and beating yourself up about it—or letting your partner beat herself up about it—is a complete waste of time and energy.

- Learn. Ask your doctors every question you can think of, and read everything you can get your hands on. But be careful to consider the source. Because infertility brings out the desperation in many couples, you'll find no shortage of "guaranteed" schemes that will separate you from your money, get you all optimistic, and then leave you worse off than before when they don't work.

- Get ready for the ups and downs. It's natural to get excited right before any procedure, and just as natural to feel devastated if it's unsuccessful. Typically, the more expensive and complex the procedure, the more stress couples experience.

- Have a little fun. Set aside some time to see a movie, have dinner together, hit the gym. Take advantage of the downtime between treatments to have wild, passionate sex in the backseat of your car. Don't let your entire lives revolve around treatments. You've got to give yourself some breaks from the routine.

- Set some limits. Is there a maximum amount of time you're willing to devote to trying to have a baby? A maximum budget?

- Listen, talk, then listen some more. Ask your partner what she needs from you. Tell her what you need from her. Be prepared to just listen. Although it might work in other situations, trying to solve her problems now may do more harm than good.

Give Yourself a Hand

If you and your partner aren't able to conceive within a year, her OB may suggest fertility treatments. The first step—because it's the easiest—is to do a semen analysis. The lab will be looking for a number of things, including count (how much semen is produced and how many sperm per milliliter it contains), morphology (size, shape, and appearance of the individual sperm), and motility (how quickly and how straight the sperm swim).

There are a variety of ways to collect semen (either for analysis or artificial insemination), almost all of which involve masturbation. In many cases, the festivities will happen at your partner's OB's office. Chances are they have a room that's outfitted with at least a few raggedy porn magazines (though hopefully the pages won't be stuck together), where you'll be expected to masturbate into a clean collection cup. Your partner will not be invited to assist. And keep in mind that any feeble attempts at humor, such as asking the nurse whether she'd give you a hand, won't go over well. Especially if your partner finds out about it. If you need any other visual aids, you can download plenty of them onto your PDA or smartphone.

If you'd rather not produce your sample in the doctor's office, you may be able to do it at home, as long as you can get the fresh sample there within an hour. The at-home approach gives you a few other options as well. You could do it yourself. Or your partner could help by bringing you to orgasm any way she wants and collecting the sample in the cup. Or you could have sex and collect the sample by withdrawing before climaxing or using a special condom that the doctor will give you.

- Stay away from places where there are going to be lots of people with children. Of course, that's not always going to be possible, but don't be shy about turning down invitations (or backing out of obligations) if you think it would be better for your mental health.
- Keep your mouth shut. Whether you choose to tell people about your infertility is your choice. Some couples want to keep it to themselves, others feel better talking about it. But one thing is certain: there is absolutely no upside to telling anyone whose "fault" it is.
- Get some support. People who have never had to deal with infertility have no idea how devastating it is. Consider joining a support group so you can connect with others in your situation. If you don't want to do it in person, take a look at some of the options in the Resources appendix.

Resources

To paraphrase Dorothy in *The Wizard of Oz*: My! Resources for expectant and new dads come and go so quickly. And because they do, this is by no means a comprehensive list (in fact, there are more resources on our website, www.resources fordads.com). To create a truly comprehensive list, we could really use your help. If you know of a resource that can benefit dads and their families, let us know. The constantly evolving list will live on the website.

Adoption

Adoption.com provides information on all aspects of adoption for those who wish to place a child for adoption, for those who want to adopt, for adoptees and birth parents who are searching, and for those who want to adopt internationally; support information; and much more.

adoption.com

Adoptuskids.org offers a national photo listing of children from across the nation and provides links to a variety of websites throughout the U.S.

tel: (888) 200-4005
email: info@adoptuskids.org
www.adoptuskids.org

National Adoption Center offers a great list of questions to ask adoption agencies; addresses single-parent, tax, and legal issues; provides photos of kids waiting to be adopted, book reviews, lists of state and local contacts, and links to other adoption-related organizations.
Tel.: (800) TO-ADOPT
email: nac@adopt.org
www.adopt.org

African American Fathers

African American Male Leadership Institute
ddce.utexas.edu/aamri/

Black Dads
blackdadconnection.org/

Baby Names

Baby Namespedia
www.babynamespedia.com/resources

BehindTheName.com provides the etymology and history of names.
www.behindthename.com/

GodChecker.com contains info on nearly 4,000 "weird and wonderful Gods, Supreme Beings, Demons, Spirits and Fabulous Beasts" from legend, folklore, and mythology all over the world.

www.godchecker.com/

Social Security Administration Top Baby Names

www.ssa.gov/OACT/babynames/

Blogs

Alltop Dads is a listing of many dad blogs.

dads.alltop.com

DadBlogs features tons of blogs by, for, and about dads.

www.dad-blogs.com

Breastfeeding

Kelly Mom

kellymom.com/

La Leche League International provides information and mother-to-mother support through La Leche League's network of lay leaders and professional experts. In addition to attending local meetings, any new mother may call a local leader for assistance, contact a national breastfeeding hotline, email the national office for help, search LLLI's database of research articles, visit the Ask the Experts columns, or join an online computer chat for answers to her breastfeeding questions.

www.lalecheleague.org/

Medications and Mothers' Milk

www.medsmilk.com/

United States Breastfeeding Committee. Its goal is to improve the nation's health by working collaboratively to protect, promote, and support breastfeeding.

tel: (202) 367-1132
email: office@usbreastfeeding.org
www.usbreastfeeding.org/

Childbirth, Assistance

American College of Nurse-Midwives accredits midwife education programs, establishes standards, and provides information and referrals to midwives in your area.

www.midwife.org

American Congress of Obstetricians and Gynecologists (ACOG)

www.acog.org

DONA International provides resources and referrals to doulas near you.

www.dona.org

International Childbirth Education Association is a professional organization that supports educators and other health-care providers who believe in freedom to make decisions based on knowledge of alternatives in family-centered maternity and newborn care.

www.icea.org

Child Care and Daycare

Child Care Aware (also known as National Association of Child Care Resource and Referral Agencies, or NACCRRA) is a nationwide organization to help parents identify quality child care in their communities. Great source of local referrals.

tel: (800) 424-2246
www.childcareaware.org

International Nanny Association is a nonprofit association for nannies and those who educate, place, employ, and support professional in-home child-care providers. Provides links to placement agencies and more.

www.nanny.org

The National Resource Center For Health and Safety in Child Care and Early Education is a wonderful general resource. Plus, it has a listing of child-care regulations for all 50 states.

tel.: (800) 598-KIDS
email: info@nrckids.org
nrckids.org/

Cord Blood Banking/ Stem Cell Research

Cord Banking offers information about cord blood banking, cord blood donation, and umbilical cord research and technology. The organization looks at this topic from the eyes of parents and provides answers to important practical and ethical questions.

cordbanking.org/

Cord Blood Banking Guide

www.bankingcordblood.org/resource-center

Parents Guide to Cord Blood Foundation

parentsguidecordblood.org/

Death and Grief

American SIDS Institute

www.sids.org

Fathers Grieving Infant Loss Blog

fathersgrievinginfantloss.blogspot.com/

First Candle offers resources on how to survive SIDS and stillbirth and also guides you through decisions you need to make during this difficult time.

www.firstcandle.org/

The Miscarriage Manual is a guide for parents who have experienced the death of a child through miscarriage, stillbirth, or other perinatal loss.

www.inciid.org/miscarriage-manual

MISS Foundation is a nonprofit organization that provides immediate and ongoing support to grieving families.

tel: (888) 455-MISS
email: info@missfoundation.org
www.misschildren.org/

Family-Friendly Employers

50 Best Small & Medium Workplaces List

www.greatplacetowork.com/best-companies/best-small-a-medium-workplaces

100 Best Corporate Citizens

www.thecro.com/content/100-best-corporate-citizens

Fathers and Fatherhood, General

Boot Camp for New Dads is a father-to-father, community-based workshop that inspires and equips men of different economic levels, ages, and cultures to become confidently engaged with their infants, support their mates, and personally navigate their transformation into dads.

www.bootcampfornewdads.org/

MrDad.com is my website. You can get information there about pretty much every aspect of pregnancy, childbirth, and fatherhood; find out more about my other fatherhood books; and send me questions and comments.

mrdad.com

National Center For Fathering has resources designed to help men become more aware of their own fathering style and then work toward improving their skills.

tel.: (800) 593-DADS
email: dads@fathers.com
www.fathers.com

Fathers, Divorced or Single

American Coalition For Fathers and Children is dedicated to promoting equal rights for all parties affected by divorce or the breakup of a family. Chapters nationwide.

tel.: (800) 978-3237
email: info@acfc.org
www.acfc.org

Dad's Divorce offers divorce information and resources about alimony, child support, and child custody for men and fathers at any stage of divorce.

dadsdivorce.com/

Making Lemonade is an online resource community for single parents. Find support, information, referrals to experts, and a good laugh.

www.makinglemonade.com

Single Fathers Due to Cancer is dedicated to the thousands of fathers who lose their spouses each year to cancer and must adjust to being sole parents.

email: singlefathersduetocancer @unc.edu
www.singlefathersduetocancer.org/ home.do

Fathers, Groups

City Dads Group is a growing national organization dedicated to helping fathers socialize and support one another.

www.citydadsgroup.com/

Just a Dad 247 has an amazingly comprehensive map of dads groups all around the world—not just at-home-dad groups, but all of them.

justadad247.com/map-of-dad-groups/or goo.gl/bUIC9i

Fathers, Older

Older Fathers Blog
olderfathers.blogspot.com/

Fertility and Infertility

American Society of Reproductive Medicine is an excellent source of information on a broad range of topics, including fertility, contraception, menopause, and sexuality. Patients will find articles and fact sheets that explain an extensive list of subjects in a clear and thorough manner.

tel: (205) 978-5000
email: asrm@asrm.org
www.reproductivefacts.org/

Path2Parenthood (formerly American Fertility Association) focuses specifically on issues of family building. It provides education, advocacy, and support for couples who are struggling to have children. Patients can find general information about such topics as reproductive health, fertility treatments, and adoption, as well as relevant news articles and a nationwide support network.

tel: (888) 917-3777
email: info@path2parenthood.org
www.path2parenthood.org

Society For Assistive Reproductive Technology provides information about procedures, success rates, candidacy, and medications for fertility patients who are interested in learning more about ART.

tel: (205) 978-5000, x 109
email: kjefferson@asrm.org
www.sart.org

Finances (College Savings, Financial Planning, Insurance, and so on)

American Council of Life Insurers (ACLI) provides basic information on the spectrum of life insurance products and operates the National Insurance Consumer Helpline, which can give you referrals to local agents.

www.acli.com

College Savings Plans Network offers great information on all of the state-sponsored college savings plans, including head-to-head comparisons and referrals to the ones in your state.

www.collegesavings.org

Financial Planning Association provides information on financial planning and referrals to certified financial planners in your area.

www.plannersearch.org/pages/home
.aspx

National Association of Personal Financial Advisors provides referrals to fee-only (as opposed to commission-based) planners.

www.napfa.org

Gay Parents

Gayfamilysupport.com has an abundance of information and resources dedicated to assisting families support their LGBT children.

www.gayfamilysupport.com

Gay Parent Magazine is for gay and lesbian parents and those hoping to become gay and lesbian parents.

www.gayparentmag.com/

Grandparents

AARP

www.aarp.org/relationships/friends-family/info-08-2011/grandfamilies-guide-getting-started.html

American Grandparents Association is dedicated to enhancing the lives of grandparents and their families.

www.grandparents.com/american-grandparents-association

Grandparents Raising Grandchildren

www.usa.gov/Topics/Grandparents
.shtml

Grandparents Rights Organization. Its purpose is to educate and support grandparents and grandchildren and to advocate for their desire to continue a relationship that may be threatened with loss of contact, usually following: family acrimony; a grandchild being born out of wedlock; the death of one of the grandchild's parents; or the divorce of the grandchild's parents.

www.grandparentsrights.org/

Green Parenting/ Healthy Living

Environmental Working Group's mission is to use the power of public information to protect public health and the environment.

www.ewg.org

The Green Guide is a wonderful newsletter (and website) filled with tips for healthy organic living.

www.thegreenguide.com

GreenHome explains how to create a healthy, nontoxic home environment and offers a full range of healthy, eco-friendly products for home and nursery, from paints that don't give off toxic gases to nontoxic insecticides and cleaning products.

www.greenhome.com

The Green Parent is a kid-friendly guide to earth-friendly living.

www.thegreenparent.com/category/
green-home

Healthy Child Healthy World's mission is to create a movement that inspires parents to protect young children from harmful chemicals.

healthychild.org

Health and Safety, Baby

Danny Foundation educates the public about crib dangers and advises eliminating the millions of unsafe cribs currently in use or in storage.

www.dannyfoundation.org

Kids in Danger is a nonprofit organization dedicated to protecting children by improving children's product safety.

www.kidsindanger.org

National Highway Traffic Safety Administration offers the latest info on car and car-seat safety. Includes a shopping guide for car seats, recall information, and safety literature.

www.safercar.gov/parents/index.htm

National Safety Council provides facts, information, and resources on environmental issues and accident prevention.

www.nsc.org

Parents Central provides resources for keeping kids safe when they're on the move.

www.safercar.gov/parents

U.S. Consumer Product Safety Commission provides comprehensive safety checklists, notices of recalls, and other important safety info.

www.cpsc.gov

BOOKS ON SAFETY

Mitchell J. Einzig, ed. *Baby & Child Emergency First Aid: Simple Step-By-Step Instructions for the Most Common Childhood Emergencies*. New York: Meadowbrook Press, 2011.

Christopher M. Johnson. *Keeping Your Kids Out of the Emergency Room: A Guide to Childhood Injuries and Illnesses*. Lanham, MD: Rowman & Littlefield Publishers, 2013.

Lawrence E. Shapiro, Richard L. Jablow, and Julia Holmes. *The Baby Emergency Handbook: Lifesaving Information Every Parent Needs to Know*. Oakland, CA: New Harbinger, 2008.

Morning Sickness

Morning Sickness Resources
morningsick.org/

Morning Sickness USA
www.morningsicknessusa.com/

Native American Fathers

National Indian Parent Information Center provides support, education, and encouragement for the families of Native American tribal children with disabilities or learning challenges.

tel: (855) 720-2910
email: indian.info@nipic.org
www.nipic.org/

Native American Fatherhood and Families Association is dedicated to strengthening families by responsibly involving fathers in the lives of their children, families, and communities and partnering with mothers to provide happy and safe families.

tel: (480) 833-5007
email: info@aznaffa.org
www.nativeamericanfathers.org

Native American Professional Parent Resources empowers, educates, and provides supportive services to build healthy Native American children and families.

tel: (505) 345-6289
nappr.org/

Postpartum Depression

The Online PPD Support Group
postpartumdepression.yuku.com/

Postpartum Dads
postpartumdads.org/

Postpartum Men
www.postpartummen.com

Postpartum Progress
postpartumprogress.org/

Postpartum Support International is dedicated to helping women suffering from perinatal mood and anxiety disorders, including postpartum depression, the most common complication of childbirth.

postpartum.net/Default.aspx

Preemies

PreemieParents.com offers a wealth of articles, books, links, and resources for parents of preemies.

www.preemieparents.com

Preemies Today supports families through the medical, emotional, financial, and social challenges of a premature birth to help ensure the best possible outcomes and futures for their children. It provides meaningful connections for preemies' families both in the NICU and beyond by enabling them to meet other families whose lives have been affected by premature birth.

www.preemiestoday.com/

Prematurity provides a wealth of support and information on the long-term effects of prematurity for parents of children born prematurely.

www.prematurity.org/index.html

Pregnancy and Parenting, General

There are a number of excellent Internet sites offering comprehensive pregnancy, childbirth, and parenting information, advice, resources, and products. Most have community sections where you can post questions and get advice from other parents. Most also have special sections for dads (although they usually aren't as good as the websites listed above). Among the best are:

American Pregnancy Foundation

americanpregnancy.org/

Babycenter.com

www.babycenter.com

The National Parenting Center provides comprehensive and responsible parenting advice by some of the world's most respected authorities in the field of child rearing and development (doctors, psychologists, and parenting experts/authors). The articles are targeted toward children in each stage of development.

www.tnpc.com/

Parenting 24/7. This University of Illinois website was developed to be a "one-stop" source of news, information, and advice on parenting. It provides recent news articles related to parenting and children, feature articles written for parents on a wide variety of topics, and a large number of video clips of parents and professionals discussing parenting challenges and strategies.

tel: (217) 333-2912
email: parenting247@uiuc.edu
parenting247.org

Pregnancymagazine.com is one of the leading pregnancy websites. It publishes 11 issues per year, including "The Pregnant Dad," the only pregnancy magazine issue written and edited by new and experienced fathers.

www.pregnancymagazine.com

Pregnancy, Alcohol and Drugs

Motherisk provides evidence-based information and guidance about the risk to the developing fetus or infant from maternal exposure to drugs, chemicals, diseases, radiation, and environmental agents.

www.motherisk.org/women/index.jsp

Pregnancy and Drinking Alcohol

alcoholism.about.com/od/preg/

Pregnancy and Substance Abuse

www.nlm.nih.gov/medlineplus/
pregnancyandsubstanceabuse.html

Twins (and more)

MOST (Mothers of Supertwins) provides information, resources, empathy, and support to families with triplets and more.

www.mostonline.org

Preemietwins.com is a helpful resource for parents of twins born prematurely.

preemietwins.com

The Triplet Connection

www.tripletconnection.org

The Twins Foundation is a great source for research on twins and other multiples.

www.twinsfoundation.com

Twins Magazine has print and online versions. Both offer advice, anecdotes, facts, support, and resources for parents of twins.

www.twinsmagazine.com

Work/Life Balance

Families and Work Institute is a research and advocacy organization that provides a wealth of research and resources for living in today's changing workplace, changing family, and changing community.

www.familiesandwork.org/

Fathers, Work and Family Blog

fathersworkandfamily.com/

Third Path Institute provides resources, information, and consulting to help people find a "third path"—an integrated, balanced approach to work and family. They advocate shared care at home and flexible, supportive approaches at work.

www.thirdpath.org/

We're constantly revising and updating this book and are always looking for ways to improve it. So if you have any comments or suggestions, please send an email to: **armin@mrdad.com**

Please also connect with us on social media:
• Twitter: @mrdad
• Facebook.com/mrdad
• Pinterest.com/mrdad
• Linkedin.com/in/mrdad
• plus.google.com/+Mrdad

Selected Bibliography

BOOKS

Agnew, Connie L., Alan Klein, and Jill Ganon. *Twins: Pregnancy, Birth, and the First Year of Life*. New York: HarperPerennial, 1997.

American College of Obstetricians and Gynecologists. *The ACOG Guide to Planning for Pregnancy, Birth, and Beyond*. Washington, DC: ACOG, 1990.

Aumann, Kerstin, Ellen Galinsky, and Kenneth Matos. *The New Male Mystique*. New York: Families and Work Institute, 2011.

Bainbridge, Jason. "Blaming Daddy: The Portrayal of the Evil Father in Popular Culture." In *Against Doing Nothing: Evil and Its Manifestations*, edited by Shilinka Smith and Shona Hill. Oxford, UK: Inter-Disciplinary Press, 2010.

Beal, Carole R. *Boys and Girls: The Development of Gender Roles*. New York: McGraw-Hill, 1994.

Bradley, Robert A., Marjie Hathaway, Jay Hathaway, and James Hathaway. *Husband-Coached Childbirth: The Bradley Method® of Natural Childbirth*. Fifth edition. New York: Bantam Dell, 2008.

Bryan, E. M. "Prenatal and Perinatal Influences on Twin Children: Implications for Behavioral Studies." In *Twins as a Tool of Behavioral Genetics*, edited by T. J. Bouchard Jr. and P. Propping. New York: John Wiley & Sons, 1993.

Camann, William, and Kathryn J. Alexander. *Easy Labor: Every Woman's Guide to Choosing Less Pain and More Joy During Childbirth*. New York: Ballantine, 2006.

Cath, S. H., A. Gurwitt, and L. Gunsberg, eds. *Fathers and Their Families*. Hillsdale, NJ: Analytic Press, 1989.

Caton, Donald. *What a Blessing She Had Chloroform: The Medical and Social Response to the Pain of Childbirth from 1800 to the Present*. New Haven, CT: Yale University Press, 1999.

Colman, L. L., and A. D. Colman. *Pregnancy: The Psychological Experience*. Revised edition. New York: Noonday Press, 1991.

Cowan, Carolyn Pape, and Philip A. Cowan. *When Partners Become Parents: The Big Life Change for Couples*. New York: Basic Books, 1992.

Duff, Margaret. "A Study of Labor." Ph.D. diss., University of Technology, Sydney, Australia, 2005.

Eliot, Lise. *Pink Brain, Blue Brain: How Small Differences Grow into Troublesome Gaps— And What We Can Do about It*. Boston: Houghton Mifflin Harcourt, 2009.

Glausser, Anne O. "The Placenta's Second Life." Master's thesis, Massachusetts Institute of Technology, 2009. Available online at http://dspace.mit.edu/bitstream/handle/1721.1/54572/567779304.pdf

Greenberg, Martin. *The Birth of a Father*. New York: Avon, 1995.

Haines, Helen. "'No worries': A Longitudinal Study of Fear, Attitudes and Beliefs about Childbirth from a Cohort of Australian and Swedish Women." Ph.D. diss., Uppsala University, Uppsala, Sweden, 2012. Available online at http://www.diva-portal.org/smash/get/diva2:570597/FULLTEXT01.pdf.

Harrington, Brad, Fred Van Deusen, Jennifer Sabatini Fraone, and Samantha Eddy. *The New Dad: Take Your Leave; Perspectives on Paternity Leave from Fathers, Leading Organizations, and Global Policies*. Chestnut Hill, MA: Boston College Center for Work and Family, 2014. Available online at http://www.thenewdad.org/.

Johnson, Patricia Irwin. *Launching a Baby's Adoption: Practical Strategies for Parents and Professionals*. Indianapolis, IN: Perspectives Press, 1997.

Jordan, Pamela. "The Mother's Role in Promoting Fatherhood." In *Becoming a Father: Contemporary Social Developmental and Clinical Perspectives*, edited by Jerrold Lee Shapiro, Michael J. Diamond, and Martin Greenberg, 61–71. New York: Springer, 1995.

Kitzinger, Sheila. *The New Experience of Childbirth*. Revised and updated edition. London: Orion, 2004.

Klaus, Marshall H., and Phyllis H. Klaus. *Your Amazing Newborn*. Cambridge, MA: Perseus Books, 1999.

Koukis, Marena. "Pregnancy Dreams." In *Perchance to Dream: The Frontiers of Dream Psychology*, edited by S. Krippner and D. J. Ellis, 167–80. New York: Nova Science, 2009.

Kutner, Lawrence. *Pregnancy and Your Baby's First Year*. New York: William Morrow, 1993.

Lamb, Michael, ed. *The Role of the Father in Child Development*. Fifth edition. Hoboken, NJ: Wiley, 2010.

Levene, Malcolm I., and Frank A. Chervenak, eds. *Fetal and Neonatal Neurology and Neurosurgery*. Fourth edition. London: Churchill Livingstone, 2009.

Logan, Brent. *Learning Before Birth: Every Child Deserves Giftedness*. Bloomington, IN: AuthorHouse, 2003.

May, Linda. *Physiology of Prenatal Exercise and Fetal Development*. New York: Springer, 2012.

Minnick, M. A., K. J. Delp, and M. C. Ciotti. *A Time to Decide, a Time to Heal: For Parents Making Difficult Decisions about Babies*. Fourth edition. St. Johns, MI: Pineapple Press, 1999.

Outcomes CoPIiP: Best and Promising Practices for Improving Research, Policy and Practice of Paternal Involvement in Pregnancy Outcomes. Washington, DC: Joint Center for Political and Economic Studies, 2010.

Parke, Ross, and Armin Brott. *Throwaway Dads: The Myths and Barriers that Keep Men from Being the Fathers They Want to Be*. Cambridge, MA: Houghton Mifflin, 1999.

Pederson, A., and P. O'Mara, eds. *Being a Father: Family, Work and Self*. Santa Fe, NM: John Muir, 1990.

Profet, Margie. "Pregnancy Sickness as Adaptation: A Deterrent to Maternal Ingestion of Teratogens." In *The Adapted Mind: Evolutionary Psychology and the Generation of Culture*, edited by Jerome Barkow, Leda Cosmides, and John Tooby, 327–65. New York: Oxford University Press, 1992.

Pruett, Kyle, and Marsha Kline Pruett. *Partnership Parenting: How Men and Women Parent Differently—Why It Helps Your Kids and Can Strengthen Your Marriage*. Philadelphia: DaCapo Lifelong, 2009.

Rankin, Lissa. *What's Up Down There?: Questions You'd Only Ask Your Gynecologist If She Was Your Best Friend*. New York: St. Martin's Griffin, 2010.

Rodriguez, Robert G. *An Anxious Time for Men: Pregnancy; A Research Study That Measured Anxiety, Stress, Marital Satisfaction, and Depression in First Time Expectant Fathers*. Columbus, OH: Greenborough Publishing, 2003.

Roehrich, Susan K. "Men's Perspectives on a Spouse's or Partner's Postpartum Depression." Ph.D. diss., Virginia Polytechnic Institute and State University, 2007. Available online at http://scholar.lib.vt.edu/theses/available/etd-09242007-164439/unrestricted/0907RoehrichDissertation.pdf.

Shapiro, Jerrold L. *When Men Are Pregnant*. New York: Delta, 1993.

Siegel, Alan. *Dream Wisdom: Uncovering Life's Answers in Your Dreams*. Berkeley, CA: Celestial Arts, 2003.

Tassone, Shawn, and Landherr, Kathryn. *Hands off My Belly!: The Pregnant Woman's Survival Guide to Myths, Mothers, and Moods*. Amherst, NY: Prometheus Books, 2009.

Thevenin, Tine. *The Family Bed*. Wayne, NJ: Avery Publishing Group, 1987.

Van de Carr, F. R., and M. Lehrer. *While You Are Expecting*. Atlanta: Humanics Learning, 1997.

Vanston, Claire M. "Maternal Cognitive Function in Pregnancy and Its Association with Gestation, Endocrine Factors, and Fetal Sex: A Longitudinal Study of Women from Early Pregnancy to the Postpartum Period." Ph.D. diss., Simon Fraser University, 2005.

Verny, Thomas, and Pamela Weintraub. *Nurturing the Unborn Child: A Nine-Month Program for Soothing, Stimulating, and Communicating with Your Baby*. New York: Dell, 1992; Open Road Integrated Media ebook, 2014.

ARTICLES AND PAPERS

Abel, E. L., and M. L. Kruger. "Symbolic Significance of Initials on Longevity." *Perceptual and Motor Skills* 104 (2007): 179–82.

Adams, Matthew, Carl Walker, and Paul O'Connell. "Invisible or Involved Fathers? A Content Analysis of Representations of Parenting in Young Children's Picturebooks in the UK." *Sex Roles* 65, no. 3–4 (2011): 259–70.

Alexander, G. M., T. Wilcox, and R. Woods. "Sex Differences in Infants' Visual Interest in Toys." *Archives of Sexual Behavior* 38, no. 3 (June 2009): 427–33.

Alicesteen, Rachel, and Young-ok Yum. "The Effect of Sex and Sex Talk during Pregnancy on Relationship Satisfaction." Paper presented at the International Communication Association annual meeting, New York, May 2009. Available online at www.allacademic.com/meta/p12762_index.html.

Alio, A. P., M. J. Bond, Y. C. Padilla, J. J. Heidelbaugh, M. Lu, and W. J. Parker. "Addressing Policy Barriers to Paternal Involvement during Pregnancy." *Maternal and Child Health Journal* 15, no. 4 (May 2011): 425–30.

Alio, A. P., H. M. Salihu, J. L. Kornosky, A. M. Richman, and P. J. Marty. "Feto-Infant Health and Survival: Does Paternal Involvement Matter?" *Maternal and Child Health Journal* 14, no. 6 (November 2010): 931–37.

Allen, V. M., R. D. Wilson, and A. Cheung. "Pregnancy Outcomes after Assisted Reproductive Technology." *Journal of Obstetrics and Gynaecology Canada* 28, no. 3 (March 2006): 220–50.

American Academy of Pediatrics Task Force on Circumcision. "Circumcision Policy Statement (Reaffirmed)." *Pediatrics* 130, no. 3 (September 2012): 585–86.

Anderson, David A., and Mykol Hamilton. "Gender Role Stereotyping of Parents in Children's Picture Books: The Invisible Father." *Sex Roles* 52, no. 3–4 (February 2005): 145–51.

Andersson, G., and G. Woldemichael. "Sex Composition of Children as a Determinant of Marriage Disruption and Marriage Formation: Evidence from Sweden." *Journal of Population Research* 18, no. 2 (2001): 143–53.

Arabin, B., J. von Eyck, J. Wisser, H. Versmold, and H. K. Weitzel. "Fetales Verhalten bei Mehrlingsgravidität: Methodische, klinische und wissenschaftliche Aspekte" (Fetal Behavior in Multiple Pregnancy: Methodologic, Clinical and Scientific Aspects). *Geburtshilfe und Frauenheilkunde* 51, no. 11 (November 1991): 869–75.

Autor, David H. "Skills, Education, and the Rise of Earnings Inequality among the 'Other 99 percent.'" *Science* 344, no. 6186 (May 2014): 843–51.

Badenhorst, W., S. Riches, P. Turton, and P. Hughes. "The Psychological Effects of Stillbirth and Neonatal Death on Fathers: Systematic Review." *Journal of Psychosomatic Obstetrics & Gynaecology* 27, no. 4 (December 2006): 245–56.

Barrett, Geraldine, et al. "Women's Sexual Health After Childbirth." *BJOG: An International Journal of Obstetrics & Gynaecology* 107, no. 2 (February 2005): 186–95.

Bartels R. "Experience of Childbirth from the Father's Perspective." *British Journal of Midwifery* 7, no. 4 (1999): 681–83.

Batman, P. A., J. Thomlinson, V. C. Moore, and R. Sykes. "Death Due to Air Embolism During Sexual Intercourse in the

Puerperium." *Postgraduate Medical Journal* 74, no. 876 (October 1998): 612–13.

Beaton, John M., William J. Doherty, and Martha A. Rueter. "Family of Origin Processes and Attitudes of Expectant Fathers." *Fathering* 1, no. 2 (June 2003): 149–68.

Becker, Gay, Anneliese Butler, and Robert D. Nachtigall. "Resemblance Talk: A Challenge for Parents Whose Children Were Conceived with Donor Gametes in the US." *Social Science & Medicine* 61, no. 6 (2005): 1300–1309.

Bekkers, René. "George Gives to Geology Jane: The Name Letter Effect and Incidental Similarity Cues in Fundraising." *International Journal of Nonprofit and Voluntary Sector Marketing* 15, no 2 (May 2010): 172–80.

Bélanger-Lévesque, M.-N,, M. Pasquier, N. Roy-Matton, S. Blouin, J.-C. Pasquier. "Maternal and Paternal Satisfaction in the Delivery Room: A Cross-Sectional Comparative Study." *BMJ Open* 4, no. 2 (February 2014).

Bell, John D. "Giving Birth to the New Soviet Man: Politics and Obstetrics in the USSR." *Slavic Review* 40, no. 1 (Spring 1981): 1–16.

Bellver, Jose, et al. "Influence of Paternal Age on Assisted Reproduction Outcome." *Reproductive BioMedicine Online* 17, no. 5 (November 2008): 595–604.

Bergstrom, M., H. Kieler, and U. Waldenstrom. "Effects of Natural Childbirth Preparation versus Standard Antenatal Education on Epidural Rates, Experience of Childbirth and Parental Stress in Mothers and Fathers: A Randomised Controlled Multicentre Trial." *BJOG: An International Journal of Obstetrics & Gynaecology* 116, no. 9 (August 2009): 1167–76.

Bianchi, Diana W., et al. "DNA Sequencing versus Standard Prenatal Aneuploidy Screening." *The New England Journal of Medicine* 370 (February 2014): 799–808.

Biehle, S. N., and K. D. Mickelson. "Preparing for Parenthood: How Feelings of Responsibility and Efficacy Impact Expectant Parents." *Journal of Social and Personal Relationships* 28, no. 5 (August 2011): 668–83.

Bond, M. J. "The Missing Link in MCH: Paternal Involvement in Pregnancy Outcomes." *American Journal of Men's Health* 4, no. 4 (December 2010): 285–86.

Bond, M. J., J. J. Heidelbaugh, A. Robertson, P. A. Alio, and W. J. Parker. "Improving Research, Policy and Practice to Promote Paternal Involvement in Pregnancy Outcomes: The Roles of Obstetricians-Gynecologists." *Current Opinion in Obstetrics and Gynecology* 22, no. 6 (December 2010): 525–29.

Borrelli, Francesca, et al. "Effectiveness and Safety of Ginger in the Treatment of Pregnancy-Induced Nausea and Vomiting." *Obstetrics & Gynecology* 105, no. 4 (April 2005): 849–56.

Boyce, P., J. Condon, J. Barton, and C. Corkindale. "First-Time Fathers' Study: Psychological Distress in Expectant Fathers During Pregnancy." *Australian & New Zealand Journal of Psychiatry* 41, no. 9 (September 2007): 718–25.

Brandão, Sónia, and Bárbara Figueiredo. "Fathers' Emotional Involvement with the Neonate: Impact of the Umbilical Cord Cutting Experience." *Journal of Advanced Nursing* 68, no. 12 (December 2012): 2730–39.

Breggin, Peter R., and Ginger Breggin. "Exposure to SSRI Antidepressants in Utero Causes Birth Defects, Neonatal Withdrawal Symptoms, and Brain Damage." *Ethical Human Psychology and Psychiatry* 10, no. 1 (2008): 203–7.

Brennan, A., S. Ayers, H. Ahmed, and S. Marshall-Lucette. "A Critical Review of the Couvade Syndrome: The Pregnant Male." *Journal of Reproductive and Infant Psychology* 25, no. 3 (2007): 173–89.

Brodzinsky, David, and Laureen Huffman. "Transition to Adoptive Parenthood." *Marriage and Family Review* 12 (1988): 267–86.

Bronte-Tinkew, Jacinta, et al. "Resident Fathers' Pregnancy Intentions, Prenatal Behaviors, and Links to Involvement with Infants." *Journal of Marriage and Family* 69, no. 4 (November 2007): 977–90.

Bronte-Tinkew, J., K. Moore, G. Matthews, and J. Carrano. "Symptoms of Major Depression in a Sample of Fathers of Infants: Sociodemographic Correlates and Links to Father Involvement." *Journal of Family Issues* 28, no. 1 (January 2007): 61–99.

313

Broude, Gwen J. "Rethinking the Couvade: Cross-Cultural Evidence." *American Anthropologist* 90, no. 4 (December 1988): 902–11.

Callister, Lynn Clark. "Perinatal Loss: A Family Perspective." *Journal of Perinatal & Neonatal Nursing* 20, no. 3 (September 2006): 227–34.

Cannon, M. "Contrasting Effects of Maternal and Paternal Age on Offspring Intelligence: The Clock Ticks for Men Too." *PLoS Medicine* 6, no. 3 (March 2009): 2.

Capogna, Giorgio, Michela Camorcia, and S. Stirparo. "Expectant Fathers' Experience during Labor with or without Epidural Analgesia." *International Journal of Obstetric Anesthesia* 16, no. 2 (April 2007): 110–15.

Carin, A., et al. "Correlation between Oral Sex and a Low Incidence of Preeclampsia: A Role for Soluble HLA in Seminal Fluid?" *Journal of Reproductive Immunology* 46, no. 2 (2000): 155–66.

Chang, Grace, Tay McNamara, E. John Orav, and Louise Wilkins-Haug. "Identifying Risk Drinking in Expectant Fathers." *Birth* 33, no. 2 (June 2006): 110–16.

Christenfeld, N., D. Phillips, and L. Glynn. "What's in a Name: Mortality and the Power of Symbols." *Journal of Psychosomatic Research* 47 (1999): 241–54.

Christiansen, Solveig Glestad. "The Impact of Children's Sex Composition on Parents' Mortality." *BMC Public Health* 14 (2014): 989.

Christiansen, S., and R. Palkovitz. "Why the 'Good Provider' Role Still Matters: Providing as a Form of Paternal Involvement." *Journal of Family Issues* 22 (2001): 84–106.

Condon, John T., Carolyn J. Corkindale, and Phillip Boyce. "Assessment of Postnatal Paternal-Infant Attachment: Development of a Questionnaire Instrument." *Journal of Reproductive and Infant Psychology* 26, no. 3 (August 2008): 195–210.

———. "The First-Time Fathers Study: A Prospective Study of the Mental Health and Wellbeing of Men during the Transition to Parenthood." *Australian & New Zealand Journal of Psychiatry* 38, no. 1–2 (January–February 2004): 56–64.

Cox, J. E., M. Buman, J. Valenzuela, et al. Depression, Parenting Attributes, and Social Support among Adolescent Mothers Attending a Teen Tot Program." *Journal of Pediatric & Adolescent Gynecology* 21, no. 5 (October 2008): 275–81.

Cumings, David. "The Effects of Miscarriage on a Man." *Emotional First Aid* 1, no. 4 (1984): 47–50.

Dahl, Gordon B., and Enrico Moretti. "The Demand for Sons: Evidence from Divorce, Fertility, and Shotgun Marriage." National Bureau of Economic Research Working Paper, no. 10281 (February 2004).

Daly, Mary C., and Leila Bengali. "Is It Still Worth Going to College?" Federal Reserve Bank of San Francisco Economic Letter, no. 2014-13 (May 5, 2014).

Davidson, J. R. "The Shadow of Life: Psychosocial Explanations for Placenta Rituals." *Culture, Medicine, and Psychiatry* 9, no. 1 (March 1985): 75–92.

Deave, T., and D. Johnson. "The Transition to Parenthood: What Does It Mean for Fathers?" *Journal of Advanced Nursing* 63, no. 6 (September 2008): 626–33.

Dekker, Gustaaf, et al. "Immune Maladaptation in the Etiology of Preeclampsia: A Review of Corroborative Epidemiologic Studies." *Obstetrical & Gynecological Survey* 53, no. 6 (June 1998): 377–82.

De La Rochebrochard, Elise, Ken McElreavey, and Patrick Thonneau. "Paternal Age over 40 Years: The Amber Light in the Reproductive Life of Men?" *Journal of Andrology* 24, no. 4 (July–August 2003): 459–65.

Diemer, Geraldine A. "Expectant Fathers: Influence of Perinatal Education on Stress, Coping, and Spousal Relations." *Research in Nursing & Health* 20, no. 4 (August 1997): 281–93.

The Dieringer Research Group. "Telework Trendlines 2009: A Survey Brief by WorldatWork" (February 2009). Available online at http://www.worldatwork.org/waw/adimLink?id=31115.

Doucet, Andrea. "Dad and Baby in the First Year: Gendered Responsibilities and Embodiment." *The Annals of the American Academy of Political and Social Science* 624, no. 1 (July 2009): 78–98.

Draper, J. "Men's Passage to Fatherhood: An Analysis of the Contemporary Relevance of Transition Theory." *Nursing Inquiry* 10, no. 1 (March 2003): 66–77.

Dyck, Vera, and Kerry Daly. "Rising to the Challenge: Fathers' Role in the Negotiation of Couple Time." *Leisure Studies* 25, no. 2 (April 2006): 201–17.

Elliott, Stuart. "Campaigns for Challenging Times Put Children and Mothers First." *New York Times*, March 16, 2009.

Engeland, Anders, et al. "Prescription Drug Use Among Fathers and Mothers before and during Pregnancy: A Population-based Cohort Study of 106,000 Pregnancies in Norway 2004–2006." *British Journal of Clinical Pharmacology* 65, no. 5 (May 2008): 653–60.

Eriksson, Carola, Pär Salander, and Katarina Hamberg. "Men's Experiences of Intense Fear Related to Childbirth Investigated in a Swedish Qualitative Study." *The Journal of Men's Health & Gender* 4, no. 4 (December 2007): 409–18.

Erlandsson, Kerstin, A. Dsilna, I, Fagerberg, and K. Christensson. "Skin-to-Skin Care with the Father after Cesarean Birth and Its Effect on Newborn Crying and Prefeeding Behaviour." *Birth* 34, no. 2 (2007): 105–14.

Erwin, P. G. "First Names and Perceptions of Physical Attractiveness." *The Journal of Psychology* 127, no. 6 (November 1993): 625–31.

Fagan, J., and R. Palkovitz. "Unmarried, Nonresident Fathers' Involvement with Their Infants: A Risk and Resilience Perspective." *Journal of Family Psychology* 21, no. 3 (September 2007): 479–89.

Fägerskiöld, Astrid. "A Change in Life as Experienced by First-Time Fathers." *Scandinavian Journal of Caring Sciences* 22, no. 1 (March 2008): 64–71.

Field, Tiffany, et al. "Pregnancy Anxiety and Comorbid Depression and Anger: Effects on the Fetus and Neonate." *Depression and Anxiety* 17, no. 3 (2003): 140–51.

Field, T., et al. "Prenatal Depression Effects on the Fetus and the Newborn." *Infant Behavior & Development* 27, no. 2 (May 2004): 216–29.

Field, T., et al. "Prenatal Paternal Depression." *Infant Behavior & Development* 29, no. 4 (December 2006): 579–83.

Finnbogadóttir, H., E. Svalenius, and E. Persson. "Expectant First-Time Fathers' Experiences of Pregnancy." *Midwifery* 19, no. 2 (June 2003): 96–105.

Flaxman, S. M., and P. W. Sherman. "Morning Sickness: A Mechanism For Protecting Mother and Embryo." *Quarterly Review of Biology* 75, no. 2 (June 2000): 113–48.

Fletcher, R., S. Silberberg, and D. Galloway. "New Fathers' Postbirth Views of Antenatal Classes: Satisfaction, Benefits, and Knowledge of Family Services." *Journal of Perinatal Education* 13, no. 3 (Summer 2004): 18–26.

Fox, Douglas. "Gentle Persuasion." *New Scientist* 173, no. 2329 (February 2002): 32.

Friedewald, Mark, Richard Fletcher, and Hedy Fairbairn. "All-Male Discussion Forums for Expectant Fathers: Evaluation of a Model." *Journal of Perinatal Education* 14, no. 2 (Spring 2005): 8–18.

Ginath, Y. "Psychoses in Males in Relation to Their Wives' Pregnancy and Childbirth." *The Israel Annals of Psychiatry and Related Disciplines* 12, no. 3 (September 1974): 227–37.

Gipson, Jessica D., Michael A. Koenig, and Michelle J. Hindin. "The Effects of Unintended Pregnancy on Infant, Child, and Parental Health: A Review of the Literature." *Studies in Family Planning* 39, no. 1 (March 2008): 18–38.

Glazebrook, Cristine, Sara Cox, Margaret Oates, and George Ndukwe. "Psychological Adjustment during Pregnancy and the Postpartum Period in Single and Multiple In Vitro Fertilization Births: A Review and Preliminary Findings from an Ongoing Study." *Reproductive Technologies* 10, no. 2 (March 2000): 112–19.

Goldbach, Kristen R. C., et al. "The Effects of Gestational Age and Gender on Grief after Pregnancy Loss." *American Journal of Orthopsychiatry* 61, no. 3 (July 1991): 461–67.

Golombok, Susan, et al. "Children: The European Study of Assisted Reproduction Families: Family Functioning and Child Development." *Human Reproduction* 11, no. 10 (1996): 2324–31.

Goodman, J. H. "Becoming an Involved Father of an Infant." *Journal of Obstetric, Gynecologic, & Neonatal Nursing* 34, no. 2 (March–April 2005): 190–200.

Goodwin, T. M. "Hyperemesis Gravidarum." *Obstetrics & Gynecology Clinics of North America* 35, no. 3 (September 2008): 401–17.

Green, R. F., et al. "Association of Paternal Age and Risk for Major Congenital Anomalies from the National Birth Defects Prevention Study, 1997–2004." *Annals of Epidemiology* 20, no. 3 (March 2010): 241–49.

Grube, M. "Pre- and Postpartal Psychiatric Disorders and Support from Male Partners: A First Qualitative Approximation." *Der Nervenarzt* 75, no. 5 (2004): 483–88.

Gruenert, S., and R. Galligan. "The Difference Dads Make: Young Adult Men's Experiences of Their Fathers." *E-Journal of Applied Psychology* 3, no. 1 (2007): 3–15.

Habib, Cherine, and Sandra Lancaster. "The Transition to Fatherhood: Identity and Bonding in Early Pregnancy." *Fathering* 4, no. 3 (2006): 235–53.

Hagen, Edward. "The Functions of Postpartum Depression." *Evolution & Human Behavior* 20 (September 1999): 325–59.

Hammarberg, K., J. R. W. Fisher, and K. H. Wynter. "Psychological and Social Aspects of Pregnancy, Childbirth, and Early Parenting after Assisted Conception: A Systematic Review." *Human Reproduction Update* 14, no. 5 (September–October 2008): 395–414.

Hanson, Suzanne, Lauren P. Hunter, et al. "Paternal Fears of Childbirth: A Literature Review." *Journal of Perinatal Education* 18, no. 4 (Fall 2009): 12–20.

Hay, D. A., and P. J. O'Brien. "Early Influences on the School Social Adjustments of Twins." *Acta Geneticae Medicae et Gemellologiae: Twin Research* 36, no. 2 (1987): 239–48.

Henley, K., and K. Pasley. "Conditions Affecting the Association between Father Identity and Father Involvement." *Fathering* 3, no. 1 (Winter 2005): 59–80.

Hepper, Peter G. "Fetal 'Soap' Addiction." *The Lancet* 331, no. 8598 (June 1988): 1347–48.

Hepper, Peter G., and Sara Shahidullah. "Development of Fetal Hearing." *Archives of Disease in Childhood* 71, no. 2 (September 1994): F81–87.

Hinton, Lisa, Louise Locock, and Marian Knight. "Partner Experiences of 'Near-Miss' Events in Pregnancy and Childbirth in the UK: A Qualitative Study." *PLoS ONE* 9, no. 4 (2014)

Hjelmstedt, Anna, and A. Collins. "Psychological Functioning and Predictors of Father-Infant Relationship in IVF Fathers and Controls." *Scandinavian Journal of Caring Sciences* 22, no. 1 (March 2008): 72–78.

Hjelmstedt, Anna, et al. "Personality Factors and Emotional Responses to Pregnancy Among IVF Couples in Early Pregnancy: A Comparative Study." *Acta Obstetricia et Gynecologica Scandinavica* 82, no. 2 (2003): 152–61.

Holditch-Davis, Diane, et al. "Beyond Couvade: Pregnancy Symptoms in Couples with a History of Infertility." *Health Care for Women International* 15, no. 6 (November–December 1994): 537–48.

Holopainen, D. "The Experience of Seeking Help for Postnatal Depression." *Australian Journal of Advanced Nursing* 19, no. 3 (March–May 2002); 39-44.

Hook, J. L., and C. M. Wolfe. "New Fathers? Residential Fathers' Time with Children in Four Countries." *Journal of Family Issues* 33, no. 4 (April 2012): 415–50.

Hossain, Z., T. Field, J. Gonzalez, et al. "Infants of 'Depressed' Mothers Interact Better with Their Nondepressed Fathers." *Infant Mental Health Journal* 15, no. 4 (Winter 1994): 348–57.

Howell-White, Sandra. "Choosing a Birth Attendant: The Influence of a Woman's Childbirth Definition." *Social Science & Medicine* 45, no. 6 (September 1997): 925–36.

Humphrey, M., and R. Kirkwood. "Marital Relationships Among Adopters." *Adoption & Fostering* 6, no. 2 (July 1982): 44–48.

"Information for Moms-to-Be about the New Full-Term Pregnancy Definition." National Child Maternal Health Education Program. Available online at https://www.nichd.nih.gov/ncmhep/terms/Pages/MomsToBe.aspx.

Johansson, Margareta, Ingegerd Hildingsson, and Jennifer Fenwick. "Important Factors Working to Mediate Swedish Fathers' Experiences of a Caesarean Section." *Midwifery* 29, no. 9 (September 2013): 1041–49.

Johnson, Erin. M., and M. Marit Rehavi. "Physicians Treating Physicians: Information and Incentives in Childbirth." National Bureau of Economic Research Working Paper, no. 19242 (2013).

Jordan, Pamela. "Enhancing Understanding of the Transition to Fatherhood." *Interna-*

tional Journal of Childbirth Education 22, no. 2 (June 2007): 4–6.

———. "Laboring for Relevance: Expectant and New Fatherhood." Nursing Research 39, no. 1 (January–February 1990): 11–16.

Jove, Chelsea Ivy-Rose. "The Portrayal of Men in the Media." Undergraduate Research Journal for the Human Sciences 9 (2010). Available online at http://www.kon.org/urc/v9/jove.html.

Kao, Bi-Chin, Meei-Ling Gau, et al. "A Comparative Study of Expectant Parents' Childbirth Expectations." Journal of Nursing Research 12, no. 3 (September 2004): 191–202.

Knoester, C., and D. Eggebeen. "The Effects of the Transition to Parenthood and Subsequent Children on Men's Well-Being and Social Participation." Journal of Family Issues 27, no. 11 (November 2006): 1532–60.

Koren, Gideon, Svetlana Madjunkova, and Caroline Maltepe. "The Protective Effects of Nausea and Vomiting of Pregnancy against Adverse Fetal Outcome—A Systematic Review." Reproductive Toxicology 47 (August 2014): 77–80.

Kotila, L. E., S. J. Schoppe-Sullivan, and C. M. Kamp Dush. "Boy or Girl? Maternal Psychological Correlates of Knowing Fetal Sex." Personality and Individual Differences 68 (October 2014): 195–98.

Kurki, T., L. Toivonen, and O. Ylikorkala. "Father's Heart Beat Responds to the Birth of His Child." Acta Obstetricia et Gynecologica Scandinavica 74, no. 2 (February 1995): 127–28.

Leddy, M. A., M. L. Power, and J. Schulkin. "The Impact of Maternal Obesity on Maternal and Fetal Health." Reviews in Obstetrics & Gynecology 1, no. 4 (Fall 2008): 170–78.

Lee, Chih-Yuan, and William Doherty. "Marital Satisfaction and Father Involvement during the Transition to Parenthood." Fathering 5, no. 2 (Spring 2007): 75–96.

Leighton, B. L., and S. H. Halpern. "The Effects of Epidural Analgesia on Labor, Maternal and Neonatal Outcomes: A Systematic Review." American Journal of Obstetrics & Gynecology 186, no. 5, Supplement (May 2002): S69–S77.

LeMoyne, E. L., D. Curnier, S. St-Jacques, and E. Ellemberg. "The Effects of Exercise during Pregnancy on the Newborn's Brain: Study Protocol for a Randomized Controlled Trial." Trials 13 (May 2012): 68.

Levy-Schiff, Rachel, Ora Bar, and Dov Har-Even. "Psychological Adjustment of Adoptive Parents-to-Be." American Journal of Orthopsychiatry 60, no. 2 (April 1990): 258–66.

Li, De-Kun, Teresa Janevic, Roxana Odouli, and Liyan Liu. "Hot Tub Use During Pregnancy and the Risk of Miscarriage." American Journal of Epidemiology 158, no. 10 (2003): 931–37.

Lis, A., A. Zennaro, C. Mazzecchi, and M. Pinto. "Parental Styles in Prospective Fathers: A Research Carried Out Using a Semi-Structured Interview during Pregnancy." Infant Mental Health Journal 25, no. 2 (March–April 2004): 149–62.

Luke, B., N. Mamelle, L. Keith, et al. "The Association between Occupational Factors and Preterm Birth: A United States Nurses' Study." American Journal of Obstetrics & Gynecology 173, no. 3, Part 1 (September 1995): 849–62.

Lumley, Judith. "Sexual Feelings in Pregnancy and after Childbirth." Australian and New Zealand Journal of Obstetrics and Gynaecology 18, no. 2 (May 1978): 114–17.

Lund, Najaaraq, Lars H. Pedersen, and Tine Brink Henriksen. "Selective Serotonin Reuptake Inhibitor Exposure In Utero and Pregnancy Outcomes." Archives of Pediatric and Adolescent Medicine 163, no. 10 (October 2009): 949–54.

MacCallum, Fiona, Emma Lycett, Clare Murray, Vasanti Jadva, and Susan Golombok. "Surrogacy: The Experience of Commissioning Couples." Human Reproduction 18, no. 6 (June 2003): 1334–42.

Mackeen, A. D., et al. "Suture Compared with Staple Skin Closure after Cesarean Delivery: A Randomized Controlled Trial." Obstetrics & Gynecology 123, no. 6 (June 2014): 1169–75.

Manrique, Beatriz, et al. "A Controlled Experiment in Prenatal Enrichment with 684 Families in Caracas, Venezuela: Results to Age Six." Journal of Prenatal and Perinatal Psychology and Health 12, nos. 3–4 (Spring 1998), 209–34.

Martin, Laurie T., Michelle J. McNamara, et al. "The Effects of Father Involvement during Pregnancy on Receipt of Prenatal

Care and Maternal Smoking." *Maternal and Child Health Journal* 11, no. 6 (November 2007): 595–602.

Matthews, Fiona, Paul Johnson, and Andrew Neil. "You Are What Your Mother Eats: Evidence for Maternal Preconception Diet Influencing Foetal Sex in Humans." *Proceedings of the Royal Society B* 275, no. 1643 (July 2008): 1661–68.

May, Katharyn A. "Factors Contributing to First-Time Fathers' Readiness for Fatherhood: An Exploratory Study." *Family Relations* 31, no. 3 (July 1982): 353–61.

———. "First-Time Fathers' Responses to Unanticipated Caesarean Birth: An Exploratory Study." Unpublished report to University of California San Francisco (1982).

———. "Three Phases of Father Involvement in Pregnancy." *Nursing Research* 31, no. 6 (November–December 1982): 337–42.

May, Katharyn A., and Deanna Tomlinson Sollid. "Unanticipated Cesarean Birth from the Father's Perspective." *Birth* 11, no. 2 (Summer 1984): 87–95.

McIntyre, Matthew H., and Carolyn Pope Edwards. "The Early Development of Gender Differences." *Annual Review of Anthropology* 38 (October 2009): 83–97.

Mennella, J., A. Johnson, and G. K. Beauchamp. "Garlic Ingestion by Pregnant Women Alters the Odor of Amniotic Fluid." *Chemical Senses* 20, no. 2 (April 1995): 207–9.

Mercer, R. T. "Relationship of the Birth Experience to Later Mothering Behaviors." *Journal of Nurse-Midwifery* 30, no. 4 (July–August 1985): 204–11.

Michaels, Paula. "Childbirth Pain Relief and the Soviet Origins of the Lamaze Method." The National Council for Eurasian and East European Research (2007). Available online at http://www.ucis.pitt.edu/nceeer/2007_821-10g_Michaels.pdf.

Miller, W. E., and S. Friedman. "Male and Female Sexuality during Pregnancy: Behavior and Attitudes." *Journal of Psychology & Human Sexuality* 1, no. 2 (1989): 17–37.

Mozurkewich, E. L., B. Luke, M. Avni, and F. M. Wolf. "Working Conditions and Adverse Pregnancy Outcome: A Meta-Analysis." *Obstetrics & Gynecology* 95, no. 4 (April 2000): 623–35.

Nelson, Leif D., and Joseph P. Simmons. "Moniker Maladies: When Names Sabotage Success." *Psychological Science* 18, no. 12 (December 2007): 1106–12.

Olsen, Sjurdur F., et al. "Milk Consumption during Pregnancy Is Associated with Increased Infant Size at Birth: Prospective Cohort Study." *American Journal of Clinical Nutrition* 86, no. 4 (October 2007): 1104–10.

Omranifard, Victoria, and Ghorbanali Asadollahi. "Association between Paternal Age at Birth Time and the Risk of Offspring Developing Schizophrenia." *American Journal of Applied Sciences* 6, no. 1 (2009): 179–81.

Osterman, Michelle J. K., and Joyce A. Martin. "Primary Cesarean Delivery Rates, by State: Results from the Revised Birth Certificate, 2006–2012." *National Vital Statistics Reports* 63, no. 1 (January 23, 2014). Available online at http://www.cdc.gov/nchs/data/nvsr/nvsr63/nvsr63_01.pdf.

Palazzari, Kari. "The Daddy Double-Bind: How the Family and Medical Leave Act Perpetuates Sex Inequality across All Class Levels." *Columbia Journal of Gender & Law* 16, no. 2 (June 2007): 429–70.

Palkovitz, Rob, and Glen Palm. "Transitions within Fathering." *Fathering* 7, no. 1 (Winter 2009): 3–22.

Pauleta, J. R., N. M. Pereira, and L. M. Graça. "Sexuality during Pregnancy." *Journal of Sexual Medicine* 7, no. 1, Part 1 (January 2010): 136–42.

Pelham, Brett W., Matthew C. Mirenberg, and John T. Jones. "Why Susie Sells Seashells by the Seashore: Implicit Egotism and Major Life Decisions." *Journal of Personality and Social Psychology* 82, no. 4 (April 2002): 469–87.

Pinzur, Laura, and Gary Smith. "First Names and Longevity." *Perceptual and Motor Skills* 108, no. 1 (February 2009): 149–60.

Piontelli, Alessandra. "A Study on Twins before and after Birth." *International Review of Psycho-Analysis* 16, no. 4 (1989): 413–26.

Plantin, L., A. A. Olukoya, and P. Ny. "Positive Health Outcomes of Fathers' Involvement in Pregnancy and Childbirth Paternal Support: A Scope Study Literature Review." *Fathering* 9, no. 1 (2011): 87–102.

Polman, E., M. M. H. Pollmann, and T. A. Poehlman. "The Name-Letter-Effect in Groups: Sharing Initials with Group Members Increases the Quality of Group Work." *PLoS ONE* 8, no. 11 (November 2013).

Powdthavee, N., S. Wu, and A. Oswald. "The Effects of Daughters on Health Choices and Risk Behaviour." Department of Economics, University of York, Discussion Papers, no. 10/03 (2010). Available online at http://www.york.ac.uk/media/economics/documents/discussionpapers/2010/1003.pdf.

Premberg, A., and I. Lundgren. "Fathers' Experiences of Childbirth Education." *Journal of Perinatal Education* 15, no. 2 (Spring 2006): 21–28.

Price, Bradley B., Saeid B. Amini, and Kaelyn Kappeler. "Exercise in Pregnancy: Effect on Fitness and Obstetric Outcomes—A Randomized Trial." *Medicine & Science in Sports & Exercise* 44, no. 12 (December 2013): 2263–69.

Quinn, Suzanne M. "The Depictions of Fathers and Children in Best-Selling Picture Books in the United States: A Hybrid Semiotic Analysis." *Fathering* 7, no. 2 (Spring 2009): 140–58.

Ramchandani, P., et al. "Paternal Depression in the Postnatal Period and Child Development: A Prospective Population Study." *The Lancet* 365, no. 9478 (June 25, 2005): 2201–5.

Righetti, P. L., M. Dell'Avanzo, M. Grigio, and U. Nicolini. "Maternal/Paternal Antenatal Attachment and Fourth-Dimensional Ultrasound Technique: A Preliminary Report." *British Journal of Psychology* 96, Part 1 (February 2005): 129–37.

Roscoe, Joseph A., and Sara E. Matteson. "Acupressure and Acustimulation Bands for Control of Nausea: A Brief Review." *American Journal of Obstetrics & Gynecology* 186, no. 5, Supplement 2, (May 2002): S244–S247.

Sayle, A. E., D. A. Savitz, J. M. Thorp Jr., I. Hertz-Picciotto, and A. J. Wilcox. "Sexual Activity during Late Pregnancy and Risk of Preterm Delivery." *Obstetrics & Gynecology* 97, no. 2 (February 2001): 283–89.

Schoen, E. J., M. Oehrli, et al. "The Highly Protective Effect of Newborn Circumcision against Invasive Penile Cancer." *Pediatrics* 105 (March 2000). Available online at http://pediatrics.aappublications.org/content/105/3/e36.full.

Senkul, T., C. Iseri, B. Sen, et al. "Circumcision in Adults: Effect on Sexual Function." *Urology* 63, no. 1 (January 2004): 155–58.

Shahidullah, Sara, and Peter G. Hepper. "Frequency Discrimination by the Fetus." *Early Human Development* 36, no. 1 (January 1994): 13–26.

Shayeb, A. Ghiyath. "Male Obesity and Reproductive Potential." *The British Journal of Diabetes & Vascular Disease* 9, no. 1 (January–February 2009): 7–12.

Sheldon, Sally. "Reproductive Technologies and the Legal Determination of Fatherhood." *Feminist Legal Studies* 13, no. 3 (2005): 349–62.

Simkin, P. "Just Another Day in a Woman's Life? Part I: Women's Long-Term Perceptions of Their First Birth Experience." *Birth* 18, no. 4 (December 1991): 203–10.

———. "Just Another Day in A Woman's Life? Part II: Nature and Consistency of Women's Long-Term Memories of Their First Birth Experiences." *Birth* 19, no. 2 (June 1992): 64–81.

Skjærven, Rolv, et al. "Recurrence of Pre-Eclampsia Across Generations: Exploring Fetal and Maternal Genetic Components in a Population Based Cohort." *British Medical Journal* 331, no. 7521 (October 2005): 877.

Skotko, Brian G. "With New Prenatal Testing, Will Babies with Down Syndrome Slowly Disappear?" *Archives of Disease in Childhood* 94, no. 11 (November 2009): 823–26.

Stainton, M. C. "The Fetus: A Growing Member of the Family." *Family Relations* 34 (July 1985): 321–26.

Storey, Anne E., Carolyn J. Walsh, Roma L. Quinton, and Katherine E. Wynne-Edwards. "Hormonal Correlates of Paternal Responsiveness in New and Expectant Fathers." *Evolution & Human Behavior* 21, no. 2 (March 2000): 79–95.

Stotland, N. E., P. Sutton, J. Trowbridge, D. S. Atchley, J. Conry, et al. "Counseling Patients on Preventing Prenatal Environmental Exposures—A Mixed-Methods Study of Obstetricians." *PLoS ONE* 9, no. 6 (June 2014). Available online at http://journals.plos.org/plosonearticle?id=10.1371/journal.pone.0098771.

Sutton, P., T. J. Woodruff, J. Perron, N. Stotland, J. A. Conry, M. D. Miller, and L. C. Giudice. "Toxic Environmental Chemicals: The Role of Reproductive Health Professionals in Preventing Harmful Exposures." *American Journal of Obstetrics & Gynecology* 207, no. 3 (September 2012): 164–73.

Tang, C. H., M. P. Wu, J. T. Liu, et al. "Delayed Parenthood and the Risk of Cesarean Delivery: Is Paternal Age an Independent Risk Factor?" *Birth* 33, no 1 (March 2006): 18–26.

Teichman, Y., and Y. Lahav. "Expectant Fathers: Emotional Reactions, Physical Symptoms and Coping Styles." *British Journal of Medical Psychology* 60, no. 3 (September 1987): 225–32.

Thorn, Petra. "Understanding Infertility: Psychological and Social Considerations from a Counselling Perspective." *International Journal of Fertility & Sterility* 3, no. 2 (August–September 2009): 48–51.

Triche, Elizabeth W., et al. "Chocolate Consumption in Pregnancy and Reduced Likelihood of Preeclampsia." *Epidemiology* 19, no. 3 (May 2008): 459–64.

Vahratian, A., J. Zhang, J. Hasling, et al. "The Effect of Early Epidural versus Early Intravenous Analgesia Use on Labor Progression: A Natural Experiment." *American Journal of Obstetrics & Gynecology* 191, no. 1 (July 2004): 259–65.

Vanston, Claire M., and Neil V. Watson. "Selective and Persistent Effect of Foetal Sex on Cognition in Pregnant Women." *NeuroReport* 16, no. 7 (May 2005): 779–82.

van Tilburg, Wijnand A. P., and Eric R. Igou. "The Impact of Middle Names: Middle Name Initials Enhance Evaluations of Intellectual Performance." *European Journal of Social Psychology* 44, no. 4 (June 2014): 400–11,

Vilska, S., et al. "Mental Health of Mothers and Fathers of Twins Conceived via Assisted Reproduction Treatment: A 1-Year Prospective Study." *Human Reproduction* 24, no. 2 (February 2009): 367–77.

Wakefield, Melanie, Yolande Reid, Lyn Roberts, Robyn Mullins, and Pamela Gillies. "Smoking and Smoking Cessation among Men Whose Partners Are Pregnant: A Qualitative Study." *Social Science & Medicine* 47, no. 5 (September 1998): 657–64.

Waller, Maureen, and Marianne P. Bitler. "The Link Between Couples' Pregnancy Intentions and Behavior: Does It Matter Who Is Asked?" *Perspectives on Sexual and Reproductive Health* 40, no. 4 (December 2008): 194–201.

Wayne, Julie Holliday, and Bryanne L. Cordeiro. "Who Is a Good Organizational Citizen? Social Perception of Male and Female Employees Who Use Family Leave." *Sex Roles* 49, no. 5–6 (September 2003): 233–46.

Williams, Edith, and Norma Radin. "Effect of Father Participation in Child Rearing: Twenty-Year Follow-Up." *American Journal of Orthopsychiatry* 69, no. 3 (1999): 328–36.

Williams, Kristi, and Debra Umberson. "Medical Technology and Childbirth: Experiences of Expectant Mothers and Fathers." *Sex Roles* 41, no. 3–4 (1999): 147–67.

Wolfberg, Adam J., et al. "Dads as Breastfeeding Advocates: Results from a Randomized Controlled Trial of Educational Intervention." *American Journal of Obstetrics & Gynecology* 191, no. 3 (September 2004): 708–12.

Wong, Cynthia, Barbara Scavone, et al. "The Risk of Cesarean Delivery with Neuraxial Analgesia Given Early versus Late in Labor." *The New England Journal of Medicine* 352, no. 7 (February 2005): 655–65.

Yogman, M. W., D. Kindlon, and F. Earls. "Father Involvement and Cognitive/Behavioral Outcomes of Preterm Infants." *Journal of the American Academy of Child & Adolescent Psychiatry* 34, no. 1 (January 1995): 58–66.

Zayas, Luis H. "Psychodynamic and Developmental Aspects of Expectant and New Fatherhood: Clinical Derivatives from the Literature." *Clinical Social Work Journal* 15, no. 1 (Spring 1987): 8–21.

———. "Thematic Features in the Manifest Dreams of Expectant Fathers." *Clinical Social Work Journal* 16, no. 3 (Fall 1988): 282–96.

Zuk, Marlene. "Essay Review: The Case of the Female Orgasm." *Perspectives in Biology and Medicine* 49, no. 2 (Spring 2006): 294–98.

Acknowledgments

When the first edition of this book came out, I was a wet-behind-the-ears, first-time author and I couldn't have imagined how well it would be received—or that it would completely change my life. I also had no idea how many people it takes to put a book together—so many, in fact, that it's nearly impossible to thank them individually. But I'll try. Andrea Adam read all the early drafts, encouraged me, and helped hone my ideas while adding a few of her own. David Cohen and Jackie Needleman and Matt and Janice Tannin also contributed stories, recipes, advice, and friendship to the first edition. Keri Schwab and Megan Lee, research assistants extraordinaire, helped come up with some of the most amazing studies. Certified financial planners Joe Pitzl (pitzlfinancial.com) and Jackie Mazur (Weitzberg) (guidemyfinances.com) reviewed the sections on finances and made some great suggestions.

In previous editions, the team at DrSpock.com and, in particular, Marjorie Greenfield, M.D., reviewed everything and anything medical. For later editions, I had a whole medical review board, well-stocked with OBs and fertility specialists: Elan Simckes, Saul Stromer, Susan Warhus, Saul Weinreb, and especially Lissa Rankin. All took the time—a lot of it—not only to fact-check chapters, but also to add their own insights, wisdom, and stories.

Behind the scenes, Bob Abrams and Cynthia Vance Abrams at Abbeville Press have championed *The Expectant Father* and helped turn a book from a first-time author into a best-selling series. Jackie Decter edited the first edition, correcting my mistakes and massaging my prose while leaving my ego intact. She passed the baton to Susan Costello, who did an equally masterful job of keeping me on track, and then came back for this edition without missing a beat. Celia Fuller,

Misha Beletsky, and Ada Rodriguez are the brains behind the wonderful design. Nicole Lanctot did a fine job keeping everything in line, and Louise Kurtz expertly handled the production. Nadine Winns somehow manages to keep our customers happy. Jim Levine (lgrliterary.com) and Arielle Eckstut (www.thebookdoctors .com) were there from the beginning and facilitated the early connection with Jennifer, which ultimately made the whole thing possible. Ever since then, Melissa Rowland and Miek Coccia have kept all the paperwork (you can't imagine how much) straight. And of course, my mom and dad, who with the exception of a very brief "have-you-thought-about-what-this-whole-writing-thing-will-do-to-your-career?" period, have been tirelessly supportive.

But even with all that help, this book would not be here today if it weren't for the thousands of expectant and new dads (and plenty of new moms, too) who contacted me with their suggestions, comments, complaints (usually constructive), and anecdotes. And finally, a special thank you to many, many dads who reviewed chapters, made suggestions, and much more. They include Whit Honea (@whithonea; www.whithonea.com), Chris Grady (@Lunarbaboon; www.lunar baboon.com), "Blogless" Joel Willis (tallsprout.com), and especially Pat Jacobs (@justadad247; justadad247.com).

Armin Brott

Index

ILLUSTRATION CREDITS

ABOUT THE AUTHORS

A nationally recognized expert on parenting, **Armin A. Brott** is also the author of nine critically acclaimed books for fathers. Titles include *The Expectant Father: The Ulitmate Guide for Dads-to-Be*, *FAQ for Expectant Fathers*, and *FAQ for New Fathers*. He has also written on parenting for the *New York Times Magazine*, the *Washington Post*, *Sports Illustrated*, and *Newsweek*, among many other publications, and he has been a speaker at the Dad 2.0 Summit. He writes the popular nationally syndicated column "Ask Mr. Dad" and hosts "Positive Parenting," a weekly syndicated talk show. Brott lives with his family in Oakland, California. To learn more, visit his website: mr.dad.com.

Jennifer Ash is the author of *Tropical Style: Private Palm Beach*. She also writes regularly for *Veranda* magazine and *Town & Country* magazine. Her articles have appeared in numerous publications, including the *Washington Post* and the *Palm Beach Daily News*. She and her husband, Dr. A. Joseph Rudick, live in New York City with their two children, Clarke and Amelia.

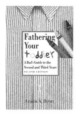
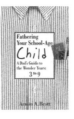
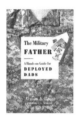
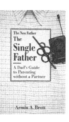
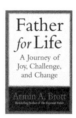
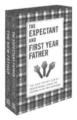
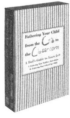

OVER 1,000,000 FATHERHOOD BOOKS IN PRINT!

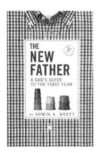

THE NEW FATHER
THIRD EDITION
A Dad's Guide to the First Year
By Armin A. Brott
Paper · 978-0-7892-1177-4 · **$13.95**
Hardcover · 978-0-7892-1176-7
$19.95

An indispensable, month-by-month handbook on all aspects of fatherhood during the first year—now fully updated and expanded—by the author of *The Expectant Father*. Incorporating a wealth of knowledge from top experts, the latest scientific research, and the author's and other fathers' personal experiences, *The New Father* presents invaluable information and practical tips on such issues as:

- Charting the baby's physical, intellectual, verbal, and social development
- Understanding your own emotional and psychological development
- Planning your finances and choosing the right life insurance policy
- Understanding how your partner is feeling and dealing with changes in your relationship
- How to understand what your baby is telling you

FAQ is an informative Q&A series for new dads and dads-to-be, from the best-selling author of *The Expectant Father*. On one page is a fill-in-the-blank statement, along with four multiple choice answers. Test yourself, then turn the page to find some helpful advice drawn from the expertise of top practitioners, as well as Brott's own background as a father of three and the real-world experience of thousands of others.

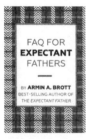

FAQ FOR EXPECTANT FATHERS
By Armin A. Brott
Paper · 978-0-7892-1269-6 · **$9.95**

With chapters on each of the 9 months of pregnancy, as well as sections on labor and delivery and infertility, this book features topics guys need to know—changes to men's hormones during pregnancy—and doesn't shy away from topics guys want to know—sex during pregnancy—all of which is told with the authority and honesty of an informed buddy.

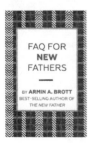

FAQ FOR NEW FATHERS
By Armin A. Brott
Paper · 978-0-7892-1270-2 · **$9.95**

With chapters on each of the 12 months in baby's first year, this book features topics guys need to know—baby blues—and doesn't shy away from topics guys want to know—work/life balance—all of which is told with the authority and honesty of an informed buddy.

For more information on the *New Father* series and a complete list of titles,
visit **www.abbeville.com/newfather**

*Available from your favorite bookstore, online retailer,
or by calling* 1-800-Artbook